THE SECRETS OF THE
AUDITORY SYSTEM

BRIDGING
AUDIOLOGY
AND
PSYCHOLOGY

© Carlos Alós Alcalde, 2020
www.audiopsychology.com

Author correspondence: audioneival@gmail.com
                        carlos.alos@audiopsychology.com

Original Spanish title: AUDIOLOGÍA Y PSICOLOGÍA – Descubriendo los secretos
del sistema auditivo

First edition: November 2020

Revision and correction: Elena Alós
Graphic design and layout: Pere Mola
Cover illustration: Dreamstime (Putra Novembria Candra Kusuma)
Translation: Stuart Dyke and Julie Graham
Printed by Amazon

Register of intellectual property: B-1536-20

CARLOS ALÓS

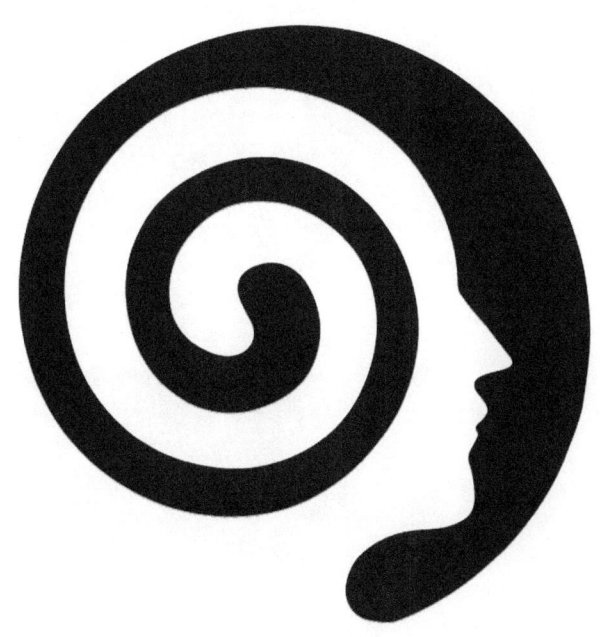

BRIDGING AUDIOLOGY AND PSYCHOLOGY

THE SECRETS OF THE AUDITORY SYSTEM

Acknowledgements

The best part of this book is undoubtedly its bibliography. I would like to express my sincere gratitude to the many researchers who have contributed to unravelling some of nature's countless enigmas. Their tenacious work has inspired me to write this essay. I am also grateful to my patients, who have been my greatest teachers. Without them, I would never have asked myself the right questions.

Fortunately, many people have helped me in the long process of turning ideas into printed text. Some collaborated with me directly. Others, no less important, provided me with means and support when needed.

I feel especially indebted to Alba García, who organized the bibliographic citations, to Pere Mola, a graphic designer who has infinite patience, and above all to my daughter Elena, whose contribution to the correction of the original Spanish text was essential.

Stuart Dyke and Julie Graham not only translated the book into English, but also provided valuable comments; as did my sister Elisa, Teresa Feliu, Anabel Pérez, Jesús Blanquet and Fernando Sánchez. Ralph Gerhardt, a good friend of mine for forty years now, is responsible for the German version and for many improvements to the original manuscript.

Aida Faura, Ramón Olomí, Mercè Comellas, M. Cruz Domínguez, Luciana Tirolli, Enrique de Juan, Tairé Paredes and Antonia Crevillén encouraged me to organize training courses which were the starting point for this project. My wife Inma and my daughter Silvia shared hours of work and were able to fill them with positive emotions.

To all of them, my most sincere recognition and gratitude.

To Inma Santamaría and my colleagues in the Neival team—Coral Ruiz, Mónica Gallerani and Mercè Reigosa—and also to those in Sint-Truiden, with whom I shared so many experiences, and to all those who help to build a better world each day, spreading around smiles, values and warm humanity.

CONTENTS

In the presence of a scientific object, if you want to get at the truth, it is not enough to learn what the "good" authors have said: you have to go and see for yourself. Scientific endeavor involves an initial rebellion against established science.

ALFRED TOMATIS

The most exciting phrase to hear in science, the one that heralds new discoveries, is not "Eureka!" but "That's funny..."

ISAAC ASIMOV

INTRODUCTION

A round 1991 I started to get interested in the hearing system. This is a bit strange for a psychologist who studies behavior and learning, but I met Alfred Tomatis, an unconventional ENT physician whose work goes beyond the frontiers of audiology, diving into the domains of psychology.

In today's scientific literature I can see a growing interest in exploring those limits as well. I have had the opportunity to read numerous scientific articles that are very close to Tomatis's ideas and which I have collected in order to write this book. I hope this comprehensive bibliography will arouse curiosity among health experts and inspire future research.

I will discuss little-known aspects of the ear, venturing into the mysteries of a structure that does not behave only as a sensory organ, but is involved in numerous metabolic processes, in our mental health, language and learning. I will speak of an unusual and yet real ear, able to achieve a spectacular, immediate remission of the symptoms of a stroke or psychotic break and play a major role in the maintenance of bone mass, muscle tone and posture, and which is linked to multiple other functions: Circadian cycles, hormonal balance, kidney function, detection of blood oxygen levels and cardiovascular health. I will raise more questions than answers, but there is nothing like a good question for moving things forward.

Although the subject is somewhat complex, I have tried to use a language suited to any reader with minimal training in these matters and I have included a glossary of terms to make the text easier to understand. If you are not used to the basic audiological concepts, I recommend you consult an introductory paper first. [1,2]

To bring the reader closer to these meta-audiological concepts I will first give a brief account of Tomatis's life. It will help to explain why we must place the ear at the center of our physical and psychological health. I will then reflect on the role that the auditory system has played in the evolution of the species and of the human being itself, since the origin of life, and I will describe its diagnostic and therapeutic possibilities in the light of modern science.

A.N.: Whenever the word "Tomatis" appears in this work, it refers to Alfred Tomatis, never to the trademark, with which the author is not associated in any way.

---

[1] **Soto, E. et al.** *Fisiología de la audición: la cóclea.* Puebla : Instituto de Fisiología, Univ. Aut. de Puebla, 2004. p. 17.

[2] **Moore, B.C.J.** *An Introduction to the Psychology of Hearing.* Bingley, UK : Emerald Group Publishing Limited, 2012.

A GREAT OBSERVER

1

W<!-- -->e met Tomatis almost by chance. Nobody had told us about his work at the university, but in our daughter's school his techniques were being applied, so we wanted to know a little more. We were lucky that at that time, around 1990, Tomatis himself was giving a course in Barcelona and I signed up for it.

A few minutes of listening to him talk were enough for me to realize that this was an exceptional person, an innovator. Gifted with a great memory and enormously cultured, he was able to find amazing links between seemingly independent elements.

He related hearing to psychology and motor development, explained that the main role of the auditory system was to imbue the neural network with energy, spoke about the therapeutic effects of the intrauterine maternal voice, the hormonal and psychological effects of sounds, and much more.

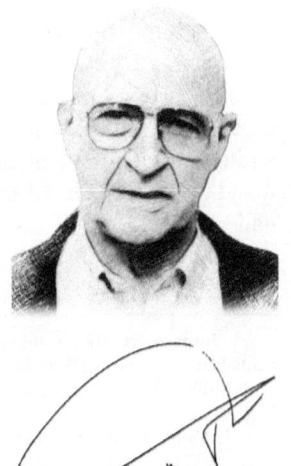

My mind never once wandered from that absolute torrent of new ideas, always delivered in a clear, logical fashion and drawing on his extensive clinical experience, of treating thousands of patients. As I listened, his reasonings sounded self-evident, to the point that I asked myself: Why didn't I think of that before?

By the end of that morning I was already exhausted, overwhelmed by so many new ideas. And the course had only just begun. Under Tomatis's influence my professional life took a new turn and I went on to study audiology, audio techniques and neuropsychology.

AN ATYPICAL DOCTOR

I will recount some of the key points in the life of this unique French ENT physician, in order to bring him closer to the reader. I would also suggest reading his autobiography, *The Conscious Ear.*[3] Other colleagues have also written about his work,[4] [5] so I will just mention the parts that I consider most relevant to the objectives of this book.

Alfred Ange Auguste Tomatis was born in the old Nice of 1920, just a few meters from the Opera House and Matisse's workshop. Very soon he showed an interest in medicine and, when still a child, his parents allowed him to move to Paris to study. His university education was to coincide with the Second World War. by the end of which he had become an experienced doctor.

In his early days, he studied the hearing pathologies of aeronautical workers and published several studies describing the audiometric profile of occupational deafness. Unlike today, around 1940 very little was known about hearing loss, there were hardly any audiometers and it was not easy to get one.[6] The first commercially available audiometer appeared around 1920 in the United States, manufactured by Western Electric. It cost about the same as a house: 1,500 current dollars. Reference zero for the calibration of audiometric equipment, as we know it today, first appeared in 1937 and had to wait until 1951 to be internationally approved.[7]

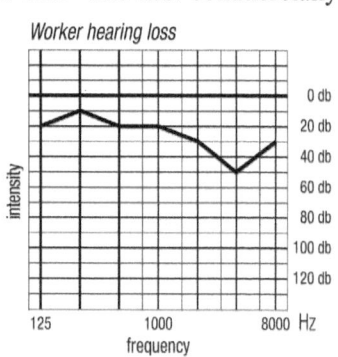

Worker hearing loss

---

[3] **Tomatis, A.** *The Conscious Ear.* Phoenix: Station Hill Press, 1991 (originally published in French as *L'Oreille et la Vie*, Editions Robert Laffont, 1977)

[4] **Sollier, P.** *Aprende a escuchar para tu bienestar.* Madrid : Grupo Editorial Sial Pigmalión, 2016.

[5] **de Voigt, M. and Vervoort, J.** *Listen to live Our Brain and Music.* s.l. : MBL Tomatis Network, 2018.

[6] *Relations entre l'audition et la phonation.* **Tomatis, A.** July, 1956, Annals of Telecommunications, Vol. 11, pp. 151-158.

[7] *The Clinical Audiogram Its History and Current Use.* **Vogel, D.A. and McCarthy, P.A.** 2, Communicative Disorders Review, Vol. 1.

A STRANGE COINCIDENCE

While still working in the hangars, Tomatis began to receive patients with voice disorders, referred by his father, Humbert Tomatis, a renowned opera singer. He soon realized that the usual treatments for the pathologies of the singing voice yielded little success.

Looking for another way to deal with these disorders and since he had an audiometer, he decided to explore the hearing of these patients, obtaining, to his surprise, audiograms that looked much like those of the aeronautical employees, with their characteristic fall in the region of 4,000 Hz (occupational deafness). Later he was able to see that a tenor can emit intensities of over 100 dB, as high as 120, measured in his own ear. He is subjected to an acoustic pressure comparable to working a short distance from the turbines of aircraft engines. Only a refined technique and training prevent hearing damage.

By the way, there are privileged ears that seem to resist anything. Not all the workers in the hangars suffered from hearing loss, despite being constantly assailed by infernal noises.

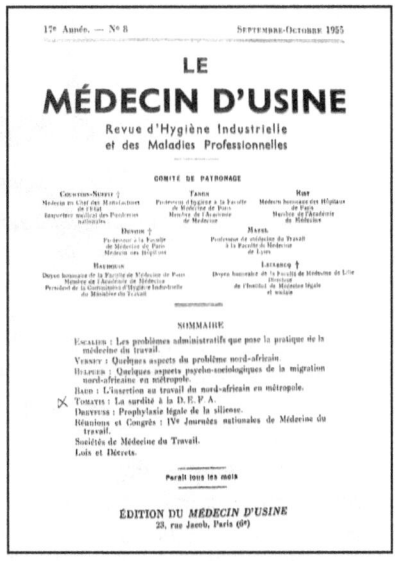

Cover of the occupational medicine journal in which Tomatis published his first articles, 1955

Tomatis then suspected that singing voice problems could be related to the inability to hear certain sounds correctly. He thought that perhaps the voice could not be emitted correctly and precisely if the ear had difficulties in capturing certain frequencies, and he was right.

AUDIOMETRY, A TEST OF THE VOICE

The study of the singers' voices and hearing highlighted the close relationship between the two. For Tomatis, audiometry (analysis of hearing) and sonograms (analysis of emitted sound) were equivalent tests. If the audiometric curve falls within a certain frequency range, the harmonics lose energy in the vocal emission, in exactly the same range of the spectrum. Remember that harmonics are the sounds that go with the note being sung (pitch), and which determine the color and quality of the voice.

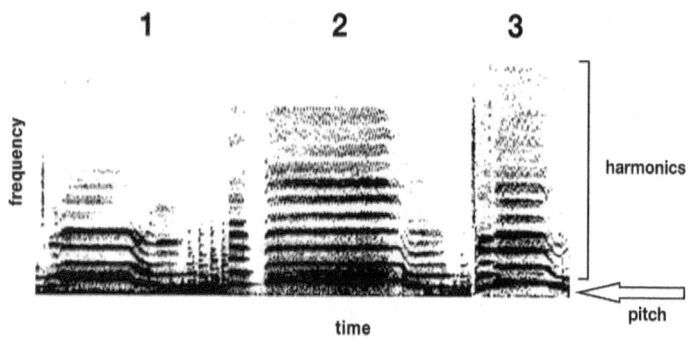

Sonogram of the same note sung by three famous sopranos.
Observe the harmonics distribution. Number 2 stands out for its density
It corresponds to Maria Callas.

When the first electronic spectrum analyzers appeared, he was able to subject the singers to different acoustic conditions by means of filters and thus observe the alterations that arose in the voice as a result of these manipulations.

In the example below, on the left is the audiogram of a normal-hearing person. On the right, a picture of his normal speaking voice (with the frequencies on the horizontal axis and the intensity on the vertical axis):

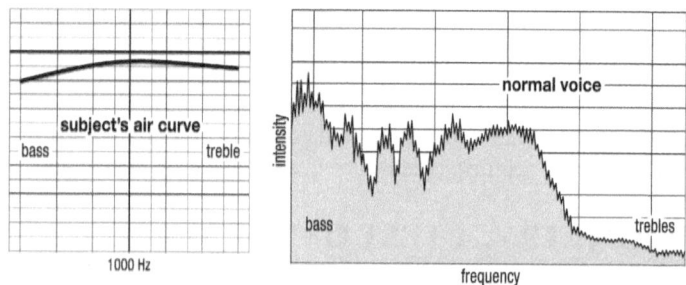

After imposing a low pass filter on the subject, which eliminates high frequencies, the voice does not change pitch but loses its high-frequency harmonics. We can see this by comparing the power spectrum graphs:

This work features in the first book by A. Tomatis: *The Ear and Language,*[8] published in 1969. Forty-four years later, Tourville, Reilly and Guenther decided to examine what was happening in the brain when artificially altering voice pitch.[9] The people being studied tried

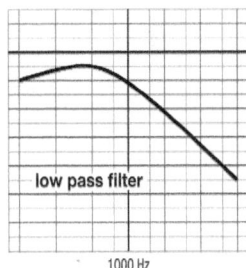

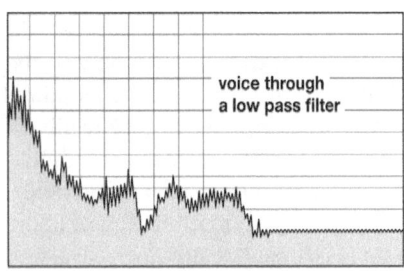

to compensate for the altered feedback. When they heard themselves in a higher pitch than normal, they lowered their voice pitch; and vice versa: they spoke in a higher-pitched voice if they heard themselves in a lower pitch than expected. It took them very little time to try to adapt their voice production to what they were hearing: about 135 msec.

The brain images showed that, during the experiment, the left hemisphere was in charge while these subjects were pronouncing the words normally. When the pitch of voice was manipulated, however, the right hemisphere was activated. The left-brain controls language and, at the same time, the right manages prosody, the music with which we envelop our speech.

The same study has been done with children with impaired language development, who tended not to compensate, directly adopting the modified speech as their own,[10] which points to hearing being involved in the disorder.

The authors suggest that there may be specific neurons that compare what the brain expects to happen with what has actually happened, and these are excited if the two do not match, generating a sequence of motor commands for the system to reset itself.

We do not always correct our voice in an attempt to compensate for altered listening. If we like what we hear, we integrate it. In a

[8] **Tomatis, A.** *L'oreille et le langage.* Paris : Éditions du Seuil, 1963.

[9] *Neural mechanisms underlying auditory feedback control of speech.* **Tourville, J.A., Reilly, K.J. and Guenther, F.H.** 3, 2008, Neuroimage, Vol. 39, pp. 1429-1443.

[10] *Auditory feedback perturbation in children with developmental speech sound disorders.* **Terband, H. et al.** 2014, J Commun Disord., Vol. 51, pp. 64-77.

study done in Canada, in which university departments of music and language collaborated, they modified the listening of a group of singers so that they heard their own voice nasalized. Quickly, the singers tried to remedy the unpleasant effect by denasalizing their voices even more than normal. However, when they were allowed to listen to their denasalized voices, they took these as their own, because they liked them just the way they sounded.[11]

Children are not as skilled as adults in developing compensatory responses to modified auditory feedback.[12,13] They are still developing their motor control. In dyslexic adults, these difficulties remain.[14] In some cases, the appearance of nodules or polyps on the vocal cords may be related to a malfunction of auditory feedback.[15]

The classic conception of sensory organs that send information to a brain that processes the data is very logical and convincing, but it does not seem to respond to reality. The Spanish neurophysiologist Álvaro Pascual Leone, a professor at Harvard University, talks, on the contrary about a brain that anticipates what is going to happen and makes us live in a virtual, imagined world.[16] The information captured from the outside by our senses is constantly being cross-checked against our brain's fantasy. If they do not match, a warning signal is given, attention is increased and the necessary correction mechanisms are put into action. If we were not constantly anticipating reality in this way it would be very difficult to carry out the simplest of tasks. Driving would become a dangerous activity and watching a tennis match would bore anyone because of its slowness and inaccuracy.

Our brain also takes the initiative in the auditory system. For example, speech is preceded by a contraction of the stirrup muscle, adjusting intralabyrinthine pressure before the sound of our voice reaches the inner ear.[17]

---

[11] *Influence of Altered Auditory Feedback on Oral-Nasal Balance in Song.* **Santoni, C. et al.** Aug, 2018, Journal of voice.

[12] *The developmental trajectory of vocal and event-related potential responses to frequency-altered auditory feedback.* **Nichole E. Scheerer, N.E., Liu, H. and Jones, J.A.** 2013, European Journal of Neuroscience, Vol. 38, pp. 3189-3200.

[13] *Sensoriomotor Learning in Children and Adults: Exposure to frequency-altered auditory feedback during speech production.* **Scheerer, N.E., Jacobson, D.S. and Jones, J.A.** 2016, Neuroscience, Vol. 314, pp. 106-115.

[14] *Deficient Response to Altered Auditory Feedback in Dyslexia.* **van den Bunt, M.R. et al.** 2018, Developmental Neuropsychology.

[15] *Vocal fold nodules: A disorder of phonation organs or auditory feedback?* **Lee, S.H. et al.,** Aug, 2019, Clin Otolaryngol.

[16] **Pascual Leone, A.** Nit Quántica TV3. *Singulars.* Dec 8, 2009.

[17] *The Activity of the Stapedius Muscle in Man During Vocalization.* **Borg, E. and Zakrisson, J.E.** 3-6, 1975, Acta Oto-Laryngologica, Vol. 79.

SINGING WITH THE RIGHT EAR

Tomatis's observations revealed other phenomena. He found that modification of the right ear's hearing automatically triggered distortions in the singing voice, which was not the case with the left one. As far as professional singers were concerned, the right ear was key.

Using sound overload techniques, he came up with empirical proof of this. He sent loud white noise (which contains all audible frequencies at equal intensity) for a few minutes to the singer's right ear. In this way, the ear was incapacitated for a few seconds, during which voice testing was carried out.

The voice suddenly lost all its qualities, making the singer sound like an amateur. On the other hand, if the targeted ear was the left one, the voice did not undergo negative changes. It even improved sometimes.

These observations coincide with what neuropsychologists who use music to explore brain plasticity tell us. While the right hemisphere is strongly involved in musical analysis, changes produced by learning, such as playing an instrument, are observed above all in the auditory areas of the left hemisphere.[18] In a nutshell, we could say that, in non-musicians, the right hemisphere is predominant with respect to musical activity while, in professionals, both hemispheres work together on equal terms.

Tomatis also observed that the movements of the singers' faces changed during the white noise experiment.

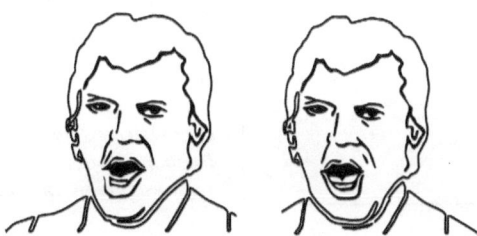

If we focus on their facial expressions, in particular, the lower lip, we see that it points either to the right or to the left depending on the imposed auditory conditions. In the first picture, right control. In the second, left control.

Since the stirrup muscle and all of the face (except the eyelid elevator) are governed by the seventh cranial pair (the facial nerve),

---

[18] *The music in the brain hemispheres* . **Gizzi, G. and Albi, E.** 4, 2017, The EuroBiotech Journal, Vol. 1.

Tomatis suspected that they moved in unison. In this way, the part of the face with the greatest mobility would signal the auditory laterality. Tomatis claimed he had never found a good left-sided singer and that, although they existed, they were never celebrities. They had a very restricted audience: in turn, left-eared listeners!

These observations led him to conclude that *the voice contains only the sounds that the ear can perceive* and that the leading ear is the right one. If it is the left one, control over the voice is lost.

In March 1957, a friend of Tomatis, Dr Husson, presented the *Tomatis Effect* to the Academy of Sciences in Paris, empirically demonstrating that changes in hearing cause instant changes in the harmonics of the voice. Using different procedures, this experiment has been replicated several times with similar results.[19]

Modifications Phonatoires d'origine auditive et applications physiologiques et cliniques

par M. Raoul HUSSON
Docteur es-Sciences
Maître de Recherches au C.N.R.S

Extrait du Bulletin de l'Académie Nationale de Médecine
Tome 141, n° 19 et 20

(Présentation faite par M. Moulonguet)

I. — INTRODUCTION.

1° Tomatis a signalé, en 1954 (1), un fait du plus haut intérêt : si un sujet émet une voyelle devant un microphone, dont la tension passe dans un filtre qui en supprime une certaine bande de fréquences avant d'être retournée à des écouteurs placés sur les oreilles du sujet, la bande considérée se trouve également supprimée de la voix du sujet. Selon le même processus, et, toujours d'après le même auteur, la voix d'un sujet atteint de scotome auditif est amputée des harmoniques qui seraient contenus dans l'îlot total supprimé. Tomatis a concrétisé ces faits dans la formule : « La voix ne contient que les harmoniques que l'oreille est susceptible d'entendre. »

The three components of sound: intensity, frequency and duration, are affected in the voice when its auditory perception is modified. A person with headphones on immediately speaks louder. If we distort temporal perception, delaying feedback, we cause stuttering. (Try the "idiotizer" app and you will verify this.) Tomatis demonstrated that the change in frequency perception was reciprocated in the vocal emission.

Husson explains in detail the reaction of the vocal cords to acoustic stimulation:[20]

- *If the stimulation is weak and only affects one ear, it affects the ipsilateral vocal cord; if its intensity increases, it affects both cords.*

---

[19] *The Tomatis Effect with Professional Opera Singers: A pilot study.* **Coppola, W.** 2016, Gestalt Theory, Vol. 38.

[20] *Acoustique et physiologie phonatoires.* **Husson, R.** Sup 3, Le Journal de physique et le radiium physique apliquée, Vol. 18, p. 23A.

- *If the stimulation is homorhythmic, when emitted, it stabilizes the laryngeal vibration.*
- *If the frequency alteration produced is little different from that emitted by the vocal cords, their vibration can be disturbed in various ways.*
- *If the disruptive sound is low-pitched (below 500 Hz), the tone of the glottic sphincter decreases; if it is high-pitched (above 2,000 Hz), the tone of the laryngeal sphincter increases, as demonstrated by the Tomatis experiments [...]*

Subsequently, the *Tomatis Effect* was presented by M. Moulonguet at the French National Academy of Medicine, in two sessions, in 1957 and 1960.[21]

When the ear is disturbed by noise or by modifying the auditory signal received, alterations are observed in all auditory competences. The modification of listening affects all motor control in general, to the point of distorting proprioception.[22] In an experiment performed in Italy, athletes were tricked during a hurdles race. By means of an electronic device, they heard the noise of their strides with a slight delay. That was enough to make them run more slowly.

Auditory feedback is used in rehabilitation, facilitating muscle exercises. At the University of Hanover, they tried it to help in executing knee movements. Depending on the angle of extension, patients heard different frequencies. This supplementary information made it easier for them to do the exercise and helped the physiotherapist.[23] Conversely, if we disturb the ear, by using noise or plugging the ear canal, the opposite effect occurs. Postural control is reduced, for example.[24]

LEARNING FROM CARUSO

This voice-hearing correspondence allowed Tomatis to describe how the hearing of the great tenor Caruso evolved, in each of his

---

[21] *Modifications phonatoires d'origine auditive et applications physiologiques et cliniques.* **Husson, M.R.** Paris : s.n., 4 de June de 1957, NuméroBulletin de l'Académie nationale de médecine Académie nationale de médecine (France), pp. 393-398.

[22] *Auditory reafferences: the influence of real-time feedback on movement control.* **Kennel, C. et al.** 69, 2015, Frontiers in Psychology, Vol. 6.

[23] *Auditory Proprioceptive Integration: Effects of Real-Time Kinematic Auditory Feedback on Knee Proprioception.* **Ghai, S. et al.** 142, 2018, Frontiers in Neuroscience, Vol. 12.

[24] *Auditory influence on postural control during stance tasks in different acoustic conditions.* **Anton, K., Ernst, A. and Basta, D.** Aug, 2019, Journal of Vestibular Research.

professional stages, based on his recordings on disc. The process of obtaining the data was extremely complex, as there were still no electronic devices capable of analyzing the sound spectrum. Tomatis used carbon paper cylinders, as was typical in phonetics studies at the time: curious artifacts that allowed frequencies to be recorded for two and a half seconds. The analyses that computers run today, with a single click, needed weeks of work then. This is how Tomatis explains the procedure:

> *"the Gramophone Company gave me the masters and I was able to experiment to my liking. I took 4,000 pictures of Caruso's voice. I photographed all his long, sustained notes. Doing that with a (cylinder) analyzer was a lot of work. There were no oscilloscopes. Analyses were done by frequency, not by band. Ten photos had to be taken for each note".*[25]

According to him, before 1902 Caruso's curve had the ideal shape, with a gradient of 6 dB/octave. After 1902, the curve doubled its gradient. The reason for the change is unknown. Tomatis believed that he had suffered some kind of injury, perhaps due to surgery he underwent in Spain, which paradoxically benefited his vocal qualities, but this has not been documented.

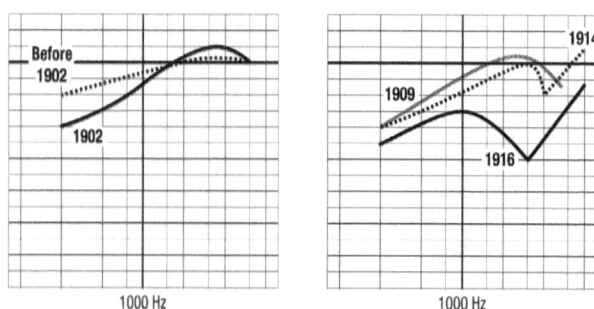

In 1909 the curve still maintained its properties, with a slight fall in the treble region. By 1914, the auditory scotoma in the high frequencies was very clear, and even more so two years later (1916).

Caruso's voice is extraordinary. To understand just how extraordinary, we have sought out some of the most beautiful voices that opera has offered us. In this case, Mario del Monaco, in *Nessun Dorma*. Let's compare their harmonic distribution:

---

[25] **Tomatis, A.** Unpublished papers.

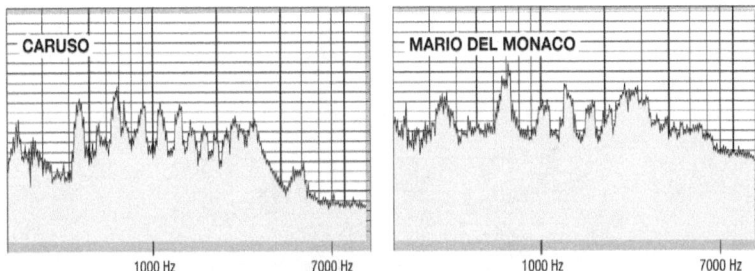

In both voices the richness of frequencies is remarkable and although Mario del Monaco's voice is beautiful, the acoustic analysis for Caruso stands out, with a rich, very well-defined harmonic sequence. His vocal imprint when at his prime is unmatched. He stands out among the best-known singers. Sometimes Caruso seems to outdo even himself. In a brilliant 1906 *Martha*, he succeeds in reaching some notes with this profile:

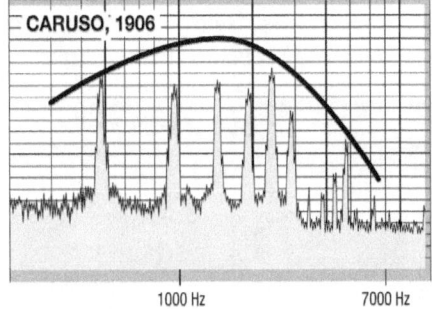

A clear distribution of harmonics, more typical of a musical instrument than of a human voice.

We can perfectly distinguish even the 13th harmonic in the series, as if these were the note of a violin:

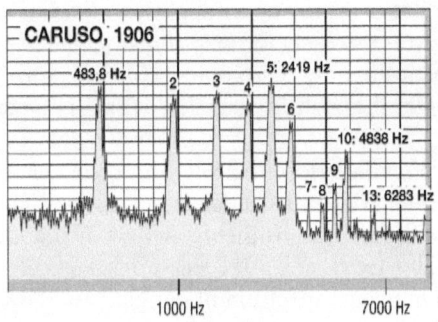

To find anything comparable we have to look to *la divina* Maria Callas, who delights us with marvelous notes in this example from the *Barber of Seville:*

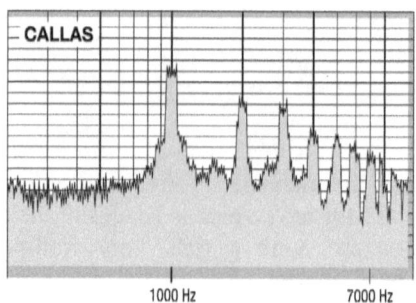

As Tomatis described, the decline of the Italian tenor's vocal qualities is noticeable at the end of his career. Its glorious frequency range fades, especially from 4,000 Hz on. Sometimes, however, a flash of the lost voice appears. Below is a sample of his voice from 1920, singing *The Jewess,* a French opera by Scribe.

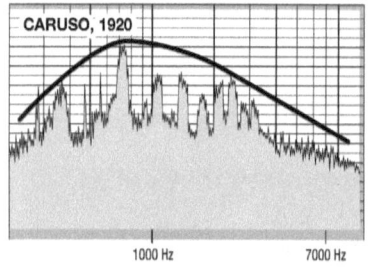 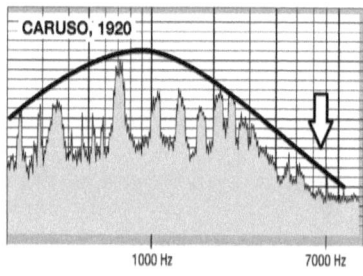

At some points in his performance, Caruso manages to show off his qualities once more. In the sonogram, we see him soar powerfully to 3,000 Hz before dropping away slightly: a fleeting echo of his best registers. However, this lasts for only a few tenths of a second. In the rest of the recording the harmonics tail off from 4,000 Hz on, revealing a loss in the high frequencies, which is typical of his voice at that time.

Older people's voices lose their high frequencies in a similar way, becoming duller and duller, as happened to Caruso. Those of you who work in hearing-aid adjustment will be familiar with this phenomenon. The frequencies the ear no longer controls gradually disappear from the vocal spectrum of our patients:

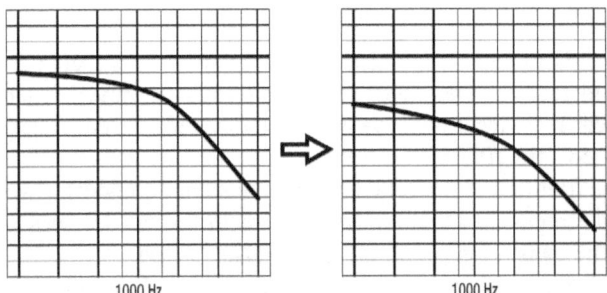

Typical progression of hearing loss

However, singers are not made great by complex sound analyzers, but by their audiences. Some aficionados prefer Plácido Domingo, others Pavarotti: there is no unanimity. Whether or not we connect with their voices does not depend on their qualities alone. Our ears are different and the way we listen determines our musical preferences to a great extent.

Once, Tomatis received a renowned singer in his office, whom he calls "T". He took the opportunity to enthusiastically show this man the progress of one of his patients, whose voice reminded him of the great Caruso, but that did not seem to impress his guest at all. Tomatis was baffled:

> *"I went to look for an album by Caruso, one of the warmest, one of the richest in frequencies: Verdi's Luisa Miller. He recorded it in 1914, at a time when he was no longer the great Caruso of maturity, although his voice still had an extraordinary range. I put it on the record player without saying anything to T.*
>
> *"Who's that?" he asked me after a few moments.*
>
> *"Caruso" I said.*
>
> *"That's exactly what I thought!" he shouted. "Ah, truly, I will never understand how that lad could get the whole world talking about him! Listen, just listen to him! How awful! He's unbearable!"*
>
> *He was furious. I had great difficulty in calming him down. I promised him he would never hear about Caruso in my house again.*
>
> *When I was left alone in my office, I meditated at length on that incident. Could it not be that he did not hear in the same way as me? I quickly built a filter to listen just like him. And indeed, in those conditions, Caruso became unbearable to me as well!"* [26]

---

[26] See note 3

UNEXPECTED EFFECTS

Tomatis thought that if ear and voice were so integrated, perhaps he could recover the singer's voice through improved listening. He designed a device (what we would today call an equalizer) which, using acoustic filters, restored the frequencies affected by hearing loss. He tried it and it worked. When the singer could hear well again, his voice regained its color, but only with the headphones on. Once out of the consulting room, the magic disappeared.

From that moment on, Tomatis concentrated on achieving stable improvement. Reading Pavlov and studying Caruso's technique, he considered the possibility that his patients' ears could be conditioned by repeatedly switching between their normal, defective hearing and corrected hearing, leaving enough preparation time for the auditory system to adjust, just before the vocal emission. He called this pause *delay*.

Tomatis was inspired again by Caruso's voice in setting this key parameter. The following sonograms correspond to the first scene of the third act of *The Force of Destiny*, by Verdi, when Álvaro sings:

"I miei parenti sognaro un ____trooooooooono"

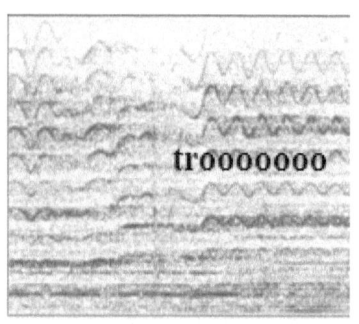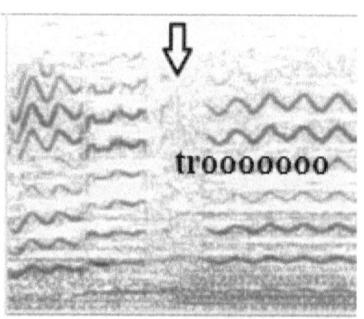

The sonogram on the left corresponds to Mario del Monaco singing this passage. On the right, Caruso. Note the sharp pause that the latter introduces before the powerful vocal emission, which, according to Tomatis, prepares the ear for capturing the next sound.

He incorporated this Carusian technique into his electronic device, thus achieving lasting effects. First, he tried it manually, using levers that changed the signal filtering. Later, when diodes appeared, he was able to build a device that automatically alternated between one or another listening mode: the singer's own and the corrected one. In

FACULTÉ DE
MÉDECINE DE PARIS

PREMIER COURS INTERNATIONAL DE

PHONOLOGIE

ET DE

PHONIATRIE

Semaine du 2 au 8 MARS 1953

1954 he patented his first "Electronic Ear". The invention won a gold medal at the International Exhibition in Brussels in 1958 (when the famous Atomium, now one of this city's landmarks, was inaugurated). Helped by this device, he achieved remarkable and permanent improvements. It did not take long for him to achieve fame as a phoniatrician, with the finest opera singers of the day among his patients.

At the age of 33, he was one of the five speakers at the first International Course in Phonology and Phoniatrics, held in Paris in 1953, joining such major figures as Ajuriaguerra, Borel-Maisonny, Negus or Perelló.

His awards bear witness to the recognition of his work:

- Chevalier de la Santé Publique (1951)
- Médaille d'Or de la Recherche Scientifique Bruxelles (1958)
- Grande Médaille de Vermeil de la ville de Paris (1962)
- Prix Clemence Isaure (1967)
- Médaille d'Or de la Société académique "Arts, Sciences et Lettres" (1968)
- Commandeur du Mérite Culturel et Artistique (1970)

The press took an interest in his research. Two months after the phoniatrics conference, on 29 May 1958, the Spanish newspaper *La Vanguardia Española*, based in Barcelona, published an article signed by P. Vila San-Juan, entitled *La Prisa*, (*Haste*) which I partially reproduce below:

"The event that motivates this chronicle is the following: Doctor Alfred Tomatis, director of the acoustics laboratory of the French Air Ministry, in Salille-sos-Bois [sic], has cured by means of his invention "the electronic ear" the famous tenor Nicole Courcel [sic], who had completely lost his voice and was suffering from terrible deafness. But in order to do this—and here is the essence of his invention—the

sound of constantly playing discs had to be applied directly to the patient's brain. Doctor Tomatis, in view of the tenor's characteristics, chose Caruso's voice, and now—prodigiously—Nicole Courcel sings exactly the same as the famous Italian who astonished the world with the power of his art. Sounds—says Doctor Adrian Selam, an Erkman-Chatrian character—work on the molecules of a liquid to produce infinite combinations, with the difference this time that, since such molecules are movable, the figures that result from them are animated beings. It is what physicists call "equivocal creation."

Indeed, the voice of Caruso has been installed in the vocal cords of Nicole Courcel. And no sooner was this scientific prodigy made known, than two clients approached Tomatis who are symbolic of the present day. One is old—the bass singer Humberto Tomatis, the doctor's father—who only aspires to recover his lost voice. The other is young, very young, and this lad, who has not lost anything, nor suffers from any illness, wanted the doctor to "imprint" on him the voice of Anselmi or Tito Schipa, because he has a fondness for opera and—this is where the haste comes in—wishes to enter the opera world as a fully-fledged virtuoso. It was not enough that the doctor very wisely told this petitioner that neither Caruso, nor Anselmi, nor Tito Schipa had their voices—and much less the indispensable art of projecting them— at his young age, but that to their natural gifts they had added study, practice and arduously gained experience. Never has the truth been so implausible. The boy left the consultation disappointed and almost indignant because the doctor did not want— according to him—to create a star of song and stage in the space of a few minutes […]"

THE MUSICAL CURVE

"I have been able to observe innumerable larynges which were well constructed, well-muscled and yet incapable of singing. Conversely, many singers remain active, singing well, with a damaged larynx. The problem, therefore, lies elsewhere and all sorts of experiences have led me to think that it is in hearing. In order to be able to sing, the person needs to perceive his own voice in a unique way, at the moment of emitting it". A. Tomatis[27]

---

[27] *Caruso est devenu Caruso par hasard.* **Gerber, A. and Tomatis, A.** March, 1973, Son Magazine, Vol. 36.

Contrasting the audiograms with the vocal and musical features of his patients, Tomatis soon came to these conclusions:

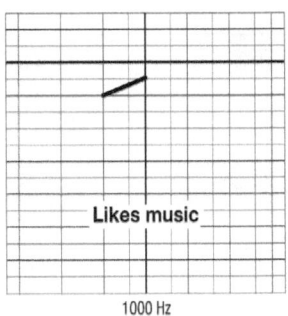

An ascending curve up to 1,000 Hz indicates that the person likes music.

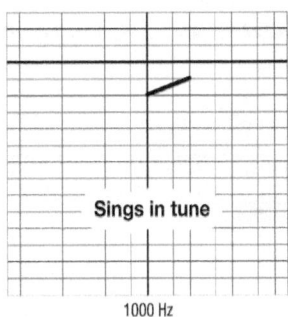

If it keeps going up to 2,000 Hz, the person also sings in tune.

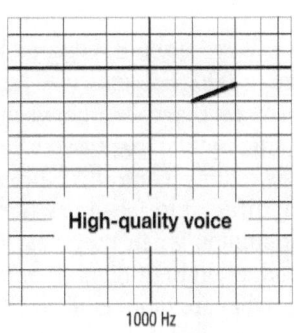

*If the curve continues to rise beyond 2,000 Hz,
the person has a pleasant voice.*

Combining the above, we would get these profiles:

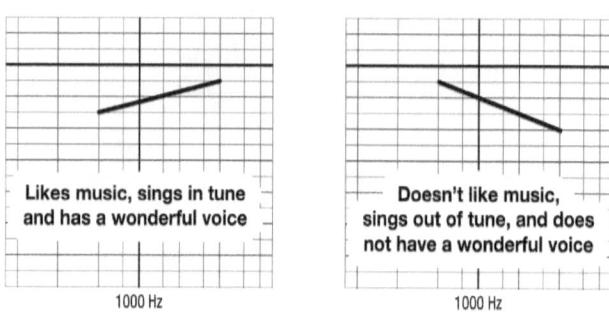

Tomatis was not alone in noticing this pattern. Mozota, an ENT specialist from Pamplona, Spain, makes similar observations in his book, *Reflejo humano otoneurofonatorio del habla (Otoneurophonatory human speech reflex).*[28] He distinguishes between a receptive ear and an expressive ear. The former is linked to the ability to appreciate music; the latter, to singing in tune.

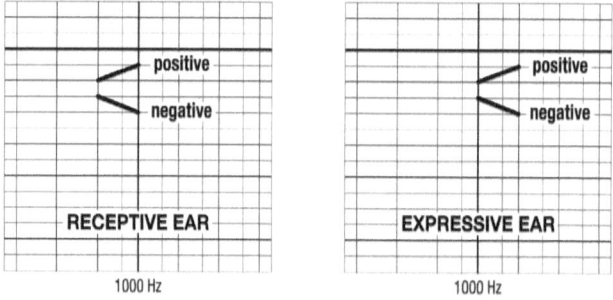

According to Mozota's research, a rising audiometric curve in the area between 500 and 1,000 Hz indicates a good predisposition towards music (receptive ear), and one between 1,000 and 2,000 Hz indicates the ability to sing in tune (expressive ear).

The singing voice is mainly controlled through bone conduction, which is why we find it difficult to recognize our voice in a recording. Singers are often disappointed when they hear themselves through a speaker, since bone conduction highlights frequencies up to 3,000 Hz, concealing some defects that are more evident in recordings.[29]

---

[28] **Mozota, M.L. et al.** *Reflejo humano otoneurofonatorio del habla.* s.l. : Palibrio, 2013.

[29] **Won, S.Y. and Berger, J.** *Estimating transfer function from air to bone conduction using singing voice.* s.l. : Center for Computer Research in Music and Acoustics, Stanford University, 2005.

Sometimes we find almost flat audiograms, close to the zero-decibel level:

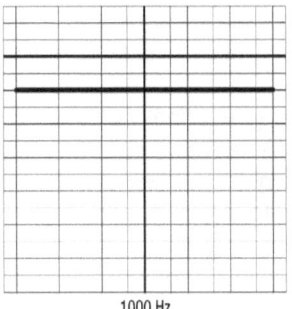

1000 Hz

Hearing all frequencies equally is not something marvelous. The (fortunately few) people with this type of audiogram lack musical qualities. This is an ear that barely analyzes, that simply reacts. Some hearing therapies seek to achieve this rectilinear profile, presumably in the belief that they should get as close as possible to the zero level on the audiogram; but this is a mistake, it is not a desirable goal. Reference zero was based on the thresholds obtained in healthy young people. It is an average of those values, not the auditory curve of any of them.

In hearing-aid adjustment, a flat curve is not the best option either. Most undesirable background noises are made up of low-pitched sounds, which have a strong masking effect, so placing them at the same level as mid-range and treble sounds is not very effective. When calibrating a hearing aid, we always favor the sounds peculiar to speech, located in the middle region.

According to Tomatis, the (utopian) ideal curve, which would represent the best ear possible and would be the goal of any auditory therapy, would resemble this one:

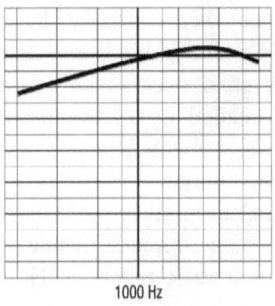

1000 Hz

TIMES OF TROUBLE

If Tomatis had confined himself to phoniatrics, his techniques would surely now be studied in universities and the electronic ear would be a medical device, but he ventured beyond the boundaries of audiology.

He was too observant to overlook the changes taking place in his patients under the effects of his therapy. In fact, they themselves explained to him that they felt different, more energetic and full of life, and were recovering from certain ailments they had been suffering from.

As their voices improved, so too did the rest of their bodies. The singers walked more upright and displayed renewed vitality. It seemed that working on the ear had inexplicable benefits. Tomatis devoted his life to investigating this matter, to understanding the relationship between the auditory system and the rest of our organism. His therapy, therefore, does not derive so much from his ideas, but from his clinical practice. His theories are largely attempts to explain phenomena that he himself did not expect to find.

As his fame and his center on Boulevard Courcelles in Paris grew, tensions with his colleagues increased. His claims were too innovative and bizarre. Scientific publications were demanded of him, while he concentrated on meticulous clinical observations (saying that the work of scientific validation was left to his successors, that he did not have time for it). Although he had the support of some physicians, the situation soon became unsustainable.

Overwhelmed by the continuous calls to order from the College of Physicians (amazingly not because of his praxis but because he was accused of advertising, something forbidden at the time), he resigned, which turned his valuable contributions into suspicious pseudoscience, a situation in which we remain today.

Despite the criticisms, however, his excellent results had not gone unnoticed. His techniques were already being used in several hospitals and medical or psycho-pedagogical centers belonging to the French public education system, such as the Villeneuve-Saint-Georges intercommunal hospital, headed by L. Fontas, the pediatric unit of Lisieux hospital, headed by Leveque, or the center in Pau, with the neuropsychiatrist Gardey in charge.

In fact, we should point out in all fairness that the story could have taken a very different turn since, on at least one occasion, Tomatis did try to carry out rigorous scientific research. He accepted an offer to lead a team in Canada to validate the application of his technique to dyslexia. The project kept getting delayed, however, for reasons beyond his control and after five years he decided that he could not devote so much time to it, returning definitively to Paris. From then on, he consistently refused to work on statistics-based research.

Validating his techniques is a very complex task. Fortunately, the Mozart-Brain-Lab institute/Atlantis Center in Sint-Truiden, Belgium has begun the arduous work of putting Tomatis back on the scientific map. They use brain maps to monitor the action of auditory therapy and collect data systematically. This is a huge challenge, consuming many resources. Someday it will be achieved.

After leaving the College of Physicians in 1974, Tomatis concentrated on developing his theories, leaving financial and administrative matters in his collaborators' hands. These were years of great expansion. When I met him, new centers were opening all over the world, which meant he had to travel most of the year, giving courses and lectures. My own impression is that, at that time, he did not surround himself with the right people. Tomatis was guided by strong ethical principles and convictions. His entourage, however, seemed more focused on other ambitions.

He finally retired in 1996, handing over his company to his son Christian, who immediately adopted a more commercial approach to the franchise: a change that was to create friction. Relations between father and son deteriorated and, finally, on May 30, 1997, Tomatis summoned all of us to a meeting in London to inform us that he was leaving Tomatis International (TISA), the network he had founded.

In fact, he created a new company that did not prosper, among other reasons because he fell ill. Subsequently, TISA closed, and the patents and trademark were transferred to a Luxembourg-based company managed by Christian Tomatis, which is still in operation.

As a result, from 1997 onwards, the international network broke up. Some centers decided to continue with Christian, but most of them went their own way, forming national associations or working independently.

During the last years of his life Tomatis remained in close contact with Jozef Vervoort, director of the Mozart-Brain-Lab, the largest center in Europe for research and development in audio-psycho-phonology. Together they developed a new electronic ear and several technical improvements. Sint-Truiden is home to Tomatis's archives and private library, which I have fortunately been able to consult extensively, thanks to his generosity.

Tomatis left us after a painful illness. A friend who lived in Carcassonne managed to alleviate his suffering with acupuncture, but this kept him a long way from Paris. He finally rented a modest apartment in Carcassonne, where he lived with his wife, Lena, until Christmas Day 2001. A few months later, his son Christian also passed away.

Alfred Tomatis left us a diagnostic and therapeutic method but, above all, a new approach to understanding the auditory system. And a lot of questions to be answered!

AUDIO-PSYCHO-PHONOLOGY

Now that we know a little about Tomatis's life, I will go deeper into his legacy, which he himself called "audio-psycho-phonology" to emphasize the relationship between ear, psyche and voice.

He published a dozen books, of which the most technical, in which he develops his ideas, are the two volumes of *Vers l'ecoute humaine (Towards Human Listening)*[30] and *Vertiges (Dizziness)*[31]. We also find a wealth of theoretical information in *La nuite uterine (The Uterine Night,*[32] *L'oreille et le langage (Hearing and Language),*[33] *Education et dyslexie (Education and Dyslexia)*[34] and *L'oreille et la voix (The Ear and the Voice).*[35]

Other volumes in his catalogue are more of general interest, some examples being *Nous sommes tous nés polyglottes (We Were All Born Polyglots),*[36] focusing on language learning, *Les troubles scolaires (Failure at School)*[37] or *Neuf mois au paradis (Nine Months in Paradise).*[38] In his last book, *Écouter l'univers (Listening to the Universe),*[39] from 1996, he reflects philosophically on hearing.

One day I asked Tomatis how he managed to find time to get through so much work and he told me what his daily routine had been for many years. He would get up at seven in the morning and

[30] **Tomatis, A.** *Vers l'écoute humaine.* Paris : ESF éditeur, 1989.

[31] —. *Vertiges.* París : Ergo Press, 1989.

[32] —. *La nuit uterine.* s.l. : Editions Stock, 1981.

[33] —. See note 8

[34] —. *Educación y dislexia.* Madrid : CEPE, 1979.

[35] —. *El oído y la voz.* Badalona : Paidotribo, 2010.

[36] —. *Nous sommes tous nés polyglottes.* Paris : Fixot, 1991.

[37] —. *El fracaso escolar.* Barcelona : Edicions La Campana, 1989.

[38] —. *Nueve meses en el paraíso.* s.l. : Biblaria, 1996.

[39] —. *Écouter l'univers.* París : Robert Laffont, 1996.

start seeing patients at eight. He went to bed at 9 p. m., getting up at midnight to work on his projects. He then went back to bed at 6, and slept for an hour, until 7 a.m.

He practiced mainly as an ear surgeon until he was 50 years old, when he left the operating theaters behind him. According to him, you should put down the scalpel while still in your prime, not when you are in decline.

ENERGY ACCORDING TO TOMATIS

2

"The ear is a dynamo. This is its main function".
A. Tomatis[40]

The courses with A. Tomatis were dense, very dense. I remember that more than once, aware of the mental fatigue of his audience, he would end his seminars with this sentence: "If, after this course, all you remember is that **the main function of the ear is to give energy to the brain**, it will have been worth it."

Therefore, the concept of *energy* in Tomatis's work is fundamental. It is not an esoteric idea. Tomatis uses this word in a very specific sense, referring to a vital need: our nervous system needs suitable, continuous stimulation in order to function. The lack of this stimulation causes disorders and, taken to the extreme, can cause irreparable damage.

And if the main source of energy is the auditory system, then the functioning of our brain depends largely on the ear. The vestibule (mainly), together with the cochlea, keeps the brain active.

This hypothesis has practical consequences. For Tomatis, excessive or insufficient supply of energy from the ear is behind some of the most common psychological disorders. He was not the only one to take note of the hearing-psyche relationship—something I will examine in detail in chapters 5 and 6.

And what happens when we are still and in silence? Does the brain stop receiving *energy*? And what about the deaf?

---

[40] *L'oreille musicale, un atout peu commun.* **Gerber, A. and Tomatis, A.** 1973, Son Magazine, Vol. 35.

THE EAR-BRAIN SYMBIOSIS

The energizing function of the ear is a concept developed by Tomatis after reading an essay by D. and K. Stanley-Jones: *The Cybernetics of Living Beings*, published in 1962, with a foreword by Norbert Wiener, the founder of cybernetics, the science of self-organizing systems.[41]

In this work, the authors introduce the concept of *nervous energy*, pointing out that animals need a minimum flow of constant stimulation to live. They point to gravitational receptors and, in particular, to the vestibular system, as being ultimately responsible for providing that circulation of *nervous energy*, since terrestrial gravity ensures constant stimulation of those sensors. Unlike light or sound, gravitational action never disappears. Tomatis was convinced that the ear is a vector of development in the course of evolution. An increasingly complex hearing system, which provides an increasing number of stimuli, requires a nervous system that develops and perfects itself in order to process that vast amount of information. He describes it to us this way:

> *Phylogenetically, (the recharge function) is the first to be established and constitutes a highly efficient energizing element. The ear can be compared to a dynamo that transforms the stimuli it receives into neural energy, which feeds the brain. This explains why an apathetic, lethargic child, who is not interested in his work, is often a child whose ear malfunctions in terms of cortical charging. In that case, the charging function of this dynamo must be restored, with the help of specially tailored techniques.[42]*

Unlike the systems that precede it in the course of evolution, the mechanical system (touch) and the chemical system (smell and taste), the sense of hearing functions at a distance, not by contact. The information transmitted is more complex, so it needs a more powerful processor to capture and analyze it. The ear and the brain need each other.

In Chapter 3 I will explain auditory phylogenesis. It is easier to understand Tomatis's concept of energy in the light of evolution.

---

[41] **Stanley Jones, D. and Stanley Jones, K.** *La cybernetique des êtres vivants.* Paris : Gauthier Villars, 1962.

[42] *Dépistage de l'enfant dyslexique a l'école maternelle.* **Tomatis, A.** s.l. : Université de Potchefstroom, 1976. Congrès National de la South African Society for Education.

ENSURING STIMULATION

The ear-brain symbiosis has been there from the very start. Which came first: the hair cell or the neuron? It is hard to answer, since neither makes sense without the other.

The vestibule of the ear (the organ of balance) stimulates the brain constantly, whether we are moving or not. Permanent activity in the synapses of vestibular cells has been proven, even in the total absence of movement.[43] Moreover, on destroying these experimentally, the discharge frequency increases in the vestibular nuclei.[44] The lack of external stimuli is quickly compensated for by another internal mechanism.

Some vestibular fibers show regular discharge patterns and others irregular ones. The same goes for auditory hair cells, which send out pulses even without any displacement or sound to perceive. This spontaneous activity is common in the animal kingdom. It has been described in mammals, birds and lower vertebrates[45] and has been observed in deaf mice.[46] Even the ears of flies behave actively, generating oscillations of about 200 Hz in the midst of absolute silence.[47]

Eliminating the cochlea does not put a stop to this process. In 1966, Koerber and his team reported that on destroying it, the activity of the ventral cochlear nucleus ceased but the dorsal one continued to pulsate. In other words, some neurons in the auditory pathway that had stopped receiving impulses from the cochlea were able to continue firing.[48]

The dorsal cochlear nucleus receives somatosensory, as well as auditory, inputs. This flow of stimulation keeps its neurons functional, even in deaf persons. Stimulation of the fingertips, for example, enhances auditory perception in patients with cochlear implants.[49]

---

[43] *Resting Discharge Patterns of Macular Primary Afferents in Otoconia-Deficient Mice.* **Jones, T.A., Jones, S.M. and Hoffman, L.F.** July, 2008, Journal of the association for research in otolaringology.

[44] **Van de Vater, T.R. and Staecker, H.** *Otolaryngology: Basic Science and Clinical Review.* New York : Thieme Medical Publishers, 2006.

[45] **Flores, A.R. et al.** *El sistema vestibular: aspectos generales y neurodesarrollo.* Puebla, México : Universidad Autónoma de Puebla, 2001.

[46] *Homeostatic control of spontaneous activity in the developing auditory system.* **Babola, T.A. et al.** 3, 2018, Neuron, Vol. 99, pp. 511-524.

[47] *The Drosophila Auditory System.* **Boekhoff-Falk, G.** 2, 2014, Wiley Interdiscip Rev Dev Biol., Vol. 3, pp. 179-191.

[48] *Spontaneous spike discharges from single units in the cochlear nucleus after destruction of the cochlea.* **Koerber, K.C. et al.** 2, Oct, 1966, Experimental Neurology, Vol. 16, pp. 119-130.

[49] *The Stochastic Resonance model of auditory perception: A unified explanation of tinnitus development, Zwicker tone illusion, and residual inhibition.* **Schilling, A. et al.** 2020, Biorixv.

Although discharge patterns change during sleep, the hearing system remains active,[50] which is essential to the functioning of structures like the hippocampus, a control center closely involved in spatial location,[51] the circadian rhythms and memory.[52] This is a two-way regulation since, in turn, the hippocampus regulates the activity of sensory neurons in accordance with the state of the brain.[53] I suspect this is one of the reasons why, after auditory therapy, patients often report improvements: saying things like "I feel more awake" or "I remember things I didn't before".

External sound can also be an inhibiting factor. In an experiment with bats, a spontaneous discharge in the inferior colliculus of more than 80% of its neurons was observed. Immediately after an acoustic stimulation, half of them stopped firing.[54]

The number of stimuli the nervous system receives through our sensory organs is enormous. Some researchers have tried to quantify them, reaching figures of several thousand per second. Most are filtered and we are only aware of a small fraction of them. If the selection process fails (as a result of stress, for example) and too many stimuli arrive, the system becomes saturated.

Vestibular overstimulation causes metabolic and circadian-cycle imbalances. P. M. Fuller's team, from the Neurology Department of the Beth Israel Deaconess Medical Center, in Boston, USA, submitted a group of laboratory mice to 2G centrifugation (twice gravitational acceleration) for eight weeks. Their metabolism was significantly reduced: they ate less and lost weight, and their average body temperature fell sharply on the third day, breaking the usual circadian rhythm pattern. Other mice that were genetically deprived of vestibular cells underwent the same process. There were no significant effects on their metabolism. The study demonstrated the involvement of the vestibular maculae in homeostatic regulation.[55]

[50] *El sistema auditivo en el ciclo sueño-vigilia.* **Velluti, R.A. y Pedemonte, M.** 5, 2005, Rev Neurol, Vol. 41.

[51] *Long-Term Effects of Permanent Vestibular Lesions on Hippocampal Spatial Firing.* **Russell, N.A. et al.** 16, July, 2003, The Journal of Neuroscience, Vol. 23, pp. 6490-6498.

[52] *Vestibular loss causes hippocampal atrophy and impaired spatial memory in humans.* **Brandt, T. et al.** 2005, Brain, Vol. 128, pp. 2732-2741.

[53] *La información sensorial y su relación con los ritmos biológicos de vigilia-sueño y theta del hipocampo.* **Pedemonte, M.** Montevideo : s.n., 2000, Actas de Fisiología, Vol. 6, pp. 71-92.

[54] *Suppression of spontaneous firing in inferior colliculus neurons during sound processing.* **Voytenko, S.V. and Galazyuk, A.V.** 4, 2010, Neuroscience, Vol. 165, p. 1490.

[55] *Neurovestibular modulation of circadian and homeostatic regulation: Vestibulohypothalamic connection?* **Fuller, P.M. et al.** 24, 2002, PNAS, Vol. 99.

SEEKING GRAVITY

In rats gestated in space, their vestibule, deprived of stimuli, does not follow its normal course of development. Although vestibular maturation is genetically programmed, it still needs the intervention of the environment.

Under weightless conditions there is an increase in otoconia (otoliths in the vestibule) and synapses with vestibular cells. Sensors are multiplying in an attempt to perceive the absent gravity.[56,57]

The mice born in these experiments later present a whole series of disorders depending on the conditions to which they were subjected and at what time: motor alterations and alterations in primary reflexes, cerebellar function and even cognitive skills. Some of these are irreversible, as there are critical periods in development.[58,59]

According to Tomatis, the lack of recharging caused by absence of movement slows down the functioning of our brain, diminishing our cognitive abilities and compromising the sophisticated balance of the nervous system. He joked that the comforts of modern life, such as TV remotes, cars or working seated at a computer, are the perfect cocktail for reducing vestibular activity and consequently the *nervous energy* it provides. Physical exercise is recommended to maintain both bodily and cognitive health. Our brain works better if we give up our sedentary lifestyle.[60]

ACTIVATING THE EAR

We can sleep with light, or with quiet music, but not while singing or dancing. These activities together produce an excitation that is incompatible with sleep, making the hearing system work at full capacity and fill our brain with energy. This would explain, for example, the predilection of musicians for post-concert parties: the exhilaration built up while performing prevents them from sleeping.

---

[56] *Effects of prenatal spaceflight on vestibular responses in neonatal rats.* **Ronca, A.E. and Alberts, J.R.** 2000, J Appl Physiol, Vol. 89, pp. 2318-2324.

[57] *Spaceflight-induced synaptic modifications within hair cells of the mammalian utricle.* **Sultemeier, D.R. et al.** 6, June 1, 2017, J Neurophysiol., Vol. 117, pp. 2163-2178.

[58] *The development of vestibular system and related functions in mammals: impact of gravity.* **Jamon, M.** Feb 11, 2014, Frontiers in Integrative Neuroscience, Vol. 8.

[59] *Critical periods in vestibular development or adaptation of gravity sensory systems to altered gravitational conditions.* **Horn, E.R.** 2004, Archives italiannes de biologie, Vol. 142.

[60] *The effects of exercise on cognitive function and brain plasticity: a feasibility trial.* **Gomes-Osman, J. et al.** 5, 2017, Restor Neurol Neurosci., Vol. 35, pp. 547-556.

A Swiss team has discovered that auditory discrimination can predict the recovery of coma patients. Regardless of their initial state, the patients who improved auditory discrimination in their encephalography records were the ones who managed to wake up.[61] It has also been observed that those treated with music therapy make better progress.[62]

The ability of the auditory system to keep us awake is not accidental: it derives from our neurological architecture, in particular its links to the hippocampus and the reticular formation.

SENSORY DEPRIVATION

Experiments in sensory deprivation began in the 1950s. Students were paid to endure hours stuffed into special suits, floating in water, completely in the dark and without noise of any kind. The aim was to nullify their perceptive mechanisms of touch, gravity, sight and hearing to see what happened.

After a few moments of relaxation, hallucinations appeared, as if the brain, deprived of sensations, was manufacturing its own. Those who endured those conditions for a long time later suffered psychological sequelae. Prolonged sensory isolation causes disorders that can prove to be irreversible[63] but if it is controlled and used for a short time it could be beneficial.

In fact, there are isolation tanks that are used for therapeutic purposes. In the long term, however, it has devastating consequences. These techniques have been used as a form of torture, leading to intervention by the European Commission of Human Rights.

In the Quora network, Alan Koenigsberg, a psychiatrist, clearly explains the link between stimulation, mental health and hearing. In answer to the question "Why does psychosis get worse at night?", he says this:

> It is because when there is less external stimulation, there is more internal stimulation. Deprivation tanks can precipitate psychosis for this reason. I remember when I was doing my residency, I spent time on a ward with patients with chronic

---

[61] *Progression of auditory discrimination based on neural decoding predicts awakening from coma.* **Tzovara, A. et al.** 2013, Brain, Vol. 136, pp. 81-89.

[62] *Music therapy for coma patients:preliminary results.* **Sun, J. and Chen, W.** 2015, European Review for Medical and Pharmacological Sciences, Vol. 19, pp. 1209-1218.

[63] **Zubek, John P.** *Sensory Deprivation: Fifteen Years of Research.* New York : Ardent Media, 1969.

schizophrenia. One young man would tell me he walked around with headphones and listened to music most of the time, because when he listened to music, the voices diminished. When he took off the headphones, they came back.[64]

Experimental sensory deprivation is an extreme situation that fortunately does not occur in everyday life. However, we can live in similar circumstances, either because we have a sedentary existence starved of stimuli, or because our sensory organs do not work properly. Otitis[65,66] or changes in the auditory system caused by stress [67] are also a partial form of sensory deprivation.

Brain plasticity studies show that rapid changes take place in unused neural networks. Neurons are shut down or recycled for other purposes. In people who do not receive auditory stimulation, these changes are visible with current technology. Deactivated zones lose gray matter, which increases in areas where information is still collected.[68] On the other hand, after musical training, the neural density is greater.[69]

In a famous experiment, Pascual Leone taught Braille to a student with no visual problems, over a week during which she was kept permanently blindfolded.[70] The brain images obtained daily showed that in the first days, the motor cortex was activated during the lessons, while at the end of the week, the occipital cells—dealing with sight—took over. As they had remained "idle", they were immediately assigned to another task: that of learning Braille in this case.

[64]   **Koenisgsberg, A.** Quora. [Online] [Cited: Sept 12, 2019.] https://www.quora.com/Why-is-psychosis-worse-at-night.

[65] *Auditory Deprivation Caused By Early Otitis Media with Effusion.* **Salgado, M. et al.** 1, 2018, Biomed J Sci &Tech Res, Vol. 5.

[66] *Auditory Deprivation in Children with Otitis Media with Effusion and its Effect on Temporal Resolution.* **Johnston, T. and Green, W.B.** 4, 2002, Journal of speech-Language pathology and Audiology, Vol. 26.

[67] *Effects of stress on the auditory system: an approach to study a common origin for mood disorders and dementia.* **Pérez-Valenzuela, C., Terreros, G. and Dagnino-Subiabre, A.** 2018, Rev. Neurosci.

[68] *Alterations in gray matter volume due to unilateral hearing loss.* **Wang, X. et al.** May 13, 2016, Nature Scientific Reports.

[69] *Musical training intensity yields opposite effects on grey matter density in cognitive versus sensorimotor networks.* **James, C.E. et al.** 2013, Brain Struct Funct.

[70] **National Geographic.** My music brain [On line] Nov 13, 2012. [Cited: Jun 8, 2019.] https://www.youtube.com/watch?v=tR32CPKkxTA.

EAR, ENERGY AND RETICULAR FORMATION

The reticular formation, located in the brainstem, is the most archaic part of our brain and is involved in major bodily functions (over one hundred have been described). It includes the ascending reticular activator system (ARAS), which regulates sleep and wakefulness by means of cyclic discharges that are projected onto certain areas of the brain. In addition, it controls the striated (antigravitational) musculature and regulates the endocrine system, via the hypothalamus.

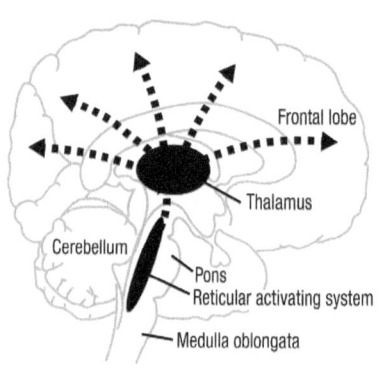

The neurons of the reticular formation become activated when receiving impulses from any of the sensory organs. This flow of *nervous energy* helps us stay awake.

When we turn off the lights, silence envelops us and we place ourselves on a soft mattress (which cushions our gravitational perception), we send fewer impulses to the reticular formation, which induces the cortex to enter the sleep phase. Compared to other senses, the action of the vestibular system on the reticular formation is tremendously powerful. We are always fighting gravity to move, and that is a source of constant stimulation. Movement gives us energy.

Most reticular neurons react to vestibular stimuli—in the medial zone more than 75% of them—while between 23% and 40% respond to acoustic stimuli.[71] Therefore, the vestibular system, in addition to controlling balance and muscle tone, also exerts a notable energizing function that modulates brain activity and gives the ear the leading role in activating the reticular system. According to Tomatis:

> *"The human ear supplies a large part of cortical energy. It intervenes in a proportion of 60% in relation to the other sensory organs. If we add to this the responses of the skin, whose sensory function is phylogenetically linked to the auditory function and if*

---

[71] *Behavioral functions of the Reticular Formation.* **Siegel, J. M.** [ed.] Elsevier. 1, 1979, Brain Research Reviews, pp. 69-105.

we also consider the sensory-muscular and sensory-articulatory responses, which arise from differentiated sensors that share their auditory origin, we reach a percentage of 90% as regards the energy attributed to the cochleo-vestibular apparatus, which is a considerable figure ".[72]

From an audiological perspective, we should emphasize that the reticular formation is also involved in the control of the stapedial reflex and the filtering of ambient noise.[73]

Tomatis also pointed out the importance of one's own voice as a recharge source. The richness of harmonics offered by good radio announcers attracts the audience's attention and at the same time activates the speaker's own nervous system. Depending on the quality of their voice, people can get either tired or exultant after talking: an effect that can last for several hours.

In the audio-vocal courses organized by Tomatis, some at his home in Carboneras, in the south of Spain, he taught us how to emit "energizing" sounds with our mouths shut: a kind of humming sound that causes a vibration in the cranium, like a resonator. He told us it was a good exercise to send energy to the brain and keep it fit. He recommended practicing it several times a day. What a surprise it was when I discovered years later that a similar technique is recommended to schizophrenics to reduce their auditory hallucinations, saturating the brain with this internal stimulus.[74]

As I will describe in the following chapters, phylogenesis, ontogenesis and physiology reveal an ear that quickly ensures the necessary stimulation is present. The close link between hearing and health, both physical and mental,[75] will appear repeatedly in every chapter of this book. It is a relationship that goes back to the very origin of life.

---

[72] See note 42

[73] **Giacomelli, F. and Mozzo, W.** *An experimental an clinical study on the influence of the brainstem reticular formation on the stapedial reflex.* s.l. : Padua University, 2005.

[74] *Auditory hallucinations in schizophrenia: Does humming help?* **Green, M.F. and Kinsbourne, M.** 5, 1989, Biological Psychiatry, Vol. 25, pp. 633-635.

[75] *Auditory deprivation and health in the elderly.* **Cherkoa, M., Hicksonb, L. and Bhuttac, M.** 2016, Maturitas, Vol. 88, pp. 52-57.

EAR
PHYLOGENETICS 3

In the course of evolution, the brain and the senses were built in parallel, in a symbiosis that especially involves the auditory cells. To understand the real role of the ear in our organism, it is indispensable to examine it through the prism of phylogenetics. It gives us the clues we need to understand its real functions.

First, we need to be clear that the ear does not arise with the purpose of listening but of perceiving gravity. That links it initially to movement, not sound: hearing is a function that is constructed later on.

Since the animal needs to interact with its environment to survive, sensory receptors appear that provide it with information about the outside world, to detect food or the presence of a predator. In unicellular organisms, the receptors located in the membrane regulate traffic, allowing some substances to pass and rejecting others. They also warn of a hostile environment, causing the cell to react, in an attempt to get away from danger. In multicellular living beings, some cells specialize, forming tissues, whose function is to analyze the information from the exterior. These will go on to form the sensory organs.

The predator needs to move in the right direction if it wants to eat. And if it holds back, the prey flees. Moving confers a major competitive advantage and, therefore, animals have developed different locomotion systems, which need at least two elements:

-   A propulsion mechanism
-   A steering mechanism

The first propellants that appear are the cilia: tiny "hairs" placed on the membrane that act as oars. The cell, always in a liquid medium, moves by paddling.

But where is it going? For what purpose?

If motor skills are based on cilia, locomotion is not precise. This system is not very useful either for the predator or for the prey. They both need to locate food or danger at a certain distance, which means rapidly developing:

- better propulsion mechanisms (which means fighting against gravity)
- a gravity sensor: the ear
- remote detectors (of light waves, magnetic waves, sound waves, etc.)
- a nervous system capable of giving the correct motor commands, based on the information received by the sensory organs: a goal-oriented motor system
- a feedback mechanism or cybernetic loop, an element of great importance that we will analyze below.

The animal has to manage information coming from the environment and from itself. The brain must know that by moving the tail to the left, the body moves to the right or that, on closing the mouth, the tongue is not something to eat. In other words, the bodily vessel must be properly steered, knowing what is happening outside and inside the organism. To achieve this, each muscle, tendon and joint is permanently reporting on its status, to organize the next movement. This is known as *proprioception*, which allows fast and precise corrections to be made, adjusting motor action to internal and external information in order to achieve the objective.

All of our muscles have proprioceptive sensors: the muscle spindles. If these do not report accurately, dysfunctional responses are generated because they are based on erroneous data. Eye muscle spindles, for instance, are one of the keys to dyslexia, as French ophthalmologist Patrick Quercia explains.[76] Similarly, we find them in the muscles of the middle ear.[77]

---

[76] **Quercia, P. et al.** *Traitement proprioceptif et dyslexie : dysperceptions et cognition.* Beaune : AF3dys, 2008.

[77] *Observations on the number, distribution and morphological peculiarities of muscle spindles in the tensor tympani and stapedius muscle of man.* **Kierner, A.C. et al.** 1-2, Sept, 1999, Hearing Research, Vol. 135, pp. 71-77.

According to Andrew Bell (see Chapter 4), a failure of these sensors could trigger Meniere's vertigo.[78]

We always organize our motility in accordance with our position in relation to gravity. The ear thus becomes the main regulator of motion, since it is the gravity sensor. It seems to make sense, then, that when faced with motor disorders, as professionals we should always evaluate the auditory function, especially the vestibular system.

Over millions of years the ear is perfected, gathering better information about the position in space. The saccule appears after the utricle, followed by one, two, and then three semicircular canals, forming a functional group that we call the vestibule. The utricle, the first vestibular structure to appear, reports on the horizontal plane. The saccule reports on the vertical plane and the canals together form a real gyroscope.

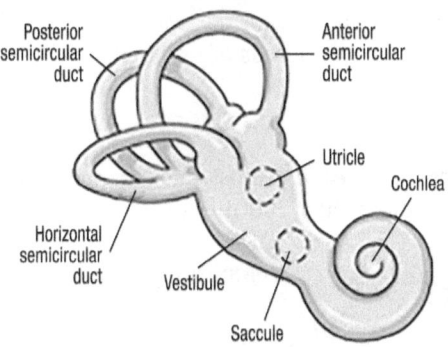

The brain grows in order to be able to process all this data. Ear and brain evolve in tandem: the ear sending information and the brain organizing responses, essentially motor ones. At first, these are reflex reactions but, as the nervous system develops, they become increasingly elaborate, automatic, oriented towards survival goals, able to reflect emotional states and tasked with carrying out our intentions. There is no doubt: movement is the protagonist of our origins.

We believe that our brain is mainly dedicated to thinking. However, as Mlodinow reminds us: "[...] *well over half of the neurons are dedicated to motor control and the five senses. On the other hand,*

---

[78] *Middle ear muscle dysfunction as the cause of Meniere's disease.* **Bell, A.** 3, 2017, Journal of Hearing Science, Vol. 7, pp. 9-25.

the part of our brain that separates us from the "lower" animals is relatively small".[79]

The close relationship between ear and brain is well exemplified in salps: marine animals that swim in their larval stage and have brains to organize their movements. However, in their adult phase as polyps, when they adhere to a rock, they get rid of their brain because they no longer need it.

Watch the video by scanning this QR code

The sensitivity of the gravity sensor enables it to be used as an acoustic detector, which will go on to reach a high degree of sophistication in mammals, with the appearance of the cochlea, in a process that takes many hundreds of millions of years.

JELLYFISH EAR

Jellyfish are some of the most ancient non-extinct animals we know, as fossils more than 700 million years old have been found. They gather information on water composition, gravity and light.

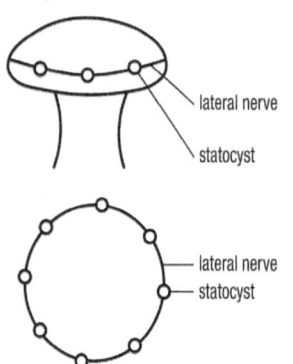

Their ear is a gravity sensor that allows them to coordinate their movements to get around. It contains a set of hair cells, located in small cavities on the surface of the jellyfish: the statocysts, through which seawater circulates. These are the ancestors of our vestibule.

Inside the statocysts we find small stones: the statoliths, whose function is the same as that of our otoliths. As the jellyfish moves, the statoliths collide with the walls and set off currents of water around them, due to their inertia, which agitate the hair cells. In this way the cells capture movement and inform their nervous system.

---

[79] **Mlodinow, L.** *Las lagartijas no se hacen preguntas*. Barcelona : Crítica, 2016.

The latter extends in the form of a network throughout the body of the jellyfish, and is sprinkled with slow-conducting neurons, though there is one area with fast-transmission fibers: the base of the bell, along the outer edge of the animal. The information gathered by the hair cells in the statocysts is transmitted through this circuit.

In the *Obelia* jellyfish for example, the ear is made up of eight statocysts along the lateral nerve, only one of which is needed to ensure the overall dynamics. If we eliminate all eight, its motor activity ceases entirely.[80]

The hair cells of jellyfish have evolved to organize themselves better and better, forming structured colonies of cells. They flood the nervous system with data, forcing it to evolve in parallel to be able to process so much information and pinpoint the position of the animal, its speed and its acceleration. However, in the jellyfish there is no grouping of neurons of any kind to sketch out a primitive brain that could centralize the information collected. Sensory impulses are disseminated through the neural network—through the lateral cord in particular.

And along that lateral line, about 200 million years after the appearance of the jellyfishes, neural ganglia arose in the flatworms. These were small clusters of neurons that we could regard as the first ever brain. In this way, the ear takes on the leading role in evolutionary neurological development.

HISTORY OF THE VESTIBULE

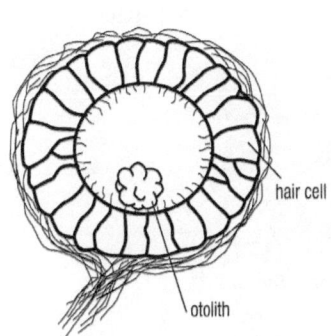

hair cell

otolith

The statocyst of the jellyfish is nothing more than the utricle of the vestibule. We have seen that its functioning is simple: a weight half-floating over the sensory cells, either solid (statolith or otolith) or viscous (statoconium or otoconium), whose inertia pushes it in the opposite direction to the movement of the animal. Always attracted by gravity, the otolith provides the positional reference.

---

[80] See note 41

When the saccule and semicircular canals appear later on, we continue to find hair cells and otoliths inside them. In other words, the design remains little changed to this day, after millions of years: our own system works on the same principles.

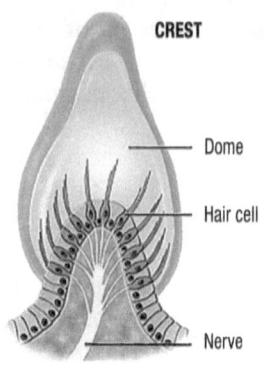

CREST

Dome

Hair cell

Nerve

In mollusks, such as the octopus or the cuttlefish, hair cells are grouped into structures called crests, constituting the first organization of the vestibular hair cells and allowing information on angular acceleration to be obtained.

In crustaceans, the statocysts are located at the base of the second antennas and remain open to the outside. Crabs place small pebbles on the statocysts using their claws. These are their otoliths. In every molt they must get new ones. If we spread iron filings on the floor of an aquarium and the crabs pick some up to use as otoliths, we can mislead them with a magnet. They will confuse the magnetic field for gravity and will base their motor functions on it.[81]

In the cyclostomes (jawless agnathan fish), which appeared 500 million years ago, and of which the lamprey and the hagfish still survive, the statocyst closes up. It stops being in direct contact with the sea, making its own inner sea: the endolymph.

The semicircular canals appear. The hagfish has one, the lamprey two. In the bony, cartilaginous fishes of the Devonian, all three take shape and so begins the perception of three-dimensional space.

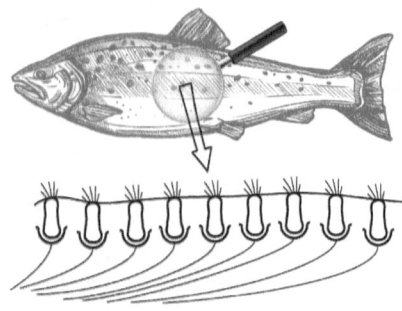

[81] **López, C. y Cussó, F.** *Fundamentos físicos de los procesos biológicos.* s.l. : Editorial Club Universitario, 2013. p. 38.

The canals are triangular shaped in reptiles, elliptical in birds and circular in mammals.

A fish's lateral line is equipped all along with hair cells, serving as a supplementary ear. It is sensitive to the flow of water around it, reporting the position of the animal in all its segments (metameric information). In addition, it can pick up sounds and water currents produced by other animals. From the appearance of the modern fish (which emerged 100 million years ago) to the present day, the vestibule has barely evolved any further.

The vestibular nuclei extend the ear's control over the entire motor apparatus, regulating muscle tone and balance. These nuclei are sets of neurons that act like a real motor brain. The first to stand out in the reticular formation are the dorsal and ventral nuclei of the lampreys.

All the neurological structures that appear later in the course of evolution connect to the pre-existing ones, including the vestibular system. In the lower vertebrates and invertebrates, the vestibulospinal bundles appear, which link the vestibule with the whole body through the spinal cord. In the upper vertebrates, the vestibular-optic pathways will allow the image to remain stable even when the head is moving, among other functions. The vestibular-cerebellar pathways will facilitate fine and precise movement management.

The cerebellum is the vestibular brain. Although it only makes up 20% of the size of the whole brain, it contains over half of the neurons and each of them connects with thousands of partners, forming a network of greater density than in the brain itself. This way, the vestibule influences any body element involved in motion, the muscles linked to locomotion and also those of vision, phonation, etc. Everything is under its control.

Later neurological development will always make connections with the vestibule. We will find its action everywhere, in the neurovegetative system, in emotions and even in cognition.[82] The *nervous energy* collected by the ear spreads throughout the entire nervous system.

In evolutionary development, the sensitivity of the hair cells will be used to capture those subtle displacements of water that are the vibrations produced by sounds and, in this way, the vestibule will go on developing to refine its acoustic perception.

---

[82] *Extending the Functional Cerebral Systems Theory of Emotion to the Vestibular Modality: A Systematic and Integrative Approach.* **Carmona, J.E. et al.** 2, 2009, Psychological Bulletin, Vol. 135.

The lagena appears in reptiles and birds and finally, in mammals, the cochlea. These structures serve to facilitate hearing, although the pattern stays the same. They are nothing more than appendages of the vestibule and, inside, we will find the same hair cells.

HISTORY OF THE MIDDLE EAR

Achieving extraordinary acoustic sensitivity is quite easy in Nature. Grasshoppers detect a considerable range of sounds: one that is wider than ours, up to almost 200,000 Hz, using tiny eardrums located on their front legs, two on each. Those of the moth, the size of a pinhead, vibrate at frequencies of up to 300,000 Hz: a record in the animal world and far beyond our own limit of 20,000 Hz. However, hearing more is not the goal. The evolutionary development of the ear has not been about expanding its frequency range or sensitivity, but selecting what we want to hear and thus obtaining relevant information.

Electronics has allowed us to manufacture small, ultra-sensitive microphones and headphones, but it has not yet been able to emulate our ability to extract sounds. Even the best hearing aid on the market is not as effective as the human ear in noisy environments, where following a conversation is tricky.

Phylogenesis shows a nervous system that quickly gets involved in the management of sounds: the efferent system, a set of neural bundles that go from the brain to the ear giving instructions, and which we have already seen on the lateral line of fish.[83] This allows perception, as opposed to mere sensation. Thus, the animal can take an active role and adjust the entry of stimuli. The great evolutionary leap of the ear occurs when animals leave the sea and settle on land. The acoustic properties of air are not those of water, so impedance matching is required. To this end, evolution will build the middle ear, equipped with active regulation mechanisms. Reptiles, for example, have a bony labyrinth that protects the ear. They will transform bones from their jaw to give them an auditory function: bones that in turn derive from fish. An elastic skin collects sound waves and transmits them to the labyrinth. The columella (the only bone in the ossicular chain) appears and in some animals there is a muscle linked to it that allows sound input to be modulated. The columella

---

[83] **Webster, D.B. and Fay, R.R.** *The Evolutionary Biology of Hearing.* s.l. : Springer Science & Business Media, 2012.

is attached to the eardrum, if there is one, or to head teguments, and it projects the sound on to the cranium.

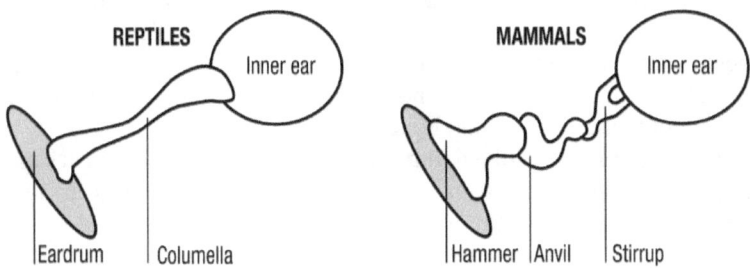

In turtles, the columella connects the inner ear to the jaw, while in snakes, it connects the inner ear to the outer bone. They receive sound through the bone. In an aerial medium snakes are quite deaf, only capturing ground vibration, but they hear well in water. They lack both an eardrum, a Eustachian tube, and an external auditory canal.

In amphibians, the columella connects the inner ear to the quadrate (lower jaw). In the urodeles (such as salamanders) there is no eardrum. Sound is captured through extratympanic pathways. The transmission of sound waves is believed to occur through the jaw, as in turtles.

Cetaceans also hear in this way, connecting the large receiving screen (the jaw and perhaps the rest of the skeleton) to the inner ear. In dolphins, as the jaw vibrates, the bone mass surrounding the auditory cells vibrates in unison, directly transmitting the information. As for humans, we have not lost the ability to listen by bone conduction. For some researchers it is a secondary pathway of sound propagation, but for Tomatis it is the main one.

In birds, there is a muscle attached to a second ossicle, the extracolumella, innervated by the facial nerve, or seventh cranial pair, and equivalent to our stapedius muscle (which moves the stirrup bone). Birdsong shows that their ear has taken an evolutionary leap forward with respect to reptiles.

The hammer and the anvil are typical of mammals and do not exist in the other vertebrates. They derive from the reptiles' square and articular bones, respectively. The stirrup comes from the latter's hyomandibular bone, which joins the jaw to the skull. The great auditory novelty introduced by mammals, apart from the cochlea, is an ossicular chain that serves to modulate sound input, with two muscles acting in synergy: the tensor tympani or hammer muscle and the stapedial or stirrup muscle.

For Tomatis and others, the middle ear is not a transmitter, but a regulator[84] of sound that makes listening possible: an active mechanism that demands participation by the hearer. The eardrum embedded in the bone does not send sound through the ossicular chain, but to the surrounding bone.

Our hearing has evolved, but we continue to share with turtles and dolphins a hearing mechanism based on the same principles. In fact, the human ossicular chain, in terms of acoustic transmission, does not have the best of designs, reaching a hydraulic gain of 19:1, a constant factor in all mammals.

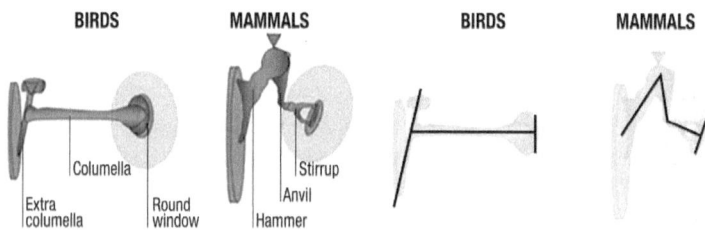

The typical structure of birds with two ossicles (columella and extracolumella) can obtain a much higher hydraulic gain.[85] There is no need to add a third element to improve impedance matching. In mammals, the design of the three ossicles in the ossicle chain does not bring greater pressure, but greater accuracy.

The middle ear is responsible for more sophisticated functions than the mere propagation of sound. In fact, it has been suggested that it was the decisive factor that led to the appearance of the cochlea.[86] Paleontologist T. Rowe of the University of Texas, using computerized X-ray tomography, has suggested that the neocortex and the mammalian middle ear evolved in parallel to each other.

Initially the ossicular chain appears as a chain of bones attached to the jaw and skull. It then separates from the jaw and positions itself behind it. The neocortex evolves simultaneously with the detachment

---

[84] See note 31

[85] **Bradbury, J.W. and Vehrencamp, S.L.** *Principles of Animal Communication.* s.l. : Oxford University Press, 2011.

[86] *Cochlear mechanisms from a phylogenetic viewpoint.* **Manley, G.A.** 22, 2000, PNAS, Vol. 97, pp. 11736-11743.

of the chain: a process that we will see repeated in ontogenetic development. First the auditory chain emerges, connected to the jaw, and then it detaches itself from it.[87]

REFLECTIONS ON PHYLOGENETICS

It may seem that the evolutionary history of the ear has nothing to do with our daily work. Quite the opposite, in fact.

I have had the opportunity to see many children with learning or developmental difficulties. In most cases, balance, the most primary function of the ear, corresponding to the vestibular system, is compromised. Balance is the forgotten sense, which we only remember when it does not work properly. A vestibular dysfunction, such as simple motion sickness in a car or a boat, causes tremors, stomach pains, sweating, and so on. In half of migraine patients, vestibular stimulation acts as a trigger.[88] I remember a friend who spent three days suffering from severe attacks of vertigo after undergoing colon hydrotherapy. That shows how far the vestibular connections reach.

Children like to move. This is how their hearing system matures. Games train their vestibule and are often accompanied by songs, thus also activating the cochlea and therefore the whole ear.

We have seen how, after balance, the ear evolves to control muscular tone, through a collection of fascicles of vestibular origin. If the tone control is problematic (hypotonic or hypertonic children), we know that the therapy will be longer than if the muscle tone is correct, adapting to each situation. Dystonia is usually accompanied by a long series of active primary reflexes.

As it is one of our oldest structures, everything links to the vestibular system in one way or another. Research has shown, for example, that it modulates hormonal secretions.[89] It is linked to the hypothalamus, the pituitary gland, the adrenal glands and, in short, to the entire autonomic nervous system, and especially to the vagus nerve (the one that projects to the eardrum, vibrating in unison).

---

[87] *Coevolution of the mammalian middle ear and neocortex.* **Rowe, T.** Aug, 1996, Science, Vol. 273.

[88] **Murdin, L.J.** Audiovestibular sensory processing in migraine. [ed.] University College London. 2010. Doctoral thesis.

[89] *Vestibular modulation of endocrine secretions – A review.* **Sai Sailesh, K. and Mukkadan, J.K.** 1, 2014, International Journal of Research in Health Sciences, Vol. 2.

Vestibular activity (e.g. sport) reduces sympathetic activity, causing a drop in blood pressure. It is involved in the production of melatonin (the sleep hormone), thyroid hormones, pancreatic hormones and cortisol, in addition to certain neurotransmitters, such as serotonin.

Tomatis emphasizes that evolution of the ear in fish, reptiles, birds and mammals coincides with a more upright posture. As the antigravity struggle is resolved, the animal's body becomes more upright. One of the singularities of the human being is its verticality, the greatest among mammals.

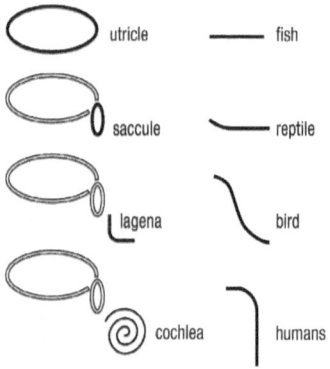

Adapted from A. Tomatis [90]

Children say their first words coinciding with the conquest of verticality. Walking and phonation require a high level of motor coordination, in which the ear is deeply involved.

In developmental disorders, verticality is often compromised. The forward-leaning neck that drags the shoulders down with it is a common feature in these cases, a sign that good control of muscle tone is missing. Mental illnesses are also often accompanied by postural and motor disorders due to the involvement of the vestibular system.[91]

NOTES ON ONTOGENETICS

The formation of the ear in the fetus is also fascinating. Between the fourth and the fifth month of gestation it is already picking up acoustic

---

[90] See note 32

[91] *Upright posture improves affect and fatigue in people with depressive symptoms.* **Wilkes, C. et al.** Auckland : s.n., 2017, Journal of Behavior Therapy and Experimental Psychiatry, Vol. 54, pp. 143-149.

vibration and, before that, it registers movements. As in phylogenetics, first the vestibule is formed, collecting motor information, and then the cochlea. The great musical pedagogue Edgar Willems senses this order when he affirms:

"From a musical point of view, rhythm precedes melody. It is a primordial element, on the same level as sensory hearing".[92]

At birth, the ossicular chain reaches almost adult size, making it a biomarker of fetal health.[93] The auditory pathways are myelinated. They are functional. Auditory precocity is universal in the animal kingdom. Almost everything is already complete at birth. Babies differentiate their mother's voice and language from any other person, and have some grammatical knowledge.[94]

Why does the fetus need a functional ear so soon? Could it not wait to mature a little later, as with vision? For Tomatis the answer is clear. The developing fetus needs stimulation, *nervous energy,* and the ear is in charge of providing it.

Ontogenesis repeats phylogenesis. Millions of years of evolution are condensed into nine months, following the same stages. The ear emerges from the branchial arches, the areas that in fish will give rise to the gills, thus retracing an ancestral path. Having been a vector of the evolution of the nervous system, the ear repeats the process in the womb.[95]

Nature is determined to keep the hearing system busy, as soon as possible, even in the absence of external stimuli. The so-called support cells seem to share this objective, making sure that the hair cells are always active.[96,97] In mice, the destruction of the Deiters cells, for example, causes severe deficiencies in postnatal maturation of hearing.[98]

In 1994, Lippe, a professor at Washington University, studying chicken embryos, observed spontaneous cyclic discharges in the

---

[92] **Willems, E.** *L'oreille musical.* Fribourg : Éditions Pro Musica, 1985.

[93] *Auditory ossicles: a potential biomarker for maternal and infant health in utero.* **Leskovar, T. et al.** Aug 21, 2019, Annals of Human Biology.

[94] *Listening to language at birth: evidence for a bias for speech in neonates.* **Vouloumanos, A. and Werker, J.F.** 2, 2007, Developmental Science, Vol. 10.

[95] See note 32

[96] *Spontaneous activity of cochlear hair cells triggered by fluid secretion mechanism in adjacent support cells.* **Wang, H.C. et al.** 6, Dec 3, 2015, Cell, Vol. 163, pp. 1348-1359.

[97] *The origin of spontaneous activity in the developing auditory system.* **Tritsch, N.X. et al.** Nov 1, 2007, Nature, Vol. 450.

[98] *Selective ablation of pillar and Deiters' cells severely affects cochlear postnatal development and hearing in mice.* **Mellado Lagarde, M.M. et al.** 4, 2013, J Neurosci., Vol. 33, pp. 1564–1576.

auditory nerve and the auditory areas of the brainstem.[99] These potentials appeared regardless of heart rate or breathing, even after removal of the ossicular chain. They changed under acoustic stimulation and did not disappear unless the cochlea was removed. To quote from Lippe's conclusions:

> *"The discharge of potentials from the afferent sensory fibers plays an important role in the development of the nervous system. The evidence for this conclusion stems in large part from the finding that manipulations that alter the amount or pattern of sensory input produce abnormalities in nerve structure."*

Lippe, however, raised doubts about whether his observations could be extrapolated to mammals, but years later, a study by Tritsch and Bergles postulated the following.

> *"Neurons in the developing auditory system fire off bursts of action potentials before the onset of hearing. **This spontaneous activity promotes the survival and maturation of the auditory neurons** [bold type added] and the refinement of synaptic connections in the auditory nuclei. However, the mechanisms responsible for initiating this activity remain uncertain".*[100]

Spontaneous discharge is now considered indispensable in the functional structuring of the auditory system, for example, to correct tonotopic distribution.[101] Although many doubts persist, it seems that the hair cells stimulate the neurons by sending glutamate into the synaptic space, weeks before the ear is ready to function. This precocity could be related to the maturation and to the very survival of the nervous tissue,[102] which fits perfectly with the role of energy captor that Tomatis ascribes to the ear.

---

[99] *Rhythmic Spontaneous Activity in the Developing Avian Auditory system.* **Lippe, W.R.** 3, March, 1994, The Journal of Neuroscience, Vol. 14, pp. 1486-1495.

[100] *Developmental regulation of spontaneous activity in the mammalian cochlea.* **Tritsch, N.X. and Bergles, D.E.** 4, 2010, J Neurosci., Vol. 30.

[101] *The precise temporal pattern of pre-hearing spontaneous activity is necessary for tonotopic map refinement.* **Clause, A. et al.** 4, May, 2014, Neuron, Vol. 82, pp. 822-835.

[102] *Spontaneous activity in the developing auditory system.* **Wang, H.C. y Bergles, D.E.** Oct, 2014, Cell Tissue Res.

Spontaneous neural firing activity has also been documented in the visual system and in other áreas of the brain, and is thought to be linked to attention and consciousness.[103]

In in vitro cultures, both the white matter (oligodendrocytes) and the grey matter (neurons) multiply their survival rate when systematic stimulation is applied to them.[104] These discoveries have already been applied to research into nerve tissue transplants for the regeneration of lesions, leading to the observation that, if the neurons are stimulated after transplantation, their survival rate multiplies, the myelinization process is accelerated and connections with muscle fibers increase.[105]

---

[103] *Residual inhibition: From the putative mechanisms to potential tinnitus treatment.* **Galazyuk, A.V. et al.** 1-13, 2019, Hearing Research, Vol. 375.

[104] *Electrical stimulation promotes the survival of oligodendrocytes in mixed cortical cultures.* **Gary, D.S. et al.** 1, Jan, 2012, Journal of Neuroscience Research, Vol. 90, pp. 72-83

[105] *Acute Stimulation of Transplanted Neurons Improves Motoneuron Survival, Axon Growth, and Muscle Reinnervation.* **Grumbles, R.M. et al.** 12, 2013, Journal of Neurotrauma, Vol. 30.

A NEW
AUDITORY THEORY 4

In 1961, Georg von Bekesy, a telecommunications engineer, received the Nobel Prize in Medicine for his description of how the ear works. Dozens of hearing theories had previously been formulated and confusion reigned.[106] Helmholtz's theory, the most widely accepted one, had not been proven. His resonators were nowhere to be found.

Bekesy presented sound empirical evidence that the scientific community immediately accepted, ignoring the objections of other researchers who in vain pointed out its inconsistencies. However, more and more doubts have set in since then and many authors now consider these to be too serious. We need to start thinking about an alternative.[107]

We know, for example, that the *travelling wave*, described by Bekesy, cannot provide the very fine frequency selectivity that we possess. A trained ear is able to distinguish a 1,000 Hz from a 1,003 Hz sound. The wave proposed by Bekesy would span the frequency zone of both, making discrimination impossible. Nor is it proven that sound passes through the ossicular chain. If a link is missing, hearing loss is only partial. The sound must necessarily follow other paths. Several publications point to the middle ear as an active regulatory mechanism, although Bekesy's theory of sound transmission through the ossicular chain is still endorsed in the textbooks.[108]

---

[106] **Bast, T.H. and Anson, B.J.** *The temporal bone and the ear.* Springfield : Charles C. Thomas Publisher, 1949.

[107] *New perspectives on old ideas in hearing science: intralabyrinthine pressure tenotomy, and resonance.* **Bell, A.** 4, 2018, J Hear Sci., Vol. 8, pp. 19-25.

[108] *Es el oído el primer filtro de selección frecuencial?* **Vallejo, L.A. et al.** 2, 2010, Acta Otorrinolaringol Esp.2010, Vol. 6, pp. 118-127.

I remember, in the school of audiologists, a series of lectures on cochlear implants, with guest speakers representing different commercial brands. In one of them, we were fortunate to hear from a person with excellent training, whom I took the opportunity to ask many questions because it is hard to understand how an implant works from within Bekesy's framework: the travelling wave disappears, and the electrodes emit electric discharges which, when passed to a loudspeaker, sound more like a broken (very broken) radio than an intelligible sound. Attempts to enhance the acoustic quality by increasing the number of electrodes have only produced even worse results, surprisingly.

As if this were not enough, the autopsies of deceased implant wearers reveal a dendritic degeneration in the first-order neurons, incompatible with correct activity in life, although it seems that they continued to miraculously transmit the information through their axon[109]. The neuron mortality observed in the autopsies is sometimes above 90% and, nevertheless, this did not prevent the implant from working well. On the other hand, one would expect better hearing thresholds in the areas of the spiral ganglion with higher neural density and, thus, greater sensitivity, but this is not the case either.[110]

I brought up another issue: a study that found vestibular damage in half of implanted subjects. However, in spite of this high rate, there were hardly any symptoms of vestibular damage after the intervention.[111] After several questions on these lines, the speaker said to me, pleasantly:

-Look, according to current auditory theory, cochlear implants shouldn't work and yet they do. It's a problem, because, as we don't know how hearing really works, our attempts to perfect these devices often fail. Is that clear?

If we could better understand the physiology of the auditory system, treatments would take a radical turn. Even if we only changed the role of the ossicular chain, from transmitting sound to regulating sound input, we would have to revise our approach to otosclerosis surgery, Meniere's disease, cochlear implants, hearing aids, prevention of hearing loss and a long etcetera.

---

[109] **Almond, M. and Brown, D.J.** The pathololgy and etiology of sensorineural hearing loss and implications for cochlear implantation. [book auth.] J.K. Niparko. *Cochlear Implants: Principles & Practices.* 2009, pp. 43-45.

[110] *Neural survival and psychophysical measures of electric hearing in cochlear implant users.* **Becken, E.T. et al.** 2, 2004, Otolaryngology - Head and Neck Surgery, Vol. 131, p. 157.

[111] *Histopathologic changes in the vestibule after cochlear implantation.* **Tien, H.C. and Linthicum, F.H.** 4, 2002, Otolaryngology - Head and Neck Surgery, Vol. 127, pp. 260-264.

We can find several articles questioning the current official theory of hearing. I will just talk about the ideas of Tomatis and Andrew Bell, a professor at the Australian National University, who has taken research in a very promising direction.

TOMATIS VERSUS BEKESY

Tomatis conceived the mechanism of hearing inversely to Bekesy. He thought that the cochlea received the sound impact by bone conduction from the tympanic ring and, as in a kettledrum, the vibration of the tympanic membrane transmitted the sound to the surrounding bone.[112] In this way, small changes in air pressure are better perceived. Nowadays nobody disputes that much of the sound is transmitted through the bone, at least in regard to our own voice.

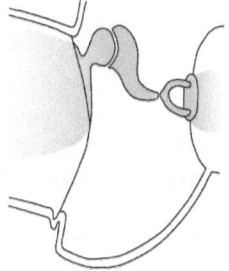

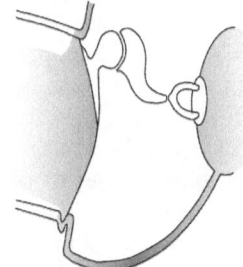

Bekesy Model:
The sound is transmitted to the cochlea through the ossicular chain.

Tomatis Model:
The sound is transmitted to the cochlea through the bone, picking up the tympanic vibration.

Even the specific weight of the air and bone conduction pathways in self-listening has been determined.[113] In nasal consonants, such as "m" and "n", bone conduction predominates. A closed mouth facilitates cranial vibration. On the other hand, the fricatives "s" or "f" are best captured by air conduction. This is, however, a generalization. If we observe in detail, we will see that for each

---

[112] See note 30

[113] *Hearing one's own voice during phoneme vocalization—Transmission by air and bone conduction.* **Reinfeldt, S., Östli, P. and Håkansson, B.** 751, Goteborg, Sweden : s.n., 2010, The Journal of the Acoustical Society of America, Vol. 128.

phoneme, certain frequencies of the spectrum are better perceived via one pathway or the other.

Furthermore, the eardrum and the bone into which it fits are not inert elements. They receive innervation from four cranial pairs: the glossopharyngeal, the trigeminal, the facial and the vagus; which suggests that our organism considers them points of special importance.

In the Tomatis model, the ossicles of the ear and their muscles are not the bridge over which sound crosses. They become modulators of the tension and shape of the eardrum, and of intracochlear pressure. Hearing thus becomes a proactive mechanism. The efferent connections to the outer hair cells complete this top-down function, which allows the brain to control the ear.[114]

Activation of the auditory muscles is ultimately decided on by the nervous system, which chooses what it wants to hear, what it does not, and how. These muscles can be trained. This is precisely the goal of Tomatis's auditory therapy.

We can read in audiology manuals that the shape of the cochlea serves to save space. According to Tomatis, its paraboloid of revolution design facilitates frequency discrimination. Its structure itself constitutes a series of filters, selectively distributing the sounds towards the hair cells: higher-frequency ones towards the base and lower-frequency ones at the tip, similarly to how sound is projected in a whispering gallery, thanks to the peculiar reflections of sound waves in its architecture. Some examples would be Saint Paul's Cathedral in London, Grand Central Terminal in New York or the Monastery of the Escorial in Madrid, where sounds can be sent to a distant listener, without other people in the room, between the transmitter and the receiver, being able to hear anything.

According to Andrew Bell, if the discrimination were carried out as Tomatis claimed, the cochlea should be elliptical and not spiral, as this would make it more efficient. Whatever the case, it seems that the snail shape responds to a functional need.

Some researchers suggest that the spiral shape helps acoustic energy to project onto the hair cells, especially in the apical zone.[115] Others believe that the cochlea's own internal structure, with its vestibular, cochlear and tympanic ramps full of

---

[114] *Sistema eferente auditivo.* **Délano P., Robles I., Robles L.** s.l. : Univ. de Chile, 2005.
[115] *Cochlea's graded curvature effect on low frequency waves.* **Manoussaki, D., Dimitriadis, E.K. and Chadwick, R.S.** 8, March 3, 2006, Phys Rev Lett., Vol. 96.

endolymph, acts as a prism, analyzing the frequency components of sound,[116] but this is still a mystery to be solved.

It has been observed that, at least in cetaceans, the frequency range can be inferred from the shape and length of the cochlea. That way, we could tell what some extinct animals could hear from their fossil remains;[117] but we do not understand why the cochlea of a guinea pig has four turns, ours two and a half, that of a whale one and a half, a horse two, a cat three, and so on. It does not seem to respond to any logic.[118]

Tomatis stresses that the difference between hearing and listening is a physiological reality. We may have serious listening problems despite having normal hearing.[119] This is the case of those who are unable to follow a conversation when there is ambient noise—typical of sensorineural hearing loss—though it also happens to people with impaired, or even with normal hearing.

According to Bekesy's theory, the stirrup muscle acts only in order to muffle noises by means of the stapedial reflex. From the perspective of Tomatis or Bell, the main function of the middle-ear muscles is to maintain optimal endolymphatic pressure in any acoustic situation, helping us to select what we want to hear. They are constantly modulating the perception of sound. Middle-ear pathology does not hinder transmission but rather the regulating function that allows us to clearly distinguish the signal that interests us, dampening background noise.

This selection begins at the eardrum itself, which does not vibrate equally over its entire length. Certain areas show a predilection for a particular frequency band and this distribution can be regulated through the muscle attached to the hammer, the tensor tympani, thus favoring certain sounds to the detriment of others.[120]

---

[116] *Frequency selectivity without resonance in a fluid waveguide.* **van der Heijden, M.** 40, 2014, Proc Natl Acad Sci U S A, Vol. 111, pp. 14548-145520.

[117] *Relationships of cochlear coiling shape and hearing frequencies in cetaceans, and the occurrence of infrasonic hearing in Miocene Mysticeti.* **Ritsche, I.S. et al.** 21, Berlin : s.n., 2018, Fossil Record, pp. 33–45.

[118] **Perelló, J., Rodríguez-González, M.A. y Serra-Reventós, M.** *Fundamentos audiofoniátricos.* Barcelona : Editorial Científica Médica, 1989.

[119] *Impaired speech perception in noise with a normal audiogram: No evidence for cochlear synaptopathy and no relation to lifetime noise exposure.* **Guest, H. et al.** 2018, Hearing Research, Vol. 364, pp. 142-151.

[120] See note 108

NEW HEARING DIAGNOSTICS

The difference between hearing and listening, which forms the core of Tomatis's conception of hearing, continues to be a subject of debate in the world of audiology. In 2005, the American Speech and Hearing Association (ASHA) established the diagnosis of auditory processing disorder (APD), which involves the impairment of acoustic signal processing, without hearing loss: identifying sounds in the presence of noise, frequency discrimination, maintaining listening over time, slowness in processing, and so on.

Hearing aid clinics are expanding their functions to offer this complementary APD diagnosis, although there is not yet consensus on which test battery should be used. The ASHA makes some recommendations without specifying how to carry out the measurements. For the moment, the lack of unified criteria and calibrated tests for each country calls these evaluations into question.

I have used some of the classic APD tests for several years, such as gap detection, dichotic listening or binaural fusion. They help to establish a diagnosis, but I am not convinced that by themselves, at least in their current version, they are a good reflection of the effectiveness of the auditory system.

When exploring listening, I am interested in knowing how it works in its entirety, at both vestibular and cochlear level. We can analyze the vestibule with tests of balance, rhythm or muscle tone, for example. At the cochlear level, in addition to the classic tests, I value other parameters: the ability to process sounds quickly and recognize them, auditory memory, listening in noise, singing in tune and the degree of listening automation (being able to listen and do something else at the same time, see p. 246).

APD tests cannot determine hearing quality by themselves. A person with no musical aptitude can easily pass an APD test battery. We therefore need to reach a consensus on what good listening means.

There are also no well-defined criteria on what to do after the evaluations. Do we train the patients by means of exercises similar to those of the test, such as sound discrimination? Should we make them sing? What about memorizing recited texts?

As long as the classical theoretical framework is maintained, it will be very difficult to advance. The theory formulated by Bekesy in the last century does not guide us towards a treatment for these deficiencies. His contributions were of great value at the time, but now we must move forward and integrate the new discoveries in otology.

ANDREW BELL'S FROG

Andrew Bell's auditory theory assigns a modulating role to the middle ear, as does Tomatis, and provides novel ideas to explain the functioning of the cochlea and other phenomena, such as the physiological origin of the musical scale.

Bell invites us to reflect on the structures of the middle ear, through the study of the frog's ear.[121] This amphibian hears equally well through water or air. How did it solve the problem of impedances to be able to hear in both media? Maybe it can give us some clues about our own hearing system.

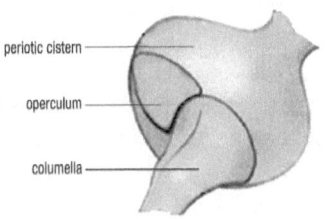

The frog has a peculiar ear. The eardrum, if it exists, is set outside, on the surface of the skin, and swells and shrinks while the frog is croaking or breathing. Its ears are interconnected directly through the skull and also connected to the throat, emitting sounds of considerable intensity: as much as 100 dB from half a meter away.

Some species of frogs lack an eardrum. However, they hear well despite being anatomically deaf. In their middle ear we find the columella (comparable to our stirrup) and next to it appears a flat structure, almost always cartilaginous, called the operculum, anchored to the shoulder of the animal and with its corresponding muscle.

Otoacoustic emissions are produced in these frogs' inner ear, but the auditory cells do not line up in a flexible basilar membrane structure as in mammals but, rather, are embedded in a rigid cartilage. They have a round window, connected to the mouth.

Numerous experiments have shown that when the cilia of the hearing cells are moved, the latter react so, it is assumed, in line with Bekesy's ideas, that the endolymph flowing between the oval window and the round window is the means by which sound is transmitted.

Andrew Bell suggests that, even so, this may not be the frogs' only means of capturing sound, as the classical travelling wave theory requires a flexible membrane. We must consider other mechanisms that allow sound waves to reach the inner ear.

---

[121] *The remarkable frog ear:implications for vertebrate hearing.* **Bell, A.** 1, 2016, Journal of Hearing Science, Vol. 6.

Until now it was believed that it was the cilia of the auditory cell that caused this transduction, converting the mechanical effect of sound into action potential, but it has been observed that one isolated hair cell—all of it—dances to the music, thanks to protein filaments that act like muscles.

Bell points out that hair cells react with high sensitivity to external pressure. The soma moves and, with it, its cilia. The hair cell is very likely to pick up sound through the pressure waves that are generated, which would explain the function of the operculum: maintaining the static pressure of the internal fluids of the ear, and so preserving the "zero" level so that any pressure variation caused by the sound can be detected.

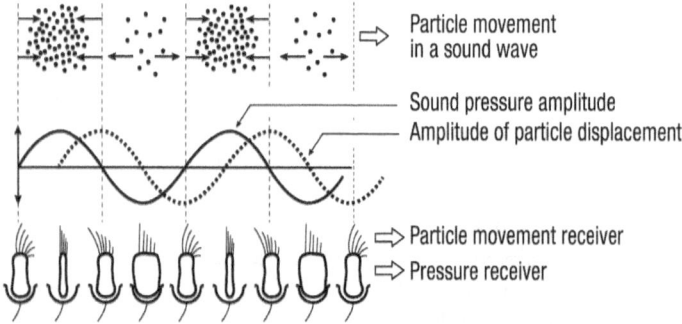

The wave has two components: pressure and displacement.
A sound wave propagated through a medium creates areas of higher particle density (compression) or lower particle density (rarefaction).
The cilia of the auditory cells can perceive the wave's displacement, while the cell body is apparently sensitive to changes in pressure.

Adapted from Bell,[122] from an original by Wehner & Gehring.

If we observe the muscle of the operculum, we will see that it relaxes and contracts to the rhythm of breathing, thus regulating the

---

[122] Ibid.

position of the columella and, consequently, the intralabyrinthine pressure, which in turn maintains hearing sensitivity, compensating for the distortion produced by breathing.

Citing Wever's experiments with evoked potentials, Bell stresses that manipulation of the operculum can vary the frog's sensitivity to sound by up to 72 dB. In salamanders, whose ears are connected, acting on one operculum automatically leads to a contralateral reaction, since the fluid flowing between the two ears is the same.

The mechanism for maintaining intralabyrinthine pressure is not exclusive to frogs. Our own stirrup performs this function so that the hair cells can capture the slightest variation in pressure. The recent discovery of piezoelectric proteins (which generate electrical discharges when subjected to pressure) in the outer hair cells supports this hypothesis.[123] Water is not easy to compress. This way, when submerged, the frog can perceive pressure waves better than in air.

The musculature of the middle ear in frogs and mammals is composed mainly of slow muscle fibers, suitable for the function of maintaining pressure but not so much for an immediate reaction, as has been assumed up to now.

RESCUING HELMHOLTZ

Bell gives a radical twist to the theory of hearing by recovering Helmholtz's ideas about resonators, which finally seem to have been found.[124,125,126,127] He suggests that the cochlea is certainly not passive, but takes the initiative in the perception of sound. It not only receives, but also emits sounds continuously, very precisely, with a frequency bandwidth below even 1 Hz. These noises can be heard through a microphone inserted into the ear canal. These are the spontaneous otoacoustic emissions.

According to Bell, otoemissions are nothing more than the sound produced by the resonators of the cochlea. But where are those resonators? Helmholtz tried to locate them but was unable to. Bell thinks that the geometric structure of the hair cells in the cochlea

---

[123] See note 107

[124] *A Resonance Approach to Cochlear Mechanics.* **Bell, A.** Nov 11, 2012, Plos One, Vol. 7.

[125] **Bell, A.** The underwater piano. Revival of the resonance theory of hearing. 2000.

[126] *How do middle ear muscles protect the cochlea? Reconsideration of the intralabyrinthine pressure theory.* **Bell, A.** 2, 2011, Journal of Hearing Science, Vol. 1.

[127] *Musical ratios in geometrical spacing of outer hair cells in the cochlea: strings of an underwater piano?* **Bell, A.**

serves a purpose. The external ones show a perfect alignment in three rows, parallel to the row of internal hair cells.

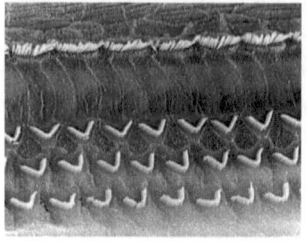 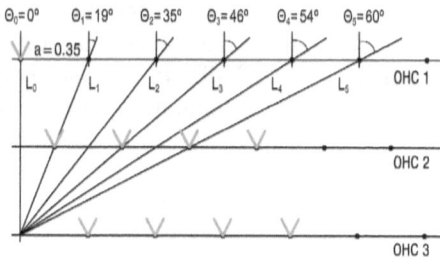

From M. Lenoir: www.cochlea.eu   *From Bell, A.* [128]

The cilia are not placed randomly, but in a peculiar W-shaped structure. By applying acoustic physics concepts to that pattern, Bell noticed that the cilia tufts were arranged in the form of resonators of different lengths, with a factor of 1.06 between them. This is very close to 1.059, which corresponds to the twelfth root of 2: the number by which a musical note must be multiplied to reach the next semitone. A sustained A3 is obtained by multiplying the A3 (440 Hz) by 1.059. That is, 466 Hz. The geometry of the hair cells practically coincides with the chromatic scale.

But why does it not match exactly? Why 1.06 and not 1.059? If we ask a group of subjects to signal exactly when they hear well-tuned octaves, we will see surprisingly that their criterion is 1.06 and not 1.059, as we tune musical instruments. The subjective octave does not exactly double the frequency in Hz; it is a little more.

Analysis of the otoacoustic emissions shows the same pattern. It is not white noise, but grouped in frequency bands separated by the same factor of 1.06.[129]

According to Bell, the arrival of the external sound activates the previously established internal tuning, similarly to the pipes of an organ. The pressure of the endolymph within the cochlea undergoes small variations that stimulate the hair cell. This cell maintains a static internal pressure, while the pressure around it is regulated by the muscles of the middle ear, through the ossicular chain. In this way, the muscles control the sensitivity of the hair cell to external sound.

---

[128] Bell, op.cit. 124

[129] *A Natural Theory of Music based on micromechanical resonances between cochlear sensing cells.* **Bell, A.** 3, 2019, J Hear Sci, Vol. 9, pp. 39-49.

Therefore, the information that the brain receives about the state of tension of these muscles, supplied by the muscular spindles, is of paramount importance.

Bell's theory offers better physiological insights and also major changes in the way of approaching the treatment of some pathologies, among them otosclerosis or Meniere's vertigo.[130] In this syndrome there are always three disorders: hearing loss, loss of balance and tinnitus.

The three can be explained by a dysfunction in the control of intralabyrinthine pressure, causing chaotic behavior of the hair cells, both vestibular and cochlear. If the external pressure is not controlled, their soma inflates or shrinks, altering their sensitivity.

Bell proposes severing the tendon of the tensor tympani muscle to treat Meniere's, reviving a procedure that was already described around 1870 by Weber-Liel.[131]

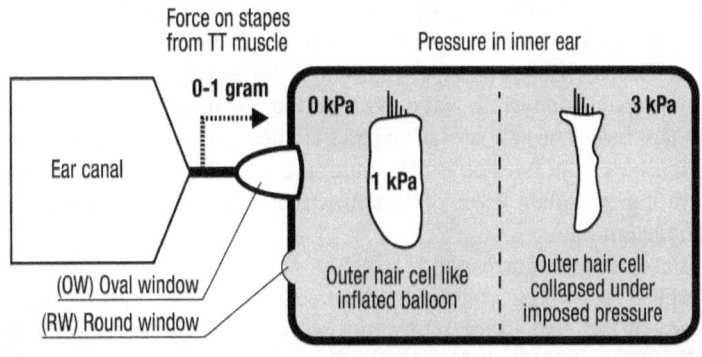

Muscle forces and fluid pressures in the otic capsule, and their effects on outer hair cells. The otic capsule is filled with incompressible fluid, so when the stapes is pushed into the oval windows (OW) by contraction of the tensor tympani (TT), the pressure increases. A force of 1 gram wt on the area of the OW (3.2 mm²) creates a pressure of 3 kPa. This pressure exceeds the internal pressure of the outer hair cells (1 kPa) and causes them to temporarily collapse. This turns down their sensitivity and the cochlear amplifier is switched off. From A. Bell[132]

---

[130] See note 78
[131] See note 107
[132] See note 78

AUDITORY NEUROLOGY ACCORDING TO TOMATIS

Tomatis developed his conception of auditory neurology over several books, mainly in Volume 2 of *Vers l'ecoute humaine.*[133] In *Vertiges*[134] and *La nuit uterine*[135] we find summaries. He divides auditory neurology into four stages, in order of phylogenetic appearance: the pre-, archeo-, paleo- and neo-labyrinth stages. Each one overlaps the previous one, configuring a more evolved ear, endowed with a more complex and competent nervous system. At each stage, an auditory and neurological anatomical novelty appears, expanding the functional range of the whole.

In the pre-labyrinth stage, the statocyst closes and the otolithic vesicle is structured. The ear is no longer in direct contact with the sea. The vestibular nuclei appear: primitive precursors of the brain that allow control of balance and muscle tone.

In the archeo-labyrinth stage the utricle, saccule and semicircular canals develop in parallel to the cerebellum, the vestibule's control center. This facilitates precise, automated movements.

In the paleo-labyrinth stage, we find the lagena and the thalamus, a relay that integrates all sensations and connects them with emotions.

Finally, in the neo-labyrinth stage, the cochlea and cortex appear, generating a higher level of organization from which listening and language emerge.

These stages correspond roughly to fish, reptiles, birds and mammals. It is the conquest of three-dimensional space through movement. At each stage motor skills are put to more elaborate and precise purposes, thanks to the concurrent evolution of the nervous system, culminating in the prodigy of neuromuscular coordination that is human phonation.

Behind the cochlea, the auditory nerve stretches from the most archaic areas of our brain to the most recent, following phylogenetic progression, carrying an acoustic signal that will be modulated in stages. Evoked potential tests inform us of each station along the way.

The neurological stages are also different levels of diagnostic examination. To simplify, we could say that when we test the primary reflexes, tone and balance we place ourselves in the pre- and archeo-levels: we are observing the automatic vestibular reactions.

---

[133] See note 30
[134] See note 31
[135] See note 32

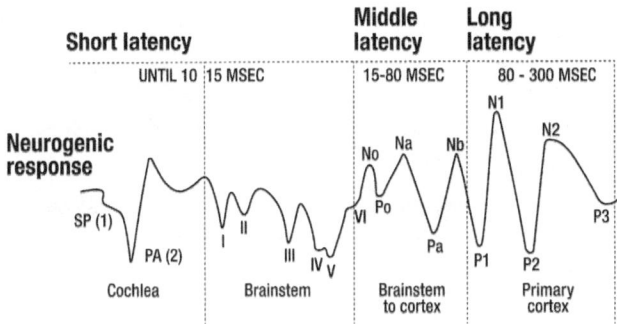

When babies cry and yell, moving their arms and legs to express the discomfort caused by hunger, sleep, cold or pain, the paleo- level is on display. There is now a connection with the emotional structures, and motility responds to desires and frustrations.

We are in the neo-stage when we are testing the praxia: gross and fine motor skills put to a particular purpose, with speech as the most highly evolved level.

In listening we also observe a similar development. Babies first react to sound on reflex. Then they grasp the emotional intention of our words, paying attention to the tone of voice that expresses our state of mind. Finally, they will understand semantics and messages will be analyzed in the cortex. As adults, we will retain all the previous stages: we will react to strange noises and the timbre and cadence of the voice will continue to be essential elements of communication.

Of course, I have had to cut a long story short here. In fact, the structures overlap and there are no clear dividing lines. Problems related to the earlier stages tend to have a worse prognosis, as they indicate disorders present in the underlying structures.

REFLECTIONS ON AUDITORY PHYSIOLOGY

We could look, for example, at the innervation of hair cells. 95% of the thickness of the auditory nerve is made up of afferent fibers (which go to the brain) and only 5% are efferent (coming from the brain). We can easily conclude from this that the afferent path is all-important—the highway towards superior levels.

However, this assumption may not be correct. In the cochlea, the hair cells are distributed in four well-ordered rows: three rows of outer hair cells and one of internal ones. The latter are the main agents responsible for sending acoustic information to the brain, and constitute most of the auditory nerve.

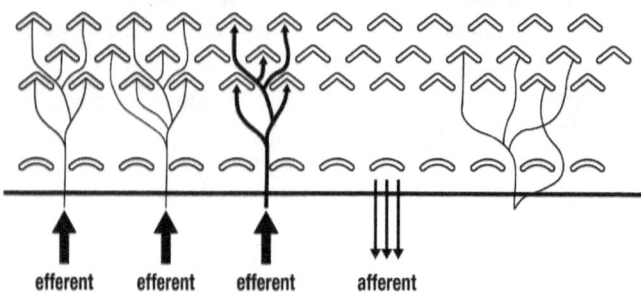

efferent   efferent   efferent   afferent

The outer hair cells, on the other hand, receive almost exclusively efferent innervation, carrying orders from the brain. As there are lines of three outer hair cells for each inner cell, efferent innervation encompasses about 75% of all brain–cochlea connections. Seen in this way, the cochlea receives more information than it sends. It is at the command of a brain that controls the three dimensions of sound: intensity, frequency and tempo.[136]

Tomatis used to say that almost all the mechanisms of the ear are paradoxically designed not to listen. The ear is ultra-sensitive. It can even react to light: the pressure differences caused by a point of light altering the temperature may be sufficient to give a sensation of sound.[137]

Patients suffering from superior semicircular canal dehiscence syndrome hear their own internal sounds in all their magnitude, even the movement of their eyes, without being able to eliminate them, which highlights the extreme sensitivity of the hair cells.

The syndrome consists of an opening in the bone overlying an area of the semicircular canal, which turns the labyrinth into a structure with three windows: the oval window, the round window and the dehiscence. This alters the functioning of the ear and highlights its extreme sensitivity when the regulation mechanisms are maladjusted. Fortunately, it can be corrected through surgery.[138]

---

[136] *The corticofugal system for hearing: Recent progress.* **Suga, N. et al.** 22, 2000, Proceedings of the National Academy of Sciences, Vol. 97.

[137] *Light-induced vibration in the hearing organ.* **Ren, T. et al.** 5941, Aug 4, 2014, Scientific Reports, Vol. 4.

[138] *Sound abnormally stimulates the vestibular system in canal dehiscence syndrome by generating pathological fluid-mechanical waves.* **Iversen, M.M. et al.** 10257, 2018, Scientific Reports, Vol. 8.

The key to good listening is to be able to select, and eliminate background noise and anything not relevant to that particular situation, such as our breathing, heartbeat, footsteps, etc. We do not fully understand how we are able to achieve good listening in adverse acoustic environments, but there are several structures involved in this process in addition to the auditory muscles, such as the olivocochlear reflex (MOCR)[139] or the mechanics of the cochlea itself.[140] Our auditory system has neurons that react not only to sound, but also to the disappearance of the acoustic stimulus.[141]

Listening and chewing

The hammer muscle or tensor tympani is activated by the trigeminal nerve, whose influence stretches to all the structures coming from the first branchial arch. This is a sensory and motor nerve, which receives sensation from the face and moves the jaw.

Speech therapists know that speech difficulties can sometimes be related to chewing habits. Children who eat only soft foods do not properly develop a musculature that is also used in pronouncing words [142] and they also tend to have listening problems. You need to repeat things to them to get them to understand, though they do not have a hearing impairment. There is a high prevalence of hearing problems in children with eating and swallowing disorders.[143]

Chewing is a way of educating the trigeminal nerve, which is also responsible for moving the eardrum. When the trigeminal does not know how to chew, it is no expert in hearing either. When we listen, we move our articulatory muscles at the same time, in perfect empathy with our interlocutor. Our tongue moves to listen.[144] While

---

[139] *A Preceding Sound Expedites Medial Olivocochlear Reflex.* **Otsuka, S., Nakagawa, S. and Furukawa, S.** 2018, Acta Acustica United with Acustica, Vol. 104, pp. 804-808.

[140] *Relationship between cochlear mechanics and speech-in-noise reception performance.* **Otsuka, S., Nakagawa, S. and Furukawa, S.** 265, 2019, The Journal of the Acoustical Society of America, Vol. 146.

[141] *When Sound Stops: Offset Responses in the Auditory System.* **Kopp-Scheinpflug, C., Sinclair, J.L. and Linden, J.F.** 10, Oct, 2018, Trends in Neurosciences, Vol. 41.

[142] *Correlation between functional disorders of the masticatory system and speech sound disorders in children aged 7-10 years.* **Grudziąż-Sękowska, J., Olczak-Kowalczyk, D. and Zadurska, M.** 2, 2018, Dent Med Probl., Vol. 55, pp. 161-165.

[143] *Prevalence of Auditory Problems in Children With Feeding and Swallowing Disorders.* **Rawool, R.W.** 5, 2017, J Speech Lang Hear Res., Vol. 60, pp. 1436-1447.

[144] *The hearing ear is always found close to the speaking tongue: Review of the role of the motor system in speech perception.* **Skipper, J.L., Devlin, J.T. and Lametti, D.R.** 2017, Brain & Language, Vol. 164, pp. 77-105.

listening, we are simultaneously speaking, in silence, repeating everything we hear, with very small, imperceptible movements. Listening activates our auditory and motor brain areas at the same time. Thanks to the work of Ignacio Calle, a specialist in dentistry and posturology, I have been able to follow the hearing development of patients in dental treatment.[145] In children with fixed orthodontics, audiometries often present distortions, especially between 125 and 1,000 Hz, and this is barely modified by auditory therapy. Once the orthodontics are removed, the curve returns to normal without any therapeutic intervention.

The relationship between the chewing muscles and the ear is well known, due to their shared origin in the first branchial arch. Dentists often come across auditory pathologies among their patients and research work on this topic is beginning to be published.[146,147,148] In future, dentists will need to work closely with other professionals. We are beginning to understand that the health of our mouth has an impact on the rest of our organism: on posture, vision, balance, etc. It is believed, for example, that gingivitis may be the cause of Alzheimer's disease.[149]

During auditory therapy patients are asked not to chew, as it mobilizes the trigeminal, interfering with the hammer-stirrup gymnastics that, according to Tomatis, takes place during the session. If we clench our jaws tightly, we will notice that we have gone a little deaf for a few seconds, the reason being that we are moving the eardrum by activating its tensor muscle. In fact, some people can contract this muscle at will. Thanks to them it has been possible to demonstrate that its contraction causes an increase in the auditory thresholds in the low-frequency region. As the muscle contracts, there is a loss of hearing via air conduction of about 20 dB and a bone-conduction hearing loss of 10 dB in the region of 250 Hz.[150] It is

[145] *Iniciación al arte de la posturología.* **Calle, J.I.** Barcelona : s.n., 2014. XIV Congreso de Sekmo.

[146] *Tensor tympani muscle: strange chewing muscle.* **Ramírez, L.M. et al.** 2007, Med Oral Patol Oral Cir Bucal, Vol. 12, pp. E96-100.

[147] *Síntomas óticos referidos en desórdenes temporomandibulares. Relación con músculos masticatorios.* **Ramírez, L.M. et al.** 2007, Rev Méd Chile, Vol. 135, pp. 1582-1590.

[148] *Tensor veli palatini and tensor tympani muscles: Anatomical, functional and symptomatic links.* **Ramírez, L.M., Ballesteros, L.E. and Sandoval, G.P.** 1, 2010, Acta Otorrinolaringológica Española, Vol. 61, pp. 26-33.

[149] *Periodontitis and Alzheimer's Disease: A Possible Comorbidity between Oral Chronic Inflammatory Condition and Neuroinflammation.* **Teixeira, F.B. et al.** 327, Oct 10, 2017, Frontiers in Aging Neuroscience, Vol. 9.

[150] *Audiometric findings with voluntary tensor tympani contraction.* **Wickens, B., Floyd, D. and Bance, M.** 2, 2017, Journal of Otolaryngology - Head and Neck Surgery, Vol. 46.

hardly surprising, therefore, that certain orthodontics can impair hearing.

Emotional muscles

Tomatis used to claim that up to 1,000 Hz an audiometry test reflects the action of the hammer muscle, while modulation of the high frequencies corresponds to the stirrup or stapedius. The structures that develop from the second branchial arch are mainly innervated by the facial nerve: the seventh cranial pair, which is responsible for moving all the muscles of the face (except the one that raises the eyelid), as well as the stapedial muscle, as has been mentioned.

We know how to recognize people's mood by the expression on their face, which highlights the link between our emotions and the tone of the facial muscles.

> "*Let's say you're a therapist or a parent, and one of your clients or children has a blank expression on their face. Their face has no muscle tone, their eyelids are drooping, and they avert their gaze. They are also highly likely to have auditory hypersensitivities and difficulty regulating their bodily state. These are common features of several psychiatric disorders, including anxiety disorders, borderline personality, bipolar disorder, autism and hyperactivity. The neural system that regulates both bodily state and the muscles of the face goes off-line. Thus, people with these disorders often show little affection in their faces and are on edge, because their nervous system is not providing them with information to calm them down*".[151]

The above quotation is from S. Porges, a professor at the University of Illinois and developer of the polyvagal theory, which I will comment on on page 90. If our emotions cause the facial nerve to change the tension of the muscles, giving the face an expression of anger, joy or surprise, will they have the same effect on the stapedial muscle? It would be strange if this nerve were to act all over its muscular territory with that one exception so, yes, they probably will.

In that case, listening must be conditioned by emotions even at the level of the middle ear, since the activity of the stapedial muscle is key to the regulation of intracochlear pressure. For

---

[151] **Dykema, R.** Don't talk to me now, I'm scanning for danger. *Nexus*. 2006.

Tomatis, the high-frequency region is the emotional part of the listening test. Sometimes I ask my patients to sing as if they were feeling different emotions: a surprising exercise. Spectral analysis reveals changes in the high-frequency harmonics. Our emotions have an effect on muscle tone, modulating the vocal emission.

Small, but essential

The stapedius is the smallest muscle in the human body, barely a millimeter long. It reacts when there is a loud sound stimulus (the so-called stapedial reflex) and it is permanently active, even during sleep, taking up 80% of movement in the REM phase.[152] It has been observed to move just before speech, thus balancing the intracochlear pressure in advance, allowing the ear to adapt to the sound that follows.[153]

This modulating effect has been proven by magnetic resonance imaging.[154] When we hear a recording of our own voice, the amplitude of the recorded magnetic fields is greater than when we are pronouncing those same words, which suggests that, as we speak, the efferent auditory system is dampening the sound of our voice. This characteristic is not exclusive to humans. Bats do the same thing to drown out their own clicks and let them identify sounds coming from echoes or other bats.

In humans, the stirrup muscle also attenuates background noise to highlight the signal so, for example, people with no stapedial reflex experience lower word intelligibility in noisy environments.[155] In laryngectomized patients, who speak through a prosthesis, the stirrup muscle does not seem to contract in anticipation, which suggests there is continuous feedback from the vocal cords.[156] In cochlear implant wearers, though, it does contract.[157]

---

[152] *Spontaneous middle ear muscle activity in man: a rapid eye movement sleep phenomenon.* **Pessah MA, Roffwarg HP.** 4062, Nov 17, 1972, Science, Vol. 178, pp. 773-6.

[153] See note 17

[154] *Modulation of the Auditory Cortex during Speech: An MEG Study.* **Houde, J.F. et al.** 8, Journal of Cognitive Neuroscience, Vol. 14, pp. 1125–1138.

[155] *The importance of acoustic reflex for communication.* **Lira de Andrade, K.C. et al.** 2011, American Journal of Otolaryngology, Vol. 32.

[156] *Measurement of stapedius contraction during vocalization effort in patients after laryngectomy or tracheostomy.* **Kawase, T. et al.** 1-2, Amsterdam : s.n., 2000, Hearing research, Vol. 149, pp. 248-252.

[157] *Stapedius reflex thresholds in cochlear implant patients.* **Stephan, K. et al.** 1988, Audiology, Vol. 27.

The physiology of the stapedial reflex raises many questions. It is triggered at the same intensities in people with impaired hearing and with normal hearing. We would expect those with hearing loss to need more decibels to activate the reflex, but this is not the case.[158]

Another peculiarity is its incredible speed. The larynx of bats produces 200 emissions per second and at this speed their stirrup muscle must contract to prevent them from being disturbed by each emitted click. These singularities make us think of a muscle that contracts instantaneously, without a motor order coming from the brain, as Bell suggests, or through some unknown anticipatory mechanism. Paradoxically, stapedial muscle fibers are of the slow type, and therefore ideal for prolonged efforts, but not for rapid reactions.

The stapedial reflex can be affected by multiple syndromes. For example, it is abnormal in hypothyroidism even when this is subclinical.[159] Alterations to the reflex have also been documented in autism,[160] which points to a hearing dysfunction in this pathology.

Ear and personality

In psychology, the terms introversion and extroversion are commonplace. They were popularized by Eysenck, an English psychologist who drew up the scale that bears his name and which measures how far we tend towards one pole or the other. This test has been widely used for decades.

Introverts and extroverts have different audiological characteristics. Introverts prefer silence or soft music. Their audiometric curves have lower thresholds than extroverts.[161] They are more sensitive.

The Israeli researcher Yair Bar-Haim, from Tel-Aviv University, found that the stapedial reflex was also different between them. Introverts could trigger the reflex more easily (so they preferred silence or soft music) while extroverts had a higher percentage of abnormal reflexes or none at all.[162]

---

[158] *A fast, "zero synapse" acoustic reflex: middle ear muscles physically sense eardrum vibration.* **Bell, A.** 4, 2017, J Hear Sci, Vol. 7, pp. 33-44.

[159] *Stapedial Reflex: A Biological Index Found to be Abnormal in Clinical and Subclinical Hypothyroidism.* **Goulis, D.G. et al.** 7, 2009, Thyroid, Vol. 8.

[160] *Quantification of the Stapedial Reflex Reveals Delayed Responses in Autism.* **Lukose, R. et al.** 5, 2013, Autism Research, Vol. 6.

[161] *Extraversion and sensory threshold.* **Smith, S.L.** 3, 1968, Psychophysiology, Vol. 5, pp. 293-9.

[162] *Introversion and individual differences in middle ear acoustic reflex function.* **Bar-Haim, Y.** 2002, International Journal of Psychophysiology, Vol. 46, pp. 1-11.

If we examine the voice instead of the ear, we find similar relationships.[163] The formant frequency of some phonemes shows high correlations with the Eysenck factors or other classical personality tests, such as the 16PF.[164]

The evoked potentials are influenced by personality traits too[165] [166]: their latency and intensity varying according to the character of the subject. This is a further indication of the close ties between psyche and hearing that are of some practical importance to the audiologist. For example, the degree of success when adjusting a prosthesis can depend on the patient's introversion/extroversion.[167] Extroverts tend to be more satisfied.

The omnipresent vagus nerve

To gain a proper understanding of the effects that auditory therapy is capable of producing, its link to the autonomic nervous system (ANS) must also be taken into account. In 1953, Seymour and Tappin observed that stress causes alterations in the endolymph and histological changes.[168] Previously, sympathetic-pathway blocking techniques had been used to treat Meniere's.

Imbalances between the sympathetic and parasympathetic systems are the cause of many of our modern diseases. This is the domain of psychosomatics: the influence of stress on health.

Generally speaking, the sympathetic system activates our glands, accelerates heart rate, and increases blood pressure and oxygen supply. It prepares us to fight or flee in the face of imminent danger. It is the basis of survival. The opposite occurs with parasympathetic or vagal activation. If we feel safe, we recover our balance.

Unfortunately, modern life exposes us to risks that never disappear, keeping us alert and on the defensive. Family, work or

---

[163] *Speech Spectrum's Correlation with Speakers' Eysenck Personality Traits.* **Hu, C. et al.** 3, 2012, Plos One, Vol. 7

[164] *Perceive one's character through his voice: The relationship between speech spectrum and personality traits.* **Chao, H. and Gen-Yue, F.** Adv Psychol Sci, Vol. 6, pp. 809-813.

[165] *Intensity Dependence of Auditory Evoked N1/P2 Component and Personality.* **Hegerl, U. et al.** 1992, Neuropsychobiology, Vol. 26, pp. 166-172.

[166] *Latency of auditory P300 correlates with self-control as measured by the Sixteen Personality Factor Questionnaire.* **Lee, H.G. et al.** 2005, Psychiatry and Clinical Neurosciences, Vol. 59, pp. 418-424.

[167] **Crandell, C.C. et al.** *Effects of personality on hearing aid/FM benefit.* Gainesville : University of Florida, 2004.

[168] *Some Aspects of the Sympathetic Nervous System in Relation to the inner Ear.* **Seymour, J.C. and Tappin, J.W.** 6, 1953, Acta Oto-Laryngologica, Vol. 43, pp. 618-635.

money problems are threats that activate our sympathetic system too often. To counteract stress, we activate the vagus nerve by practicing sports, yoga, tai-chi, meditation, etc.: techniques that help us relax.

The vagus, the tenth cranial nerve, extends over large areas of the ear, including the eardrum (Arnold's nerve), where it meets the trigeminal and glossopharyngeal nerves. In this way, sound penetrates directly into our nervous system, which explains its calming or irritating effect on us. If we observe the anatomical course of the vagus (which etymologically means *wanderer)* we see that it reaches every organ. When speaking or singing we literally "touch" our interlocutor's vagus nerve through their eardrum, and that stimulation extends throughout the body.

The vagus nerve acts on hearing and phonation. Two of its branches, the recurrent nerves, are responsible for activating the vocal cords, projecting our mood or state of health onto our voice. Other vagal fibers reach the stapedius muscle,[169] helping to regulate intracochlear pressure and thus forming an integral part of the audio-vocal circuit. We listen actively, and decide what to listen to, fortunately.

Sound invades us through the vagus, the core of the parasympathetic system. Our feelings are awoken when we hear a shout or a kind word, even if spoken in an unknown language. Other effects, such as those produced by noise pollution, take longer to appear.

Our second brain, made up of some 100 million neurons that inhabit the digestive system, has a two-way connection to the first through sympathetic and parasympathetic pathways. It is believed that 90% of our serotonin and 50% of our dopamine are located in the intestine, a figure that has put psychiatrists on alert, as these neurotransmitters are regarded as keys to mental health. Given the close relationship between the ear and the parasympathetic system, it is possible that the auditory system also influences the second brain, although this is only a hypothesis at present.[170]

Two vagus nerves

Porges has shed new light on the physiology of the vagus nerve,[171] and his discoveries help to explain the mechanism of action of Tomatis's therapy. Both have approached neurology from the angle of phylogenetics, thus furthering our understanding of our nervous system.

---

[169] **Dallos, P.** *The Auditory Periphery Biophysics and Physiology.* 1973.

[170] **Greenlaw, P. and Ruggiero, M.** *Your third brain.* Centennial : s.n., 2015.

[171] *The Polyvagal Theory: phylogenetic contributions to social behavior.* **Porges, S.W.** 2003, Physiology & Behavior, Vol. 79, pp. 503-513.

Porges points out that the traditional explanation for the fight-flight mechanism and the sympathetic-parasympathetic equilibrium does not fit anatomical and functional reality. We should be talking about two vagus nerves with their own characteristics.

Evolution has put together an ANS of overlapping structures that allow us to react to external threats. Our body first calls up the most recent, and most sophisticated, phylogenetic response. If this does not work, it uses the previous one, and so on. The most modern structure is a myelinated vagus, anatomically joined to the nerve pathways involved in communication that moves us to ask our fellows for help.

The species that require parental care to survive developed non-verbal language thoroughly: the muscular expression of emotions. In mammals and especially in humans, a part of the vagus nerve is myelinated and closely related to the cranial pairs involved in vocalization and facial expression, or in other words, with social behavior.

If we do not get the help we expect when facing danger, we will have to fight or flee, which corresponds to the second oldest level: a sympathetic activation that prepares the organism for an emergency. When this state is prolonged in time, we call it stress. The parasympathetic (vagal) system does not work as it should and the sympathetic system is triggered, causing imbalances that, in turn, generate further disorders. How many people find themselves in this state of constant anxiety, suffering from all kinds of ailments!

There is still a third possibility. When a mouse sees that it has no escape and the cat is going to catch it, it remains motionless, as if it were dead, which can turn out to be a good strategy as some predators detect moving objects better than static ones. It is the most primitive of defense mechanisms, linked to the ancient part of the non-myelinated vagus nerve.

The polyvagal theory fits in with what I tend to see in my daily practice. If parents tell me that their child has asked them for help with a particular problem, I am confident we will solve it soon. We are at the first level: the myelinic vagal response, which triggers the search for social support. Other children, though, do not ask for help. They spend their time "in flight", distracting themselves with disruptive behavior or anything else. They are a nuisance in class, and teachers ask their parents to find a solution. On the face of it, these are rebellious students, unwilling to work and learn, but in fact this is not usually the case and a thorough examination often detects learning disorders.

The most worrying children are those in the third group; those who are "absent". They do not ask for help, they do not cause disruption, but they seem to live in another reality. When they are reprimanded at school for some reason, they freeze up, not knowing how to respond. They say yes to everything. Their survival strategy is paralysis: lowering their gaze and not standing out. I wonder if selective mutism could be an expression of this non-myelinated vagus, due to the immaturity of the vagal system.

We have all used one of the three types of parasympathetic response. Who has not called for help, run away from a dangerous situation, or been completely paralyzed by fear? They are normal reactions, but sometimes the system breaks down if it is subjected, or believes itself to be subjected, to constant danger, and it falls into a spiral of stress.

Porges's theory has led to a therapeutic device to stimulate the vagus nerve, one that also acts on the ear. Vagal stimulation has recently been approved by the FDA to treat medication-resistant epilepsy and depression. The parasympathetic system is activated by electrical impulses from a device placed under the skin. This therapy is actually in fashion at the moment: similar devices are on sale to treat headaches or induce a pleasant state of relaxation by sending impulses to the rhythm of music.

The vagus nerve and the eardrum vibrate together so it would seem to make sense, given suitable acoustic stimulation, for vagal effects to occur. Tomatis used to insist that the only cutaneous innervation of the vagus is found in the tympanic membrane and constitutes its outward-facing antenna. His therapy even works at this level.

Stanley Jones, whom I have already quoted in chapter 3, postulated in 1970 that depression and mania could be at opposite ends of the imbalance in the parasympathetic system.[172] Tomatis made an observation on the same lines (see Chapter 6).

---

[172] **Stanley Jones, D.** *Kybernetics of Mind and Brain.* [ed.] Charles C. Thomas. Springfield, USA : s.n., 1970.

THE LISTENING TEST 5

The audiometric profile, according to Tomatis, reflects the way we listen to ourselves and others: our internal and external dialogue. He came to this conclusion by analyzing and questioning his patients, after thousands of observations. His approach differed from that of the conventional audiological test, as he assumed that the ear fulfils an energizing function, stimulating the nervous system. For this reason, Tomatis would always insist that he did not perform audiometric tests but listening tests, which tell us how that energy is managed, and the strengths and weaknesses that determine our physical and mental health. Ear and nervous system evolved so closely together that audiological tests also display our psychological state, with an auditory modification immediately being transferred to our nerve structure and vice versa.

EAR AND VOICE, MIRRORS OF THE SOUL

The professional audiologist is accustomed to classifying test results as either normal or pathological, and analyzing only the latter. However, those of persons with normal hearing are also very interesting. Everyone is different. Rarely are the air and bone curves parallel, and they show peaks and scotomas that have a cause.

Imagine you have the chance to regularly test people with normal hearing and collect data on their working life, emotional and health status, childhood and family relations. You will probably find that certain patterns are followed. People with psychological characteristics in common show similar audiometric profiles.

Based on my twenty-five years of experience in conducting listening tests, I agree with Tomatis on the need to consider the psychological dimension of audiometry. It reflects our whole being, not just our hearing level. I believe his observations were very accurate, although there still remains the huge task of statistically validating them.

Researchers have discovered several vocal parameters that vary according to emotional state.[173,174,175] For example, when we get angry, we increase the intensity in the speech region (between 300 and 3,400 Hz for men and between 800 and 3,400 Hz for women). Something similar happens if we feel joy, though less markedly.

Spectral analysis reveals links with personality factors.[176] The voice presents micro-oscillations that can be detected by computer to evaluate stress levels [177,178,179]. The pitch of our voice rises, while the first two vowel formants decrease in frequency. The software has achieved a high degree of accuracy in this task and some can even analyze the vocal emission to extract clinical information.

Our voice manifests our emotional state and health as well as listening, as revealed in the audiometric curve. As we have already seen (p. 25) the vocal emission is controlled by the ear through constant feedback.[180,181]

ADMINISTERING THE LISTENING TEST

In practice, there is almost no difference between conducting an audiometric test and a listening test. We use the audiometer, to measure air and bone conduction. Its calibration has been modified to better visualize the graphics, but only slightly. For example, the bone

[173] **Johnstone, T. and R., Klaus.** *The effects of emotions on voice quality.* s.l. : University of Geneve, 1999.

[174] *Vocal Indicators of Emotional Stress.* **Sondhi, S. et al.** Jul 15, 2015, International Journal of Computer Applications, Vol. 122.

[175] **Pollerman, B.Z. and Archinard, M.** Acoustic Patterns of Emotions. [aut.] E. Keller et al.(editor). *Improvements in Speech Synthesis.* 2002.

[176] See note 163

[177] **Rothkrantz, L.J.M.** *Voice Stress Analysis.* s.l. : Delft University of Technology, 2004.

[178] **Tokuno, S.** *Stress Evaluation by voice: From Prevention to treatment in mental health care.* s.l. : The University of Tokyo, 2013.

[179] *Acoustic and perceptual indicators of emotional stress.* **Streeter, L.A. et al.** 4, 1983, Journal Acoustic Society America, Vol. 73.

[180] *The Effect of Hearing Loss on the Vocal Features of Children.* **Kasbi, F. et al.** 1, Semnan, Iran : s.n., 2014, Middle East J Rehabil Health, Vol. 1.

[181] **Coelho, A.C., Medved, D.M. and Brasolotto, A.G.** Hearing Loss and the Voice, Update On Hearing Loss. [Online] Dec, 2015.

conduction thresholds have been shifted down 10 dB, so that the line does not overlap with the air conduction line.

We do not usually use soundproof cabins. We prefer to test in a similar environment to the patient's day-to-day reality (international standards set a maximum limit of 40 dB of ambient noise when measuring, but do not require a cabin). We are not testing to fit a hearing aid, but to obtain another kind of information. The test is complemented by a frequency discrimination test (selectivity) and an auditory laterality test which does not correspond to the usual dichotic listening tests. Spatialization errors are also taken into account: when the patient hears through the other ear instead of the one we are actually testing.

To make the graph easier to read, the listening test uses the color blue for air conduction and red for bone conduction, in both ears. The conventional audiometric nomenclature disappears. In this book, printed in black and white, the air curve can be easily recognized because it ranges from 125 to 8,000 Hz, while the bone curve is between 250 and 4,000 Hz and is shown with a thinner line than the air curve. Some graphs are schematic and do not correspond to real audiograms, for didactic reasons.

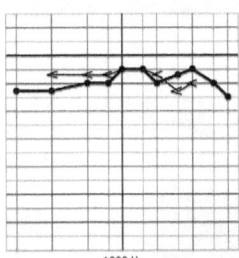

Audiogram with classical audiological nomenclature.

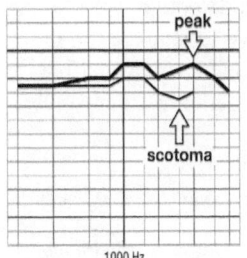

Listening test, according to Tomatis. Observe the displaced thresholds of the bone curve, facilitating visualization.

Below, I will examine audiometry as Tomatis did, based on his clinical experience. It is a promising and exciting field of study.

LISTENING TEST INTERPRETATION

To interpret the listening test, an understanding of auditory energy dynamics is needed. Our way of listening is the end result of a large number of factors, including psychological ones, sculpting it over the years. Emotions, for example, alter perception (auditory perception in this case) and vice versa, sometimes very subtly, others drastically. Any sound carries an affective charge that generates brain responses, as poets know well.[182] There is a neurological explanation for this: the extensive connections between the limbic system and the auditory system together with the omnipresence of the vagus nerve in the audio-vocal circuit. Stress causes dendritic atrophy, leading to dysfunctions at certain levels of the auditory pathway that interfere with listening.[183] If this becomes chronic, it can affect the nerve networks, making learning, creativity and reasoning difficult.[184]

Music can change our mood and that has been used, for example, to improve work performance, make shoppers buy more goods or create a festive atmosphere. In movies, it heightens the effect of the scene. If it does not match what we are seeing, the emotion dissolves.

And this can work the other way round too: emotions can affect listening. For example, we can alter the results of dichotic listening tests by asking subjects to look at certain images.[185]

The ear and the emotional brain share outbound and inbound pathways, so it is understandable that audiometry shows characteristics of our psyche. By studying it, we can infer important data about our patients. Audiometry provides us with "non-auditory" information if we are able to interpret it. Tomatis offers us some tools to achieve this.

Audiometry tells us about the person

Interpreting Tomatis's listening test resembles detective work. There is more than one way to read the data, so we have to analyze the graph and relate it to what the patient tells us, which is not easy at first but, as you gain experience, the pieces of the puzzle fit together by themselves.

---

[182] *The Sound of Words Evokes Affective Brain Responses.* **Aryani, A. et al.** 94, 2018, Brain Sci., Vol. 8.

[183] *Effects of chronic stress on the auditory system and fear learning: an evolutionary approach.* **Dagnino-Subiabre, A.** 2, Valparaíso : s.n., 2013, Rev. Neurosci., Vol. 24, pp. 227-237.

[184] **Hannaford, C.** *Aprender moviendo el cuerpo.* México : Editorial Pax México, 2008.

[185] *Mood Modulates Auditory Laterality of Hemodynamic Mismatch Responses during Dichotic Listening.* **Schock, L. et al.** 2, 2012, Plos One, Vol. 7.

Tomatis conducted numerous master-class consultation sessions, which allowed us to observe his ability to read the listening tests. He only needed to take a look at the graph to glean an extraordinary amount of information from it and then probe the patient's very essence through incisive questions. Sometimes he explained to us what kind of person was going to come through the door without having seen them before, just by looking at their test. I confess that I have never reached that level of mastery, but audiometry has served me as a guide, facilitating the interviews with my patients and helping me to find the right questions to understand the causes and possible solutions to their problems. From the Tomatis perspective we can immediately visualize possible health, postural and psychological issues, and even parts of their life story. Sometimes the graph is so explicit that both the patient and I myself marvel at the accuracy of the data reflected in the curves.

I have added an appendix to this book, containing an interview with Tomatis from 1973, on the occasion of the Third Congress of Audio-Psycho-Phonology held in Antwerp, France. In it, he sets out the guiding principles for interpreting the listening test. In later years, he revised certain points but, essentially, they have been maintained. I think it can be enriching for the reader to access the original source, in which Tomatis himself describes his methodology. It is a unique historical document, whose content does not appear in any of his books.

Next, I will describe the basic concepts of listening-test interpretation. I will address general notions to give audiologists an initial impression. Those interested in delving further into this topic should follow a training course. As an introduction, I recommend reading Tomatis's autobiography[186] and the books published by my colleagues P. Sollier,[187] and M. de Voigt and J. Vervoort.[188]

The shape

Audiometric testing is the audiologist's main tool. It allows us to assess hearing loss and adjust hearing aids with precision. The HAIC level, which defines the average number of thresholds in the central frequency region—that of language—lets us classify hearing losses as mild, moderate, severe or profound. Certain audiometric profiles are familiar to us, as they correspond to auditory pathologies: mainly

---

[186] See note 3
[187] See note 4
[188] See note 5

sensorineural and conductive hearing losses. For Tomatis, the HAIC level is relatively secondary.

The essential aspects of the audiogram are the overall shape, with its small peaks and scotomas, the comparison of both ears, discrepancies between the bone curve and the air curve, etc. The best way to begin reading audiograms from this new perspective is by examining the four curves (the two air curves and the two bone curves) as a whole. This will immediately tell us whether the profile is clean, harmonious, and smooth or, on the contrary, full of distortions.

We will also see if the four curves are similar or asymmetric, by comparing bone and air and both ears. This initial assessment gives us an overview and indicates whether the person in front of us could benefit from auditory therapy.

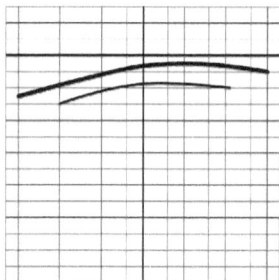 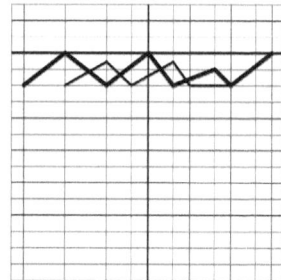

In none of the following audiograms is there noticeable hearing loss. HAIC levels are similar in both. From the Tomatis perspective, however, they are not at all alike, because what matters above all is their shape.

The graph on the left shows the ideal curve: harmonious, ascending and without distortions. It corresponds to someone who is self-confident and well-balanced. In the graph on the right, there is considerable energy depletion: this is a profile of stress. Our patient has probably lost control of his or her life, overwhelmed by adverse circumstances.

I have done thousands of audiograms in the course of my professional life and I have never seen two alike. It is as unique as a fingerprint or the auricle, whose shape is equally specific to each person.[189] The audiometric curve shows the subject in his or her entirety.

---

[189] **Curiel, A.M.** La huella de oreja como método de identificación humana. *Doctoral thesis.* s.l. : Universidad Camilo José Cela, 2009.

The air curve and the bone curve

The bone curve tells us about inner life, the vegetative functions and consciousness. It is the direct response of the auditory nerve, the cochlear reaction to sound. The air curve represents the way we listen to the outside world, to others. It involves the middle ear, with the vagal nerve extending through the eardrum, the trigeminal nerve moving the hammer muscle, and the facial nerve acting on the stapedial muscle: all regulating acoustic perception.

The air curve also registers other mechanisms that modify perception, such as any obstruction of the auditory canal. A simple wax plug compromises hearing via air conduction but leaves bone conduction intact.

Audiometric curves give us information on how we manage sound: what we want to listen to, what we do not and how. In short, it is the brain that decides on this and activates the corresponding selection mechanisms right at the entrance door: the efferent pathway sends direct orders to the cochlea and the tension of the muscles of the middle ear conditions listening. Tomatis suspected that many recurrent ear infections have a psychological cause: an attempt to block our perception. Sometimes we find perfect air curves, like this one:

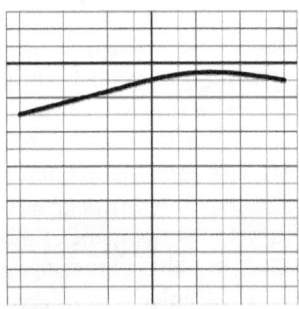

With bone curves like this:

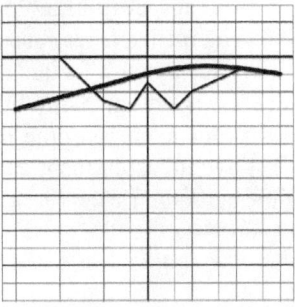

In this case, a great compensatory effort (air curve) is being made to maintain effective listening, although the auditory nerve is not perceiving signals as well as it should. While there are no symptoms, there is a considerable expenditure of energy, which cannot be maintained indefinitely. We can also find the opposite case:

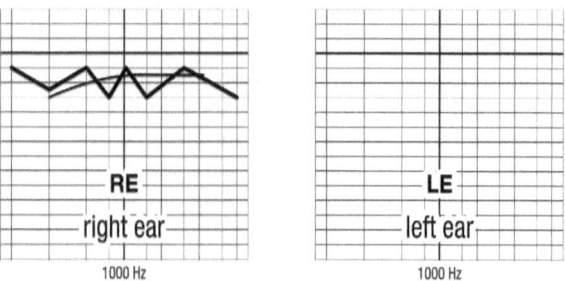

Here we see highly distorted air conduction, while the bone conduction is harmonious. This is the often the case of someone who is going through a rough patch in their life and is temporarily overwhelmed, which affects air conduction but not bone conduction. If the situation continues, the bone curve will eventually come to reflect the air curve.

Tomatis also refers to the different role of each ear. The left ear tells us about the past, the person's life story, whereas the right one tells us about the present. If we are going through a difficult situation, distortions appear more clearly in the right ear. If the problems are more long-term, stretching back into the past, they are reflected in the left ear.

The bone curve of the left ear provides the most revealing data, perhaps due to its link to the right hemisphere, less influenced by learning; or maybe due to the development of the brain hemispheres, which do not develop symmetrically. Until the age of three, the right hemisphere seems to be more active, if we compare blood flow on both sides.[190]

The listening test allows us to get to know patients better and so help them better, but we can be misled if we focus on too much detail, as the audiometric profile reflects many factors simultaneously: both psychological and physical. It is not an X-ray but rather a bird's-eye view; a global perspective, not a microscopic analysis. Taking this into account, once this first overall assessment has been made, we can explore other aspects of the audiometric curve.

---

[190] *The right brain hemisphere is dominant in human infants.* **Chiron, C. et al.** 1997, Brain, Vol. 120, pp. 1057-1065.

Analysis by sectors

According to Tomatis, each diagram can be divided into three sectors:

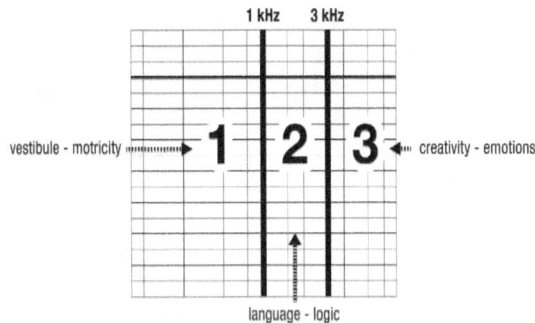

Up to 1,000 Hz we obtain information on vestibular activity, body image and motor development. Between 1,000 and 3,000 Hz we find language and communication. The high-frequency zone, from 3,000 to 8,000 Hz, shows the cortical energy charge, creativity, emotions and spirituality.

Sector 1: vestibule

It receives this name because it reflects the activity of the vestibule of the ear. It is the area of motor skills. The saccule analyzes low frequencies, up to approximately 800 Hz, being especially sensitive around 300 Hz.[191] The vestibule is even capable of capturing infrasounds, such as seismic waves.[192]

When the cochlea fails, the sensitivity of the vestibule sharpens, trying to compensate for the loss,[193] unless the saccule is damaged (it usually is damaged if the curve falls at high frequencies, without retrocochlear pathology).[194]

Michael McCue suggests in his doctoral thesis presented to the Massachusetts Institute of Technology in 1993 that, in fact, the

---

[191] *The Vestibular System Mediates Sensation of Low-Frequency sounds in mice.* **Jones, G.P. et al.** Sept, 2010, Journal of the association for research in otolaringology.

[192] *Tuning and sensitivity of the human vestibular system to low-frequency vibration.* **McAngus Todd, N.P. et al.** 2008, Neuroscience Letters, Vol. 444, pp. 36-41.

[193] *Hypersensitivity of Vestibular System to Sound and Pseudoconductive Hearing Loss in Deaf Patients.* **Emami, Seyede Faranak.** Hamadan, Irán : s.n., March, 2014, ISRN Otolaryngology.

[194] *Saccular damage in patients with high-frequency sensorineural hearing loss.* **Sazgar, A.A. et al.** 7, European archives of otorhinolaryngology, Vol. 263, pp. 608-613.

vestibule hears because it never stopped hearing. The saccule was able to analyze sounds before the cochlea, and has retained its acoustic sensitivity. According to McCue, the function of the middle ear is to protect the vestibule, to prevent sound from affecting its balance functions. His hypothesis is supported by the fact that the stapedial reflex produces a soft cushioning of the sound impact in the cochlea of about 20 dB. However, it drastically reduces the acoustic sensitivity of the vestibule.[195]

In 1976 the American Air Force commissioned a study by Miami University in Ohio to find out to what extent pilots might be affected in their maneuvers by aircraft noise. Intense sound can adversely affect the vestibular system, undermining balance, head posture and eye mobility. These effects are also produced by infrasounds.[196]

An investigation carried out with aeronautical workers (reminding us of Tomatis's first steps) confirms the link between vestibular activity and low frequencies on the audiogram. The article concerned was published in 2011, ten years after Tomatis's death, and fifty years after he described this link.

Audiograms were performed on the employees, together with a conventional vestibular test, the functional reach test. The data indicated that the worst vestibular results corresponded to the worst audiograms in the 500-1,000 Hz range.

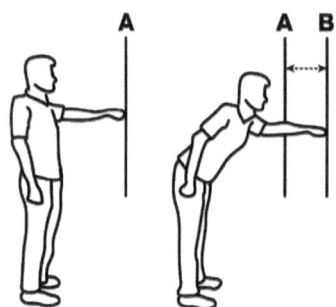

Functional reach test: the distance in cm is calculated between the furthest point the hand can reach from an upright position (A) and its maximum possible reach (B). This measure is a good indicator of the patient's balance and therefore vestibular function. The greater the distance, the better the balance.

The authors of the study only looked at the degree of hearing loss, whereas for Tomatis, the shape of the curve is the main data point to

---

[195] **McCue, M.P.** Acoustic responses from primary vestibular neurons. s.l., Massachusetts : MIT, 1993. Doctoral thesis.
[196] **Miami University.** *Effects of sound on the vestibular system.* Ohio : s.n., 1976. US Air Force.

be observed. Still, that investigation shows that there is a correlation between vestibular function and the audiogram in Sector 1.

The workers also took the Kessler 10, a psychological test. I was not surprised to read that those who showed higher rates of anxiety and depression were also the worst performers in the vestibular test.[197] Tomatis has already described this type of symptom in patients whose curve falls in Sector 1:

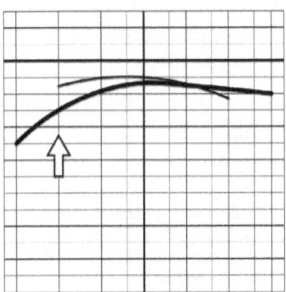

They often come to the consultation with mild depressive symptoms, but this is usually a case of incipient vestibular sensory deprivation. When they do physical exercise, they immediately bounce back and regain their good spirits.

In children under the age of seven we commonly see inverted bone and air curves in the low-frequency sector, an indicator of their psychomotor immaturity in Tomatis's view.

Gradually, the curves will run parallel, except in cases of developmental disorders. In adolescence, we will find the same phenomenon again, reflected in Sector 1 of the graph, as problems arise once more in controlling a body that is constantly changing.

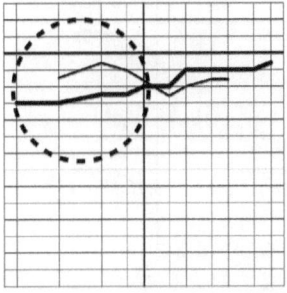

[197] *An Observed Relationship Between Vestibular Function and Auditory Thresholds in Aircraft-Maintenance Workers.* **Guest, M. et al.** 2, 2011, JOEM, Vol. 53.

In adults, these inverted bone and air curves in the low-frequency region are unusual. If they do appear, we should pay special attention and check if there is a body image disorder. They are not be confused with otitis or otosclerosis, which may have a similar profile in the early stages. In the audiograms of children with speech delay, again we tend to observe that the bone curve is more sensitive than the air curve in the low frequencies, which interferes in Sector 2.

If balance and control of muscle tone (Sector 1) are not resolved, it is difficult to achieve good competence in oral language (Sector 2), which requires great precision of movements. The connection between Sector 1 (vestibular), and Sectors 2–3 (cochlear) is also neurological: the vestibular nerve projects fibers towards the cochlear nuclei, which are auditory areas of the brainstem.[198] Furthermore, according to Tomatis:

> *"In addition, the nerve stimulations caused by the high frequencies have an effect on the vestibular system: the organ of equilibrium and, in man, upright posture. In fact, the vestibular nerve is present at all levels of the spinal column, through its junctions with the anterior roots of the medulla. The nerve stimulations caused by sounds therefore participate, through the vestibular pathway, in the control of the individual's balance, movements and verticality".[199]*

Sector 2: language

This sector lies between 1,000 and 3,000 Hz, where most speech sounds are concentrated. Therefore, it is essential to discriminate well and quickly in this frequency band. Under optimal conditions, the audiometric curve should follow an ascending path in this area:

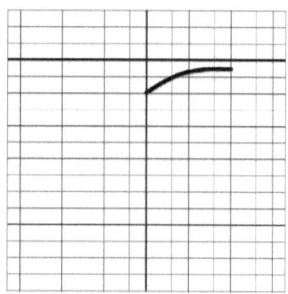

---

[198] See note 195

[199] *Musique filtrée et pédagogie psycho-sensorielle chez les enfants présentant des troubles de la communication.* **Tomatis, A.** Antwerp : s.n., 1973. III Congrès International d'Audio-psycho-phonologie.

Scotomas, peaks or a descending curve may indicate difficulties in expressing oneself correctly, lack of fluency and vocabulary, reading disorders, etc.

As language is the primary cognitive tool, it is normal for it to be associated with problems of concentration, memory or the ability to organize work and time. Dyslexic children usually have many distortions in Sector 2 and inversion of curves in Sector 1. Unsolved motor issues lie behind many language alterations.

This is the test of a seven-year-old girl who was receiving remedial school support due to her delay in learning to read. At school she worked slowly and was easily distracted:

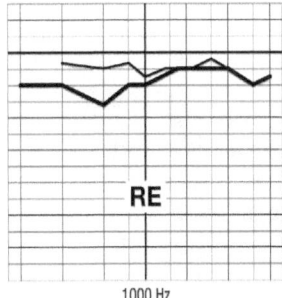
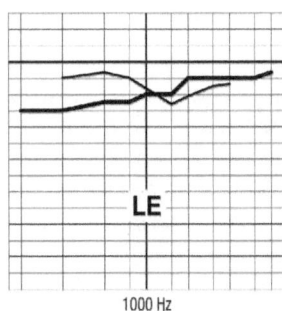

She was not very agile, and preferred quiet games. She had a history of numerous episodes of otitis but had not had one for eight months (the otoscopy and tympanometry were completely normal).

The inversion of the curves in Sector 1 is obvious. In the left ear, we can see that the bone curve also falls in Sector 2, while the air curve rises. Her school difficulties are not surprising in the light of the test. Indeed, the exploration revealed developmental disorders in motor skills and language.

Sector 2 is also the area of logic and rational thought. Those who stand out in this area, as shown in the graph, are proficient in language and orderly, methodical discourse. They often like to discuss social and political issues.

Sometimes in consultation, we see these curves described by Tomatis, in which bone and air show opposing profiles. As we have said, for Tomatis, the air curve is the appearance and the bone curve is the essence. The air curves in the graphs below indicate the person's degree of loquacity, while the bone curves refer to the quality of the discourse.

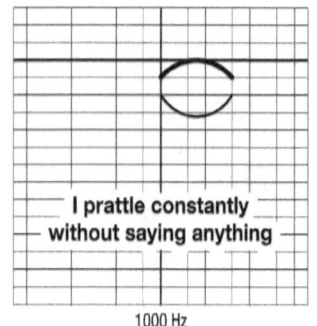

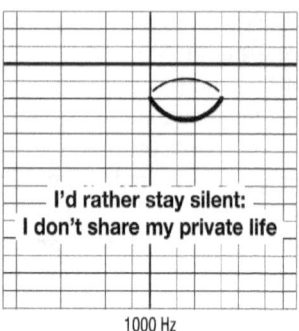

Sector 3: creativity

Tomatis placed creative capacity in the high frequencies. It is the area that stands out the most among artists.

When the curve climbs up to this area, we are dealing with a person with an emotional discourse, who is sensitive and full of ideas, although often not knowing how to carry them out. The auditory dynamo is working at full capacity, ensuring a substantial cortical recharge.

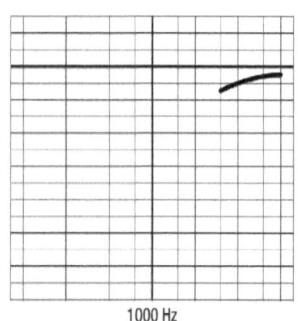

Almost all children present this curve and my experience leads me to think that their creative capacity is huge. Pilar Martín, a learning specialist, studied the development of musical talent in childhood. Before the age of 6, 18% of children showed high musical aptitude. However, that figure dropped rapidly as time passed, and by the age of 12 the percentage was almost zero. These results are thought-provoking.[200]

---

[200] *Estudio del talento en alumnos de Educación infantil y primaria.* **Martín, M.P.** 7, 2005, Revista Electrónica de Investigación Psicoeducativa, Vol. 3.

In adults we usually find this type of curve, sloping slightly in the high-frequency region:

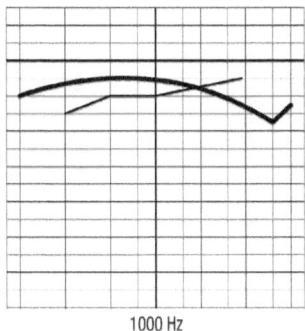

1000 Hz

This does not always point to an incipient sensorineural hearing loss. If the fall is restricted to air conduction, it can be a frustration curve—typical of people who maintain a great creative capacity (bone curve), but do not use it in their work and have no other way to express it. Perhaps they have had to accept a boring occupation because they needed the salary. If we manage to liberate this patient's artistic dimension, the air curve recovers with auditory therapy and superimposes itself on the bone curve once more, while mood improves ostensibly.

Comparing right and left ears

The two bone curves can be very different in children, but not in adults. If the bone curve of the left ear is quite similar to that of the right, the person lives a well-adjusted life, showing his/her true self.

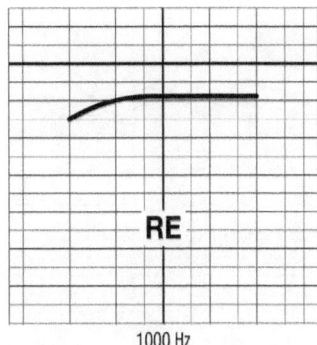

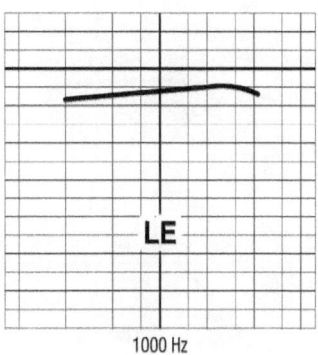

1000 Hz   1000 Hz

If they are very asymmetric, the patient's actions are highly unpredictable, as a result of a weak personality structure:

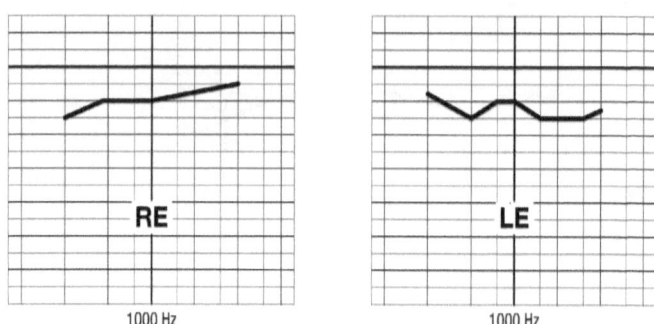

1000 Hz   1000 Hz

When we ask them how they act at work, at home or with friends, they seem to be different people in each situation. Their case history often reveals a complicated personal background.

Work or family circumstances can sometimes force people to behave differently to how they really are. In such cases, we see differences in the shape of the air and bone curves. These are always patients who are suffering, because it is exhausting to live under false pretenses all the time, even with good intentions. Generally, we tend to find a better air curve for the right ear, since they are showing their best side in the present (right ear), but they still bear their historical burden (left ear).

In the next example, the distorted curves for the left ear tell of old, long-term issues; but the air curve for the right ear, even and dome-shaped, indicates that the person has learned to face the world with some composure (in this case by controlling everything), in spite of the hidden burden.

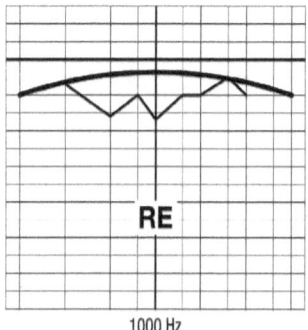 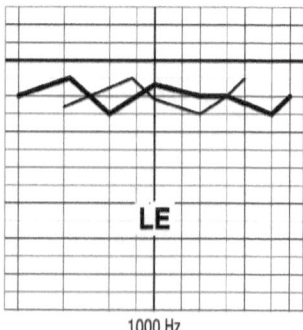

1000 Hz   1000 Hz

If it were the other way round and the uneven curve was for the right ear:

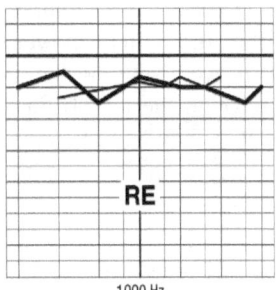 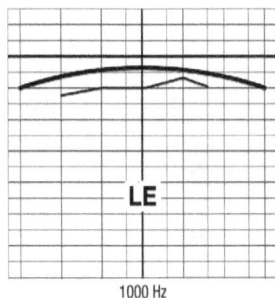

The personality structure has developed correctly. There are no distortions in the left ear, which maintains its harmonious shape. This is a favorable sign. The air curve for the right ear, however, indicates that the subject is currently experiencing difficulties of some sort.

Auditory reaction time

This is about 284 msec, almost 20% faster than visual.[201] Men generally respond faster than women to both acoustic and visual stimuli. In athletics, if a light or an image were used to start the race, everyone would arrive at the finish line later. The starting gun must also have certain characteristics. If the noise is too loud, there is a paralyzing effect and the runners take a little longer to start: very little, just hundredths of a second, but this is significant if they are trying to break a world record.[202] In sports like volleyball or tennis, the sound of the ball bouncing makes the player react before seeing it. If we put earplugs in tennis players' ears, they become slower and more imprecise when returning the serve.[203]

A study published in 1957 in which reaction time was associated with intelligence, gave rise to an intense debate among psychologists, which has lasted for decades.[204]

Today, we know that this relationship is very complex and that this data point is not in itself a good predictor of IQ.[205]

[201] *Comparison between Auditory and Visual Simple Reaction Times.* **Shelton, J. and Kumar, J.P.** 2010, Neuroscience & Medicine, Vol. 1, pp. 30-32.

[202] *"Go" Signal Intensity Influences the Sprint Start.* **Brown, A.M. et al.** Jun 6, 2008, Medicine & Science in Sports & Exercise, Vol. 40, pp. 1142-1148.

[203] *Predicting the length of volleyball serves: The role of early auditory and visual information.* **Sors, F. et al.** Dec 3, 2018, Plos One.

[204] *Relationship between intelligence and simple reacction time in mental defectives.* **Ellis, N.R. and Sloan, W.** Percept Mot Skills, Vol. 7, pp. 65-67.

In healthy people, both ears seem to perform similarly. However, if we analyze them in detail, we soon find some differences. For example, the right ear is usually faster in temporal resolution tests. If a click is sent to each ear, one after the other, in very quick succession, we perceive them better if we listen to the first one through the right ear and the second through the left. If the order is reversed, we can mistakenly conclude that they have been presented to us simultaneously.[206]

Auditory laterality

The first attempts to measure auditory laterality took reaction time to a sound stimulus as a reference, but this is no longer regarded as a suitable method. The conventional measurement is performed by means of dichotic listening tests. Pairs of words, usually numbers, are sent to both ears at once. The subject has to identify them, and the ear with the highest success rate is the dominant ear: usually the right.

Some exceptions to this rule raise new questions. If we use words with emotional content instead of numbers, those heard by the left ear are better remembered.[207] Also, blind children do not show right-side predominance in these tests and, in addition, they tend to read Braille better with the left hand.[208]

The introduction of magnetic resonance imaging has revealed dichotic auditory tests to be unreliable when response percentages do not show a huge difference in favor of one ear,[209] so we need to be cautious in assessing results.

In our daily lives the acoustic information that each of our ears receives is not exactly the same. One of them will always be closer to the sound source than the other, so the signal will arrive earlier, with differing intensity, phase and even frequency range, since the head acts as a screen, especially for high-frequency sounds. The brainstem

---

[205] *Relationship between Intelligence and Reaction Time; A Review Study.* **Khodadadi, M. et al.** 2, 2014, International Journal of Medical Reviews, Vol. 1, pp. 63-69.

[206] *Hemispheric asimmetry for auditory perception of temporal order.* **Mills, M. and Rollman, G.B.** 1979, Neuropsychologia, Vol. 18.

[207] *Emotion words are remembered better in the left ear.* **Sim, T.C. and Martinez, C.** March 2, 2005, Laterality, Vol. 10, pp. 149-59.

[208] *Absence of ear asymmetry in blind children on a dichotic listening task compared to sighted controls.* **Larsen, S. and Håkonsen, K.** March 2, 1983, Brain Lang, Vol. 18, pp. 192-8.

[209] *Determining language laterality by fMRI and dichotic listening.* **Bethmann, A. et al.** 2007, Brain Research, Vol. 1133, pp. 145-157.

compares both signals received, processing the information in less than a millisecond. That is how we locate the sound.

If we put on headphones and listen to the same music in both ears, we feel we are hearing the same on both sides. However, if we delay the signal in one ear slightly (less than a millisecond), the sound will seem to reach us through the opposing ear, which does not delay the signal. This is the time it takes for the sound wave to travel the barely 25 cm of distance between both ears. The brain concludes that if the sound comes sooner it is because it is closer to us. This very precise time calculation is made by the brainstem, without us being aware of it. If danger is approaching, we need to know immediately where it is coming from.

Neurologically, the auditory pathways and the areas where they are projected are quite asymmetrical. The area of language is found in the left hemisphere in almost the entire population.

Tomatis came to the concept of laterality through the observation of opera singers. From this perspective, the dominant ear is the one that controls the voice when speaking or singing.

"We can think of different hypotheses, but the further I go the more I think that the anatomical and cortical factors are not so important. There is no brain "inversion", contrary to what is believed. I believe (auditory) laterality happens mainly at the level of the larynx. We have two brains, but also two larynges, just as we have two ears, two nasal cavities and two mouths. One leads the other. Although we have the impression that the two sides work simultaneously, in reality, if we look closely at a person's face as they speak, we will see that they always use one side more than the other. This is an important element in the diagnosis I'm currently using".[210]

Tomatis refers here to the facial nerve, which is responsible for the mobility of both the face and the stirrup muscle. The facial expression tells us which ear is dominant.

Just as optometrists assess sensory and motor visual laterality, which do not always coincide, I believe that there are also two types of auditory laterality. The sensory one would be the one determined by dichotic listening tests and the motor one would correspond to the ear that controls the voice, as described by Tomatis; but in both cases it is most often the right ear that predominates in the general

---

[210] See note 25

population.[211] This sensorineural auditory laterality seems to be restricted to humans[212] and there is no reason to suppose it coincides with manual or visual laterality, so one can be left-handed in motor skills and right-eared, or vice versa.

The auditory efferent system is also lateralized, with the olivocochlear bundle (OCB) acting with more power in the right ear. This is composed of about 1,400 fibers that allow the brain to delimit precisely where to direct auditory attention, by acting as a frequency filter. In its final tract, it attaches to the vestibular nerve.[213]

Tomatis explained that left auditory lateralization is used as a defense mechanism. When we are not paying attention to the person talking to us, because we are in a hurry or we are not interested in what they are saying, we disconnect our right ear. After a few hours, we realize that we do not remember anything they told us.

If we use this skill too often, it may eventually become our standard way of listening and we may begin to notice its negative effects: we find it hard to express our ideas with the right words and memory fails us. We almost always find that children who hate going to school are well anchored in their left-ear hearing.

Tomatis once told me about a phenomenon that I have since been able to confirm many times: when we are giving a lecture, the audience members on our right (who are therefore proffering their right ear) pay more attention to us. Listeners on the left side (forced to proffer their left ear) have to try a little harder and show signs of fatigue sooner. In the round of questions that usually closes this type of event, the raised hands also tend to cluster to the right of the speaker as well. Knowing that, I try to address the left-side audience more often, in order to maintain their interest.

The case of Cristina

Cristina visited me in a somewhat frightened state, presenting symptoms similar to depression. The mother of a happy family, she had everything she needed to be happy, but she was not.

She was a music teacher and had been losing the desire to teach, little by little, until she reached a point where she was overwhelmed

---

[211] *Evidence of a Right Ear Advantage in the absence of auditory targets.* **Prete, G. et al.** 2018, Scientific Reports, Vol. 8.

[212] See note 28

[213] **Styles, E.A.** *Psicología de la Atención.* s.l. : Editorial Centro de Estudios Ramón Areces , 2010.

on getting up at the thought of having to go to work. She wanted to stay in bed, not from laziness, but anguish. She had been like this for a few months and things were getting worse.

Music, her great passion, no longer enthused her. She had lost the color of her voice and her guitar sat sadly in a corner. A complete medical checkup concluded that everything was fine, which reassured her, but disconcerted her. The audiometry results were quite good, with the characteristic rising profile of musicians:

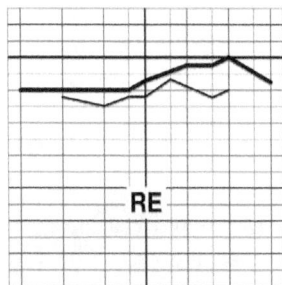 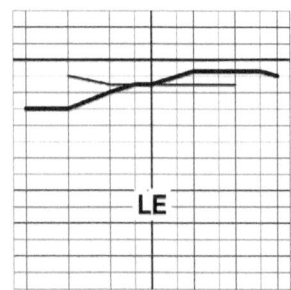

The left ear presented a curve inversion in the low-frequency region, something common in children, but in adults it warns us of problems. However, Cristina's most striking feature was her notable left-side auditory laterality. Her whole face moved to the left when speaking or singing. I proposed she should try to improve the quality of her voice by using the electronic ear to induce right-side laterality. The results were exceptional. In a matter of weeks Cristina returned to her classroom with enthusiasm.

She undertook new projects, even involving herself in activities outside the school. She did a lot of active-phase sessions in my center, singing with the electronic ear. She loved it. Her voice regained its brightness and she took up the guitar again. In a short time, her audiometric curve evolved like this:

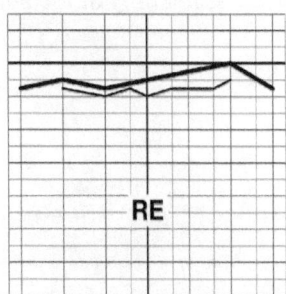 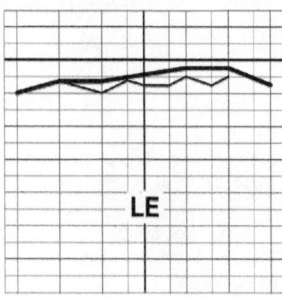

The improvement is evident, but above all she recovered right-ear laterality. That was decisive.

This is one of my favorite cases. There was a before and an after in the space of a few days, which was spectacular: a very rewarding experience for both of us. Over time, we became friends and shared great evenings with our respective families.

Several years have passed without any relapse. From time to time she still asks me to do sessions, "just in case", but I do not think she needs them. We have never known what triggered that "pseudo-depression". She does not care much either.

This case highlights the effects of auditory laterality. Cristina regained her effective neurological pathway and the consequences for her life were enormous.

What moves us

Emotions (etymologically *what moves us*) and hearing go hand in hand and this is reflected in dichotic listening tests, the results of which change depending on the person's mood.[214]

According to Tomatis, auditory laterality is unstable. In tense situations, it is possible to change the neurological circuit and go from right to left ear. At that moment, we cannot find the words and if we have to sing, our voice seems to have abandoned us. This is a slower track. The information is projected to the right hemisphere and must travel through the corpus callosum to the language area, in the left hemisphere: a considerably longer journey in neurological terms (in reality it is much more complex, as the auditory pathways are 80% contralateral and 20% ipsilateral).

Auditory laterality can even fluctuate throughout the day, as has been seen in unmedicated depression sufferers.[215] In laboratory mice, it has been possible to induce right or left motor laterality by damaging the vestibule of the ear.[216] The vestibule seems to play a prominent role in the lateralization process, not only at the auditory level.[217]

---

[214] See note 185

[215] *Auditory laterality in depression: Relation to circadian patterns and EEG sleep.* **Berger-Gross, P. et al.** 6, 1985, Biological Psychiatry, Vol. 20, pp. 611-622.

[216] *Early uneven ear input induces long-lasting differences in left–right motor function.* **Antoine, M.W. et al.** March, 2018, Plos Biology.

[217] *Does the vestibular system determine the lateralization of brain functions?* **Brandt, T. and Dieterich, M.** Oct, 2014, Journal of Neurology.

Immunized

Laterality also encompasses other systems, such as the immune or the endocrine systems.[218] In the 80s it was observed that certain lesions in the left cortex of mice caused a decrease in the immune response, but this was not the case if they occurred in the right side.

Something similar happens in humans. In an experiment, the immune response of a female group was compared according to whether they showed greater activation of the frontal cortex to the right or to the left. In the latter case there was more NK lymphocyte activity. Since the immune system is linked to the endocrine system and stress mechanisms, the role of laterality structuring in personality development and behavior has been raised.[219]

Testosterone levels (measured in saliva) are lower among left-handed individuals,[220,221] with the lowest levels having been found in those who are manual left-handers but auditory right-handers. This phenomenon is believed to be related to testosterone levels throughout pregnancy, which influence fetal development. The role of this hormone in autistic disorder is under debate.[222]

The recurrents

The vocal cords are innervated by the recurrents, the laryngeal branches of the vagus, or tenth cranial pair, the omnipresent nerve that regulates stress (being responsible for the parasympathetic system) and extends through the ear canal and eardrum.

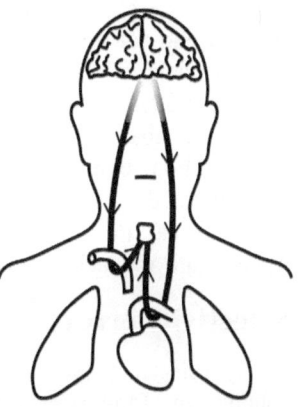

The right recurrent is shorter, so the laterality of the audio-vocal circuit is functional and anatomical. This

[218] *Frontal Brain Asymmetry and Immune Function.* **Kang, D.H. et al.** 6, Behavioral Neuroscience, Vol. 105, pp. 860-869.

[219] *Cerebral lateralization and immune system.* **Neveu, P.J.** Feb, 2002, International Review of Neurobiology, Vol. 52, pp. 303-23.

[220] *Salivary testosterone is related to both handedness and degree of linguistic lateralization in normal women.* **Gadea, M. et al.** 2002, Psychoneuroendocrinology.

[221] *Salivary testosterone levels in left and righ-thanded adults.* **Moffat, S.D. and Hampson, E.** 3, 1996, Neuropsychologia, Vol. 34, pp. 225-233.

[222] *Foetal testosterone and autistic traits in 18 to 24-month-old children.* **Auyeung, B. et al.** 11, 2010, Molecular Autism, Vol. 1.

asymmetry, said Tomatis, explains why children, when they begin to speak, utter many repeated syllables, such as *mama, dada, nana,* etc. The brain's order to make an utterance arrives first on one side and then on the other, producing this characteristic and universal syllabic duplication.

Laterality and dysphemia

A study carried out by a Japanese team analyzed the way a group of stutterers processed language, compared to a control group.[223] They gave them two tests in which they had to distinguish between two words. In the first test, they were asked to discriminate between two very similar ones (*itta–itte*), a phonetic task processed by the left hemisphere. In the second, the words were the same, but with differing intonation, such as an affirmative and an interrogative intonation (*itta–itta?*), a task linked to the right hemisphere.

In the control group, the results were as expected. They activated the left hemisphere more in the first task and the right in the second. However, the stutterers performed both tasks the same, revealing little or no hemispheric specialization. There was no lateralization.

When we hear our own voice with delay, we are unable to speak fluently and our voice resembles a stutterer's. In the middle of the last century, delayed auditory feedback (DAF) devices were tested for treating stuttering but they were not very successful and that line of work was abandoned. However, this procedure can be effective if done via bone conduction.[224]

Tomatis designed a protocol to correct dysphemia by means of the electronic ear. In his opinion, the causes lay in a deficient lateralization of language and lack of self-control via bone conduction.

Selectivity errors

By selectivity we mean the ability to discriminate between two sounds. In Tomatis's protocol, the patient's ability to distinguish between low- and high-frequency sounds is assessed by using two consecutive frequencies from the audiometer itself. If our patient makes a mistake, we draw a line above the lowest frequency of the two being compared. Taking the last error as a reference point, we regard the

---

[223] *Functional lateralization of speech processing in adults and children who stutter.* **Sato, Y. et al.** 70, 2011, Frontiers in Psychology, Vol. 2.

[224] *A new antistuttering device: treatment of stuttering using bone conduction stimulation with delayed temporal feedback.* **Stidham, K.R. et al.** 11, 2006, Laryngoscope, Vol. 116, pp. 1951-5.

selectivity as being closed from that point on. In the example below, the subject did not distinguish between 1,500 and 1,000 Hz with the left ear, nor between 750 and 500 Hz in both ears. We take closed selectivity to be from 500 Hz (as shown by the gray stripes).

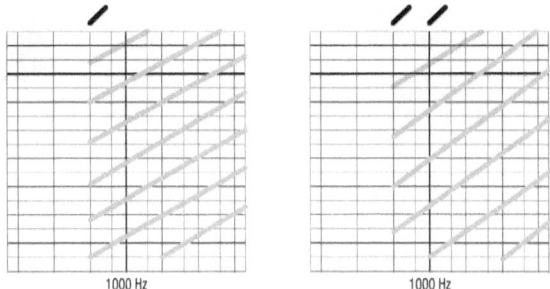

Tomatis claimed that selectivity opens up from low to high frequencies at a rate of approximately one octave per year from birth, and it seems he was right. Today, we know that the maturation of auditory discrimination of high-frequency sounds ends around the age of 10 or 11.[225,226]

If some significant event or conflict occurred during childhood, we are likely to find selectivity errors that have remained anchored ever since. By analyzing them we can reach back into the past and delve into key years in our patient's life story. This is, therefore, a very interesting test but one that still needs perfecting. Once, Tomatis admitted to me that this was the part of the listening test that most called for revising and extending. For example, a person who seems to discriminate sounds very well may start to fail spectacularly if we speed up the exercise a little, like the dyslexic children examined by Paula Tallal[227] whom I will refer to in Chapter 10.

How fast-paced should the selectivity test be in order to obtain optimal results? Is using pure sounds (which never occur in real life) the best way to test or would it be better to use musical sounds? Babies can distinguish language better than pure sounds.[228]Although the literature agrees with Tomatis that it takes about 10 to 11 years to fully develop selectivity, some data seem to contradict him regarding the

[225] *Nonsensory factors in infant.* **Olsho, L. W.** 1988.

[226] **Werner, L.A.** *Human Auditory Development.* s.l. : University of Washington, 2006.

[227] *Language learning impairments:integrating basic science, technology and remediation.* **Tallal, P., et al.** 1998, Exp Brain Res., Vol. 123, pp. 210-219.

[228] *Development of Frequency Perception in Infants and Children.* **Fenwick, K.D. and Morrongiello, B.A.** 4, 1991, JSLPA, Vol. 15.

direction of the maturation process. While Tomatis claims that this is from low tones towards high ones, other experts suggest that babies are as competent as adults in high-frequency discrimination and progressively expand these skills towards the lower tones.[229]

There is no consensus on this point. Depending on the methodology adopted, we can find conflicting results,[230] and one of the works consulted shows that children as young as one month old are capable of differentiating between 200 and 500 Hz (slightly more than one octave in the low-frequency range).

Selectivity errors indicate that certain sounds are hard to perceive. If there are many errors (closed selectivity), listening is blocked and analysis is imprecise. The resulting symptoms are numerous: problems in communication, attention, memory, relationships with others, etc. What they have in common, however, is an ear that hears without listening. The information arrives and is analyzed "a grosso modo". Learning a new language or music under these conditions can be difficult.

According to Tomatis, selectivity closure is also a defense mechanism that allows us to block listening and so distance ourselves psychologically from a conflict. The therapeutic intervention should never attempt to open selectivity abruptly, as it is necessary to do this little by little, letting patients set their own pace.

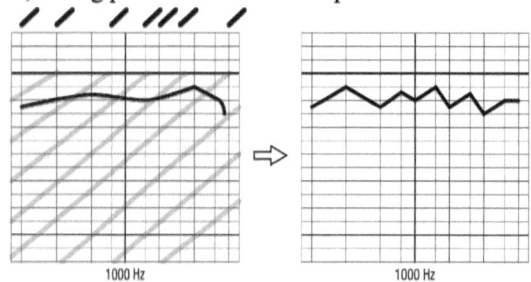

Foreseeable evolution when the selectivity opens very quickly.
The curve is disrupted, presenting many distortions.

When opened slowly, there is a smooth transition to good listening. If it is opened very quickly, another defense mechanism will appear straight away, generally in the form of a disharmonious listening curve, very far from the ideal. In these cases, the patient will surely report feeling irritable, and we will have to revise the pace and intensity of the

---

[229] **Deliege, I. and Sloboda, J.** *Musical Beginnings.* s.l. : Oxford University Press, 1996.

[230] *Pure-Tone Frequency Discrimination in Preschoolers, Young School-Age Children, and Adults.* **Rose, J. et al.** 9, 2018, Journal of Speech, Language, and Hearing Research, Vol. 61.

electronic ear program. Occasionally, selectivity may be closed in one ear but not in the other. If it is open in the right but closed in the left, this points to past affective relationships. On the other hand, closed right and open left indicate current problems in relationships and communication.

Spatialization errors

Spatialization errors are detected when the subject reports hearing with the opposite ear to the one where the sound is being presented. Except in cases of deafness, these errors indicate poor analysis in certain frequency zones, and suggest the patient should be asked about certain areas of conflict. They usually appear when testing bone conduction. We mark them with a line at the bottom of the graph.

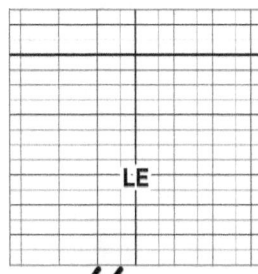

In this example, the subject responds that he hears through the right ear frequencies 500 and 750 Hz, which we have sent to the left via bone conduction.

It is less common to find them in air conduction, but it happens. It indicates unstable listening, with difficulties in locating sound in space. The spatialization errors in air conduction are marked in the graph with an asterisk. They are sometimes found in children under the age of 7, rarely after that age (with the exception of those with developmental disorders).

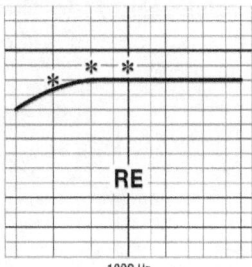
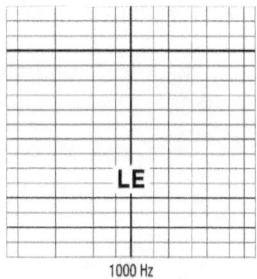

Spatialization errors via air conduction (*): sound sent through the right ear, but the patient hears from the left (frequencies 250, 500 and 1,000 Hz).

I have sometimes noticed that children who have never made such mistakes begin to do so. It lasts for a while, and then disappears again. On several occasions I have realized that this circumstance has coincided with an episode of intestinal parasites. I do not know why.

The antennas

The concept of antenna is a contribution by Jozef Vervoort, who met Tomatis through one of those personal experiences that mark a turning-point in life. Since then, he has devoted his efforts to the development of this technique.

On looking at the audiogram and paying particular attention to the bone conduction of the left ear, Vervoort explains that we can see two types of antennas: those in the bass range (*radar*) and those in the treble range (*combative*), which in turn have a positive or a negative orientation:

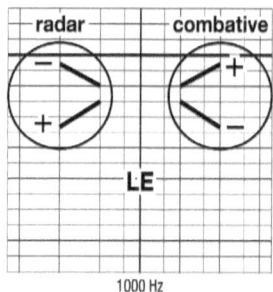

The combative antenna: fighting spirit

If the orientation is positive, this is reflected in a bone curve rising towards the high frequencies, which indicates that the person is awake, willing to fight and take on the challenges of life. On the other hand, when the curve is descending, this is a case of someone who has thrown in the towel: unmotivated and adrift.

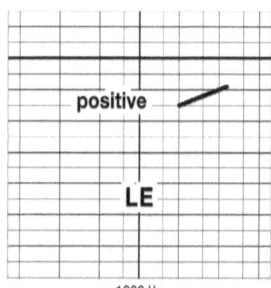
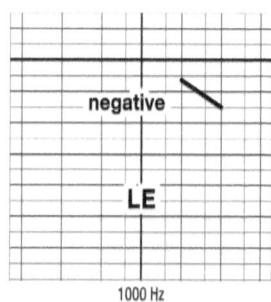

This is extremely important, as the key to any therapy process is motivation, which multiplies the odds of success. Therefore, gaining the patient's active collaboration should always be a priority.

The radar antenna

At the opposite end of the curve, in the bass range, we also check whether it is rising or falling. A descending curve indicates a person who is always on the alert, attentive to any change in the environment. It is a state that leads to stress.

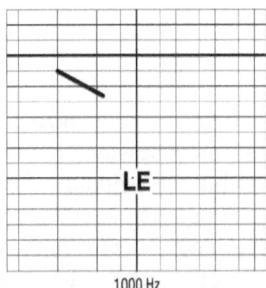

1000 Hz

In the consulting room we often receive children with this profile: always on their guard, aware of everything happening around them and worried about what will happen next. They keep asking their parents "What will we do next? When are we leaving? What's for dinner?" etc. They look at us suspiciously. It is hard to gain their trust. At school they cannot concentrate and over-dramatize quarrels with their classmates, criticism from teachers or any event that puts their low self-esteem to the test.

An article by Nils Bergman helped me understand them. Bergman (the person responsible for the good practice of immediately placing newborns in skin contact with the mother) states that the first 1,000 minutes of life are decisive for structuring the nervous system in one direction or another and the key question the system asks itself is whether it is in a safe or unsafe environment.

This polarity will determine essential aspects of our personality by activating one or other hormones. According to Bergman, cortisol, the stress hormone, accelerates different neural circuits to oxytocin, the hormone of calmness and pleasure.

I would venture to say that this must begin to happen before birth. When the fetus feels safe (probably perceiving the hormone content of the blood), its nervous system is configured differently than if it senses danger. That is why it is so important to provide tranquility and affection through contact with the mother.[231] The calm, motivated, trusting, confident child presents an ascending curve in the bass range:

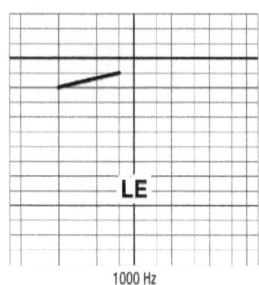

1000 Hz

Tomatis laid great emphasis on guarding against stress during pregnancy. It was almost an obsession. I guess his own story had something to do with it, but we should take his advice seriously. Stress can affect the baby's cognitive development.[232]

If you wish to delve deeper into this subject, I recommend Sapolsky's work, which describes the effects on the fetus in detail.[233] It has even been pointed out as a possible cause of the symptomatology of ADHD.[234]

AUDIOMETRY: A PERSONALITY TEST

Tomatis identified certain patterns in the audiometric curves, linked to personality traits. He then went on to classify these patterns into three main types, based on the degree of sensitivity to certain frequencies:

-vestibular or visceral: Sector 1 (125 to 1,000 Hz)
-paranoid or controlling: Sector 2 (1,000 to 3,000 Hz)
-schizoid or emotive: Sector 2I (3,000 to 8,000 Hz)

---

[231] *Early skin-to-skin contact for mothers and their healthy newborn infants (Review).* **Moore, E.R. et al.** 2012, The Cochrane Collaboration.

[232] *The Timing of Prenatal Exposure to Maternal Cortisol and Psychosocial Stress Is Associated With Human Infant Cognitive Development.* **Davis, E.P. and Sandman, C.A.** 1, 2010, Child Development, Vol. 81, pp. 131-148.

[233] **Sapolsky, R.M.**¿*Por qué las cebras no tienen úlcera* s.l. : Alianza Editorial, 2008.

[234] *Increased Risk of Asthma in Children with ADHD: Role of Prematurity and Maternal Stress during Pregnancy.* **Grizenko, N. et al.** 2, 2015, J Can Acad Child Adolesc Psychiatry, Vol. 24.

This classification is partly related to the Hippocratic temperaments: the somatotypes (endomorph, mesomorph and ectomorph), and to the Ayurvedic taxonomy of three doshas: vata, pitta and kapha. These are based on observations collected over 5,000 years, which will probably be updated in the light of epigenetics.

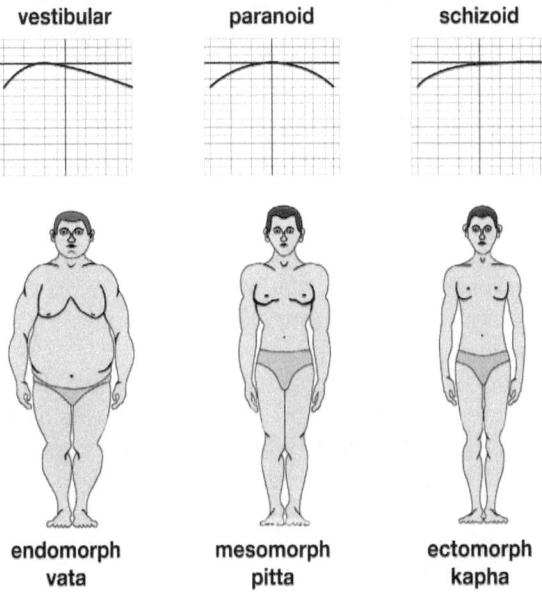

During embryonic development, the three germinal layers—endoderm, mesoderm and ectoderm—respectively generate the viscera, the muscular and skeletal system, and the skin and nervous system. Around 1940, the American psychologist W.H. Sheldon put forward the theory that the three layers do not develop equally, giving rise to the somatotypes.

The endomorph is in the Sancho Panza mold: stout and good-natured. The mesomorph takes on the appearance of an athlete: tenacious and controlling. Don Quixote would be the typical ectomorph, with a weak, lanky body and an overactive mind.

It is not easy for audiologists to notice this relationship between audiometry and personality, because of their training and because their clients are looking to solve a hearing problem, not a psychological one. Furthermore, when an auditory pathology does exist and the audiometric profile is highly impaired, it is hard to make an interpretation from the audio-psycho-phonological perspective. If the audiologist were familiar with audiograms of normal-hearing people, he would soon realize these patterns do exist.

Audiometry of the vestibular type

Vestibular curves are those presenting greatest sensitivity in the bass range, up to 1,000 Hz. They roughly correspond to individuals with the typical endomorphic build of Homer Simpson, the Ayurvedic Vata. They tend to be corpulent, likeable, funny people, lovers of good living. They make friends easily and always know how to liven up social events. They like money: not to save it, but to acquire comforts. They shy away from physical exertion. They love sports, but on TV, from the armchair, which is not

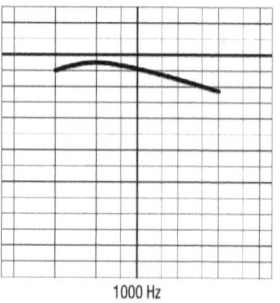

1000 Hz

good for them because, in fact, they need physical activity to feel well. After a few days of resting, their mood is usually worse. They love do-it-yourself and working with their hands in general.

According to Tomatis, this type recharges poorly in the treble range, but compensates for this by vestibular activation. However, when they become sedentary, they are at risk of succumbing to depression through lack of stimulation. They tend to respond well to therapy, but it is imperative that they regain physical activity.

A high incidence of depression and anxiety has been observed in patients with vestibular disorders. Cognitive alterations have also been documented: if both vestibules are damaged, atrophy of the hippocampus occurs, a key component in memory and spatial perception.[235]

Audiometry of the controlling type

Tomatis called them *paranoideo* (with certain traits reminiscent of paranoia). I will use the term *controlling* to avoid confusion with paranoia, a mental disorder that I am not referring to.

As good mesomorphs, their kingdom is that of reason and logic and also that of effort and discipline. They love challenges. They are

---

[235] *Does vestibular damage cause cognitive dysfunction in humans?* **Smith, P.F. et al.** 2005, Journal of Vestibular Research, Vol. 15, pp. 1-9.

fighters. In general, they seek out rational debate and demand scientific proof. Many athletes present this audiometric profile, as do social leaders, accountants, engineers, mathematicians and scientists. They are orderly, careful with money, austere and shy of taking risks: comparing prices thoroughly before making a spending decision. When choosing a restaurant, they have to analyze several menus in detail. These attitudes can be very helpful in certain circumstances, but if you are their traveling fellow and you are hungry, you will regret it. You will have a long walk ahead before finding the right place to eat.

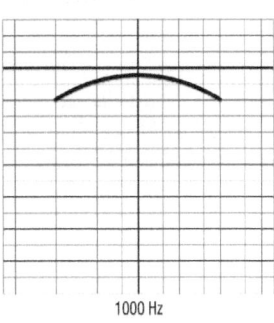

They demand rigor, effort and persistence from all those around them, because they consider these values not to be negotiable. However, they do not possess a great deal of creativity. Their effectiveness lies in knowing how to carry out the ideas of others and turn them into tangible reality. Taken to pathological extremes, these attributes lead to paranoid disorders, with their obsessive ideas, which tend not to improve with Tomatis's therapy, with some exceptions. In my opinion, when dealing with OCD (obsessive-compulsive disorder), Giorgio Nardone's brief strategic therapy is more appropriate.

The case of Manuel

This is probably the case that has impacted me the most in my career—not so much because of its clinical characteristics, but because of its circumstances. I have hesitated to include it in this book, because I am afraid it will raise suspicions, but I have finally decided to tell it as it happened.

As a young student of psychology, I used to work in a company, where I met Manuel. We became friends but, some time later, we each went our own way and lost contact.

A few years ago, my wife and I were on vacation in England. One night, I dreamt about Manuel, although I had forgotten his name. When I told Inma about my dream in the morning, she did remember his name. Around noon I got a phone call:

-Hello?

-Yes, who is it?

-Are you Carlos, the one who studied psychology and worked for the X Company?
-Yes. Who's this?
-It's me, Manuel. I used to work with you. Remember me?

The reader can understand my perplexity. I could not believe my ears. I had not heard from him in over twenty-five years!

His problems had a very unpleasant name: compulsive gambling. This is a disorder capable of annihilating not only the sufferer, but his entire family circle. In a moment of despair, he looked for my telephone number and called me. This was his initial listening test:

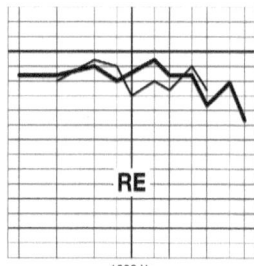 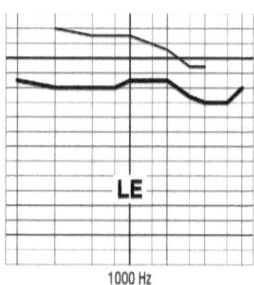

He had asymptomatic otitis in his left ear and bilateral tinnitus: in the right ear a high-pitched beep, similar to the frequency of 8,000 Hz, and in the left, of the white noise type. The distortions in the right ear are remarkable, in line with his stress levels.

For a couple of months, I devoted myself to him almost exclusively. I deployed all my resources: behavioral techniques, NLP, EMDR, auditory therapy and a large dose of inventiveness, even conducting fieldwork (or field psychology).

Fortunately, he gave up gambling. For a few years we exchanged some messages. Then we lost contact again.

Audiometry of the emotive type

Finally, we introduce the schizoid or emotive type: the Bohemian artist who takes neither food (vestibular type) nor logic (controlling type) into account. They just feel. They live without care for luxuries and comforts. They are not interested in rationality, but in artistic and spiritual debate. Their ectomorphic body is almost an afterthought to them. They are bursting with creativity but fail to put their ideas into practice. If intelligent, they surround themselves with controlling and vestibular types who will put their musings to good use and will know how to sell them, in the style of Steve Jobs.

In Spanish, when a person is very agitated, the expression *tener los nervios a flor de piel* ("having your nerves on your skin") might be used—similar to "touching a raw nerve". The phrase reflects the common ectodermal origin of both the skin and the nervous system. Children with this profile often suffer from eczema and people with psoriasis have more hearing impairments than the general population.[236]

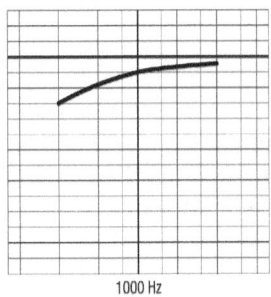

1000 Hz

Tomatis claimed that the ear is nothing more than a piece of differentiated skin, thus signaling the skin's sensitivity to sound.

Schizophrenia could be the pathological version of this type. According to Tomatis, schizophrenics suffer from an excess of cortical recharge that causes them to move away from the sensations of their physical body, living in their imagination. The therapy will consist of rooting them back, bringing them down to earthly reality. Vestibular activation tends to produce good results, combining auditory therapy with physical exercise. It would be a very helpful tool for psychiatrists. We will talk about this in Chapter 6.

Tell me how you listen, and I'll tell you who you are

When I see an audiogram, I imagine what kind of person I have in front of me. It is not infallible, but it does facilitate the interview with the patient. In spite of having seen this linkage between personality and listening test on countless occasions, it always amazes me.

In September and October consultations, patients often tell me something about their holidays. The vestibular type describe the pleasures they enjoyed: the food, the luxuries, the funny situations, and so on.

The controlling type offer a detailed account, with special mention of timetables and costs. In extreme cases, they begin their explanation with such thoroughness that after five minutes of conversation, the plane has still not taken off. If you try to suggest they sum up a little, they feel disturbed. They have set out their discourse in a certain order and it is not easy for them to improvise changes.

---

[236] *Auditory System Involvement in Psoriasis.* **Borgia, F. et al.** 2018, Acta Dermato-Venereologica, Vol. 98, pp. 655-659.

The emotive type, for their part, talk about their sensations and experiences: a sunset, the people they met and the customs of other countries. They do not care about how badly they ate or the money that someone stole from them.

However, bad food can quickly spoil the journey for the vestibular type. The same happens if the controlling type are billed incorrectly somewhere: that is enough to ruin their holidays. To the emotive type, of course, the only thing that can destroy their trip is the lack of adventures.

This ternary classification is applied in product design and advertising. When selling a car, for example, the comfort and luxuries of the vehicle are highlighted when the advertisement is aimed at the vestibular type. The controlling type are shown the wonderful technology and excellent value for money. For schizoids, the message is "the adventurous life" or "taking you wherever you want to go," accompanied by exotic images. Each car model also specializes in one of these types.

For didactic purposes I have exaggerated these profiles. In fact, we have a little of each type and, depending on circumstances, we behave more in one way or another. We tend to look for a job in the field we manage the best, although

I often see people whose audiometry results do not correspond to their work. The world is full of creative dreamers who were forced by circumstances to perform jobs that have nothing to do with their personality. In these cases, the audiometric curve breaks down. At first, the bone curve more or less maintains its shape, but the air curve

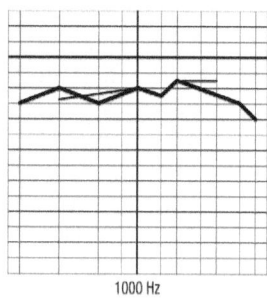

1000 Hz

tails off and is distorted. This is burnout syndrome. In today's society, artists do not easily find their place and theirs is the most frequent case of this syndrome, but any type of curve can be disrupted. Those of the controlling type can be defeated by the arrival of extremely emotive children: overwhelmed by their unpredictable behavior, not knowing what to do.

AUDIOMETRY: THE POSTURAL TEST

Tomatis noticed that his patients' posture was reflected in the bone curve shown in the audiometric test and that it changed throughout the therapy, as each frequency is linked to a particular area of the skeleton.[237]

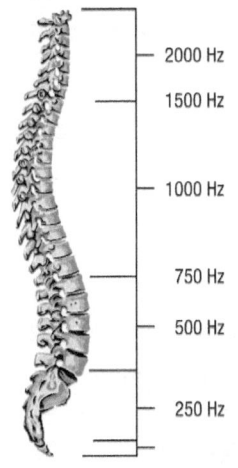

Our body vibrates when sound is applied to it and each part has its own specific resonance, as if it were a cello. Although much research is still needed, the positive effect that can be achieved in motor function by acoustic stimulation has already been documented.[238] As the auditory therapy progresses, the bone curve may become straighter and we will automatically see that the patient is more upright. However strange sounding, this in fact makes sense. Our posture depends to a great extent on our sensory captors: sight, vestibule and proprioception inform of our verticality, in opposition to gravity. If these do not work properly and the ear

2000 Hz

1500 Hz

1000 Hz

750 Hz

500 Hz

250 Hz

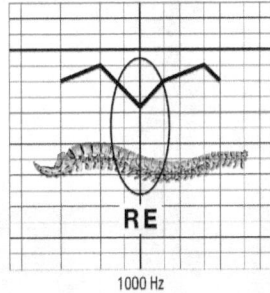

RE

1000 Hz

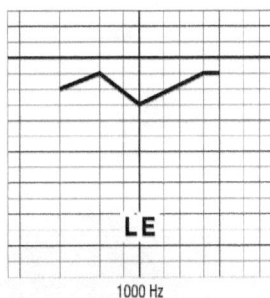

LE

1000 Hz

Probable deviation in the dorsal vertebrae

vestibules or the eyes deviate only a few tenths of a degree, the brain will regard as straight what is actually twisted, causing postural imbalances. For instance, certain idiopathic scolioses may be due to deviations in the orthogonal position of the semicircular canals in the vestibule, or to deficiencies in the integration of vestibular information.[239]

---

[237] **Sciberras, A.** Les theories de Tomatis et la scoliose. París : s.n., 1988. Thesis.

[238] *Immediate effects of different frequencies of auditory stimulation on lower limb motor function of healthy people.* **Yu, L. et al.** 2016, The Journal of Physical Therapy Science, Vol. 28, pp. 2178-2180.

[239] *Evidence for cognitive vestibular integration impairment in idiopathic scoliosis patients.* **Simoneau, M. et al.** 2009, BMC Neuroscience, Vol. 10.

Postural correction does not consist of wearing corsets, but tuning the sensory captors. These observations were made by the physicians da Cunha and Alves da Silva, founders of the Lisbon School of Posturology.[240] Back problems in adults show themselves in peaks and scotomas in the bone curve. A lack of similarity between both bone curves, right and left, can be a sign of scoliosis:

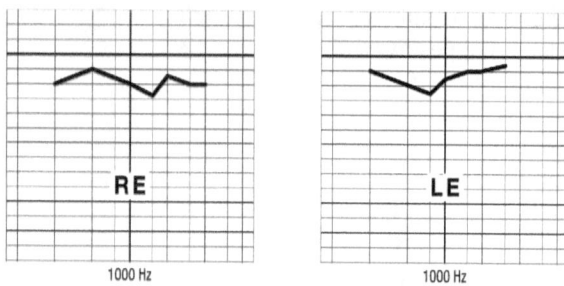

In depression sufferers, kyphosis is common, with an audiogram following the same pattern. If their posture is corrected, the symptoms improve.[241]

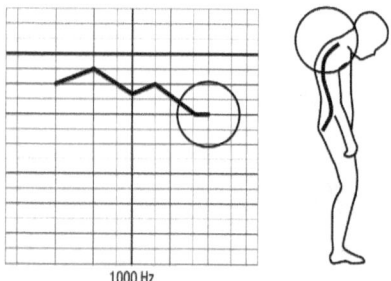

Pregnant women lower their middle ear resonance frequency during the third trimester of pregnancy.[242] Their auditory thresholds are more sensitive to the frequencies of 250 and 500 Hz, corresponding to the pelvis, which behaves like a guitar soundboard. Down there, listening, is the fetus.

According to Tomatis, the ear needs correct posture to be efficient as an energy captor. This is achieved with the back straight and the

[240] *Postural deficiency syndrome. Its importance in ophthalmology.* **Da Cunha, H.M. and Da Silva, O.A.** 11, 1986, J Fr Ophtalmol. 1986;Vol. 9, pp. 747-55.

[241] See note 91

[242] *Decrease in middle ear resonance frequency pendant pregnancy.* **Kutlu Dag, E. et al.** 147, Ankara : s.n., 2016, Audiololgy Research, Vol. 6.

head tilted forward about 30 degrees, just like a monk performing a Gregorian chant or the seated Buddha. In his training courses he insisted a lot on certain exercises to learn how to adopt that stance naturally and instantly.

Professional singers pay attention to these details. If we analyze our voice while changing posture, we will see that the harmonic distributions in the sonograms are altered. Singing involves the whole body. In an experiment, participants were asked to go up or down stairs before estimating the tone being sent to them through headphones, in Hz. After going up, they perceived a higher tone. After coming down, a lower one. In fact, it was the same.[243]

When sitting, standing, or lying on the floor, the thresholds are not exactly the same, which is why singing teachers insist so much on postural control. Guillermo González, from Barcelona, is investigating the changes that occur in singers as a result of changes in posture. It is amazing what can be achieved in the voice just by correcting the plantar support.

Susan E. Voss and her colleagues demonstrated in two articles published in 2006 and 2010 that posture also alters otoacoustic emissions and evoked potentials.[244,245] It would be a good idea to incorporate posturology into hearing aid adjustment. I would not be surprised to see results improve in this way.

A few years ago, I was successfully treated for a shoulder injury. While in the waiting room, I was able to watch a video about David Palmer, who performed the first known chiropractic maneuver in history (1895). He repositioned a vertebra for Harvey Lillard, the doorman of the building where he worked, by means of rapid, precise manual pressure. Mr. Lillard automatically recovered the hearing he had lost 17 years before, after physical exertion.

There are two remarkable things about this incident: first, and most important, that damage to a region so far from the ear could have caused deafness and, second, that the injury had not left any sequelae and, once corrected, hearing automatically came back. After that incredible success, deaf people flocked to Palmer's consulting

[243] *Reaching for the high note: judgments of auditory pitch are affected by kinesthetic position.* **Hostetter, A.B. et al.** Aug 21, 2019, Cognitive Processing.

[244]*Posture-Induced Changes in Distortion-Product Otoacoustic Emissions and the Potential for Noninvasive Monitoring of Changes in Intracranial Pressure.* **Voss, S.E. et al.** 2006, Neurocritical care, Vol. 4, pp. 251-257.

[245] *Posture systematically alters ear-canal reflectance and DPOAE properties.* **Voss, S.E. et al.** 1-2, May, 2010, Hearing Research, Vol. 263, pp. 43-51.

rooms in the hope of recovering their hearing. Most of them did not present the same clinical profile, but Lillard's case was not to be the last: several cases have been documented since then, linking the spine and hearing loss.[246]

AUDIOMETRY AS A HEALTH TEST

This is the most controversial issue, for which A. Tomatis was harshly criticized by his colleagues, not realizing that his method could be applied to all kinds of disorders.

Tomatis's goal was always to improve listening, but he discovered that when the audiometric curve is harmonized, this has several positive effects on health. His method, in short, is the sum of his clinical experience. He found air conduction to be more closely related to the viscera, while bone conduction reflected the skeleton. Scotomas indicated chronic ailments and peaks acute ones. For example, illnesses in the stomach often show up at 1,000 Hz, in the liver at 750 Hz, in the lungs at 1,500 Hz, and so on. We do not know the exact reason. Perhaps it is due to the connection of the auditory system with the vagus nerve, or a vestige of the metameric information on the lateral line of fishes. These are just hypotheses, but repeated clinical experience is a matter of fact.

The case of Miguel

Miguel was a music teacher. He came to see me because he wanted to improve his musical ear. This was his initial test:

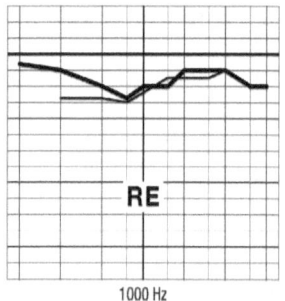

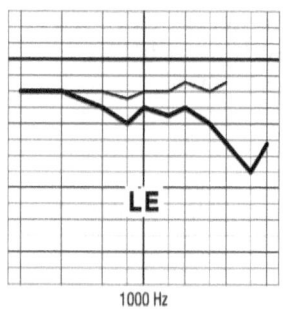

[246] *Improvement in hearing after chiropractic care: a case series.* **Di Duro, J.O.** 2, Jan 19, 2006, Chiropr Osteopat., Vol. 14.

In the right ear, the leading ear, the curve rises from 750 Hz, but not in the bass range. The left ear shows signs of an incipient process of hearing loss, despite the fact that bone conduction appears intact (audiometry with masking modified the profile of left-ear bone conduction). Several family members had suffered from hearing loss, so genetic causes were possible. The curve gradually smoothed out, but there was always a scotoma around 750 Hz:

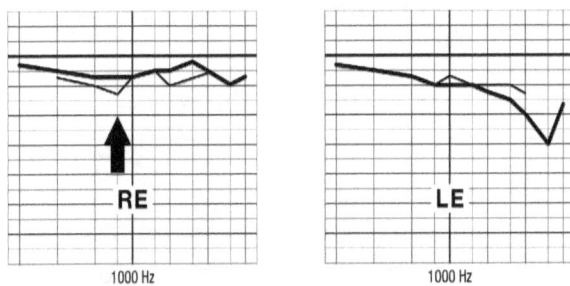

In his clinical interview he had not informed me of any illness or injury but, a few months later, I insisted:
- *Do you have a liver problem?*
- *No... But... well, yes.*
He then described to me his old history of liver disease, which I will not explain in detail in order to preserve my patient's anonymity. Finally, he said:
- *But I just had a blood test and it came out the best in years.*

Did his improvement have anything to do with the auditory therapy? Was it by chance? I cannot know, but I have experienced similar situations so many times! Here are some more examples of this audiometry–health link that Tomatis identified:

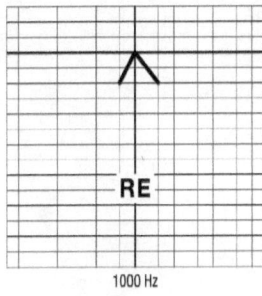

Current irritation

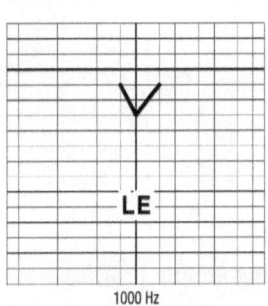

Chronic ailment

When I see this audiometric profile, it is almost certain that the person suffers from a recurring stomach problem, the stomach being their weak point, as reflected in the scotoma at 1,000 Hz in the left ear. If we find a peak in the same area in the right ear, it indicates an irritation in the present.

The link between the 1,000 Hz area and the stomach is very clear. The vagus nerve often somatizes emotions there. We have a "knot in our stomach" in stressful situations.

If the curve is of this type:

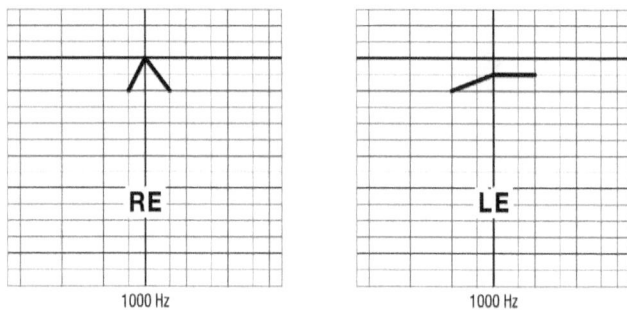

The most likely explanation is that our patient is feeling stomach discomfort right now, but not regularly, as the peak only appears in the right ear. If this were the other way round, our patient may often suffer from stomach pain, but not at this time—there is a weakness that remains asymptomatic for now:

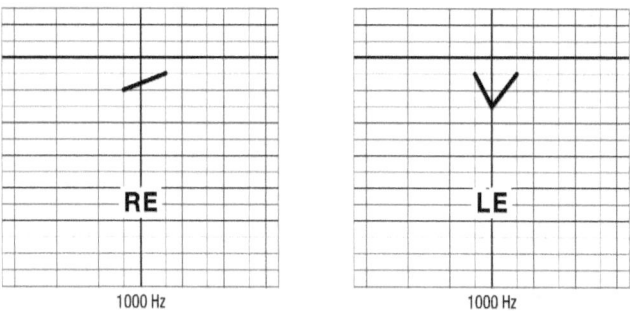

Other common profiles are:

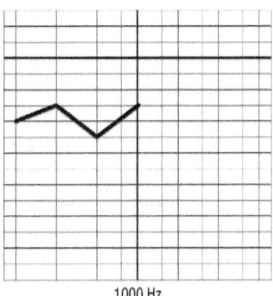

1000 Hz

Occasional diarrhea: in the right ear, the curve plunges down in the 500 Hz area, corresponding to the small intestine. If this also occurs in the left ear, the illness is probably chronic.

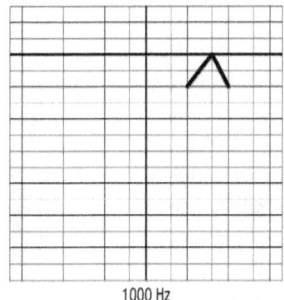

1000 Hz

Spring allergies: a peak usually appears in the air conduction curve, between 2,000 and 3,000 Hz. This is also typical of colds and sore throats. If it appears in the right ear it is sporadic. If in both ears, a recurring problem.

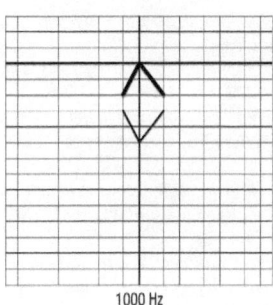

1000 Hz

When we find the bone curve and the air curve in opposition, with a scotoma in the bone curve and a peak at the same frequency in the air curve, we must ask the patient to consult the doctor.

The auditory curve usually gives advance warning of a problem, pinpointing vulnerable areas before the patient has mentioned any symptoms.

Several publications have reported on health-related variations in voice, but those exploring hearing changes are scarce. In one of them, women with polycystic ovary syndrome were found to have lower thresholds in the 8,000 to 14,000 Hz range.[247] According to the authors, perception of higher tones could be very sensitive to slight vascular problems, which would mean that we could make an early diagnosis by studying changes in sensitivity at high frequencies.

In general, the first damage to the ear occurs in the basal area of the cochlea, where the highest tones are registered, and apparently the area most vulnerable to aggressions. Extended audiometry (beyond 8,000 Hz) is proving to be an excellent diagnostic tool for detecting otological problems[248,249] and other diseases, such as rheumatoid arthritis[250] or lupus,[251] presenting a characteristic curve for each symptom. In otitis, the air conduction curve rises from 8,000 Hz.

Sensitivity increases, which is difficult to explain in terms of Bekesy's theory.[252] Otoacoustic emission testing can detect early onset of hearing damage, for instance, in diabetes.[253] Otoemissions remain even after auditory nerve degeneration.[254]

AUDIOMETRY OF STRESS

Stress is characterized by a saw-tooth pattern in the graph. There is no hearing loss. The HAIC average is usually normal, but the graph itself

[247] *Extended High Frequency Audiometry in Polycystic Ovary Syndrome.* **Kucur, C. et al.** 2013, The Scientific World Journal.

[248] *Extended high-frequency audiometry in subjects exposed to occupational noise.* **Korres, G.S. et al.** 3, 2008, B-ENT, Vol. 4, pp. 147-55.

[249] *Audiometría con extensión en altas frecuencias (9.000-20.000Hz). Utilidad en el diagnóstico audiológico.* **Rodríguez Valiente, A. et al.** 1, 2016, Acta Otorrinolaringol Esp, Vol. 67, pp. 40-44.

[250] *Early hearing loss detection in rheumatoid arthritis and primary Sjögren syndrome using extended high frequency audiometry.* **Galarza-Delgado, D.A. et al.** 2, Feb, 2018, Clin Rheumatol., Vol. 37, pp. 367-373.

[251] *Extended high frequency audiometry can diagnose sub-clinic involvement in a seemingly normal hearing systemic lupus erythematosus population.* **Lasso de la Vega, M. et al.** 2, Feb, 2017, Acta Otolaryngol., Vol. 137, pp. 161-166.

[252] *Extended High Frequency Audiometry in Secretory Otitis Media.* **Sharma, D. et al.** 2, 2012, Indian J Otolaryngol Head Neck Surg, Vol. 64, pp. 145–149.

[253] **Sambola, I.** Otoemisiones acústicas en pacientes diabéticos no insulinodependientes. [ed.] Hospital Universitari de Girona. *Doctoral thesis,* 2006.

[254] *Persistence of otoacoustic emissions in children with auditory neuropathy spectrum disorders.* **Sanyelbhaa Talaat, H. et al.** 5, 2013, Int J Pediatr Otorhinolaryngol., Vol. 77, pp. 703-6.

resembles rugged mountains. Tomatis even went so far as to define this as a fourth type of personality, the *characterial*, to be added to the other three: vestibular, controlling and emotive. Occasionally this pattern reflects a temporary state of affairs, which is why I have not previously included it among the personality types. We find it in patients who are agitated, dealing with family or work problems beyond their control. These are not

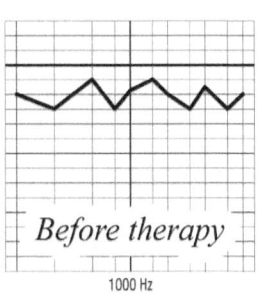

Before therapy

1000 Hz

necessarily extreme situations: what matters is how they are perceived, regardless of how serious they are when looked at objectively.

It is also common to find this type of curve in children who are unsociable and restless, whether or not they are badly behaved (if they are, they are more likely to be brought in for consultation). They often come with the ADHD label attached.

It is true that they are easily distracted, but not through a lack of attention, as often claimed, but through an excess of it, which prevents them from concentrating on just one thing. This also applies to their hearing. It is hard for them to focus on what you are saying because their attention immediately shifts elsewhere. Their learning suffers as a result, since it is not possible to understand, think or memorize when your mind is flitting from one thing to another.

This lack of control is reflected in the audiometric curve, which rises and falls like the one relating to stress. After auditory therapy, the curve relaxes, becoming smoother and more harmonious, with the peaks and scotomas fading away, and the child responds in the same way. We have only improved their listening, but the overall benefits are remarkable.

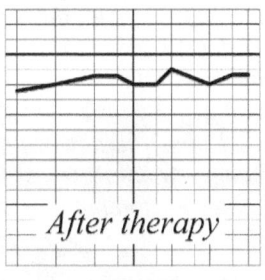

After therapy

Cochlear activity is strongly modulated by the mechanisms of stress, through the action of the glucocorticoids, which modify the cochlea's sensitivity and cause vestibular dysfunctions. Sustained stress can even atrophy dendritic connections in important nuclei of the auditory pathway. It also causes a decrease in GABA, the main neurotransmitter used by the auditory system to inform the cortex. Also, it is probably one of the causes of presbycusis.[255]

---

[255] See note 67

The Case of David

David's parents brought him to us when he was nine years old. He had school issues, specifically in learning to read. His mother was a teacher and had tried everything with no success. David's initial test came out like this:

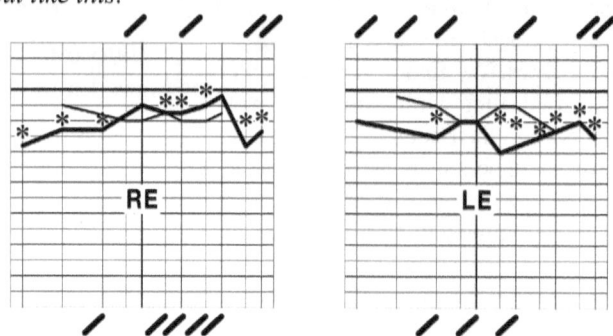

There are distortions, with curve inversion in Sector 1 in both ears. Spatialization errors appear in the air and bone conduction curves and selectivity is closed.

What struck me most about David was his apathy and lack of self-esteem: an attitude that was not restricted to schoolwork, but also caused him serious problems in his great passion: basketball. He was one of the best in his team. For his age, he handled the ball with ease and could read the game well, but he was convinced he would perform badly in matches, so he would ask the coach not to put him in. He preferred to be on the bench. Eventually, he even stopped going to see his teammates play. He just trained.

Doing therapy with no motivation is like eating without being hungry. It does not last long, no matter how hard you push. So first we set a basketball objective. After a few months, his test looked like this:

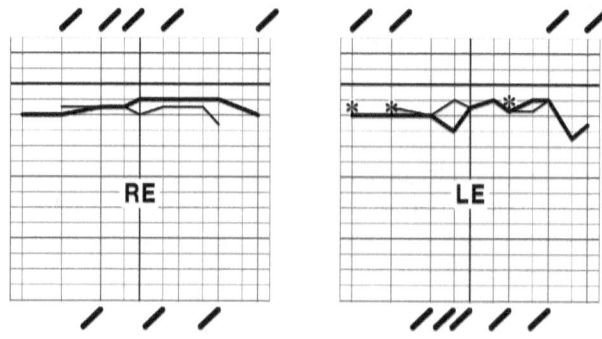

Although there were still selectivity and spatialization errors, the curve pattern had changed considerably. In those months, David began to play and went on to become the team leader and top scorer. This novel situation made him see himself in a new light. Now he was able to face up to challenges, and this renewed spirit then helped to solve his school difficulties.

AUDIOMETRY OF LANGUAGES

Having identified the link between voice and hearing in singers, Tomatis then wondered if the characteristic sounds of each language were not also a consequence of listening with specially adapted ears, which work as filters. Do English people listen in the same way as Germans or Spaniards? He did not think so.

The press soon latched onto Tomatis's work on language. In 1961 *The Times* published the article: *Training the ear to speak*, explaining the new language-learning horizons opened up by the electronic ear.[256] Later, Tomatis wrote *We were all born polyglots*, a book exploring this issue.[257]

Each language has its own preferred frequency range, within which its speakers discriminate with accuracy. The Spanish and French use the lower tones, while the English stick to the trebles, which is one of the reasons why it is so hard for the former to learn English.

	125	250	500	1000	1500	2000	3000	4000	8000	12000
German	▓	▓	▓	▓	▓					
British English						▓	▓	▓	▓	▓
Spanish	▓	▓	▓	▓	▓	▓				
French	▓	▓	▓	▓						
Italian						▓	▓	▓		
North American English				▓	▓	▓	▓	▓	▓	
Russian	▓	▓	▓	▓	▓	▓	▓	▓	▓	▓

Preferential frequency ranges of different languages, according to Tomatis

Let's look for example at the way of pronouncing the "t" for an English person and a Spanish person. The English seem to spit it out

---

[256] Training the ear to speak, hope for bad linguists. *The Times, educational supplement.* Nov 24, 1961, p. 716.
[257] See note 36

and the sound is stretched out. There is a clicking noise, full of high frequencies. Comparing the Spanish "t" with the English one, the spectral analysis shows a very different pattern. In the English "t", the density of high frequencies is greater.

If we compare the fricatives (like "f" or "s") in both languages, which are the consonants that contain the most high frequency sounds, they constitute 9.31% of the total in Spanish and 15.49% in English, almost twice as much,[258,259] and this does not take into account their length, which in English is usually greater.

When fitting a hearing aid, at least when this used to be done manually, tables were used which varied by language. The calibrations for an English patient and an American one were different, as the acoustic speech spectrums vary. According to Tomatis, North-American English uses lower tones, typical of the indigenous languages of the region.

The use of one frequency or another is determined largely by the acoustics of a place. Terrain, atmospheric pressure and humidity together produce a characteristic air impedance, which transmits some sounds better than others. Over time, the ear "focuses" on the sounds that are easier to discern. Tomatis gave the name "passing bands" to the frequency ranges the ear pays special attention to:

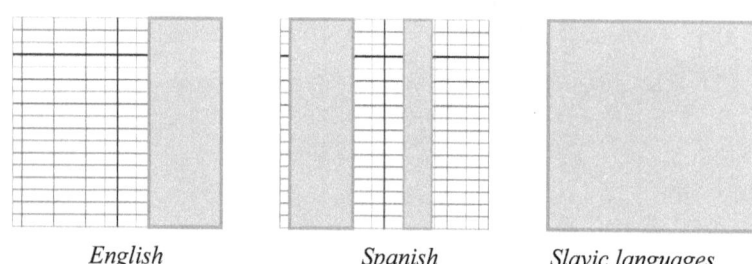

English   Spanish   Slavic languages

He offers a musical example that illustrates his theory on geographical impedances:

"I know Francescati very well, because he has participated in several of my experiments. He never wanted to play in Nice. He can't, his violin won't obey him.

[258] *Cálculo de frecuencias de aparición de fonemas y alófonos en español actual utilizando un transcriptor automático.* **Arias, I.** 1, 2016, Loquens, Vol. 3.

[259] *Power spectral entropy as an information-theoretic correlate of manner of articulation in american english.* **LlanosJoshua, F. et al.** 2017, Journal of the Acoustical Society of America, Vol. 141.

Singers also have problems in Nice. I have seen many of them in my clinic after assuring them that their larynx and ear were fine. Then they would send me telegrams saying, "I can't sing and I don't know what the problem is".

The air of Nice will not sing. Nice has an opera house by the sea, which is a replica of the Scala of Milan, though smaller. In this particular case, the house's acoustics are not to blame. I think it is a natural phenomenon in this part of the world.

The language of the people here is a very low frequency one, even more than that of the Spanish. The natives of Nice do not use their hearing beyond 500 Hz [...] it has to do with some physical phenomenon, I don't know what—maybe with the fact that Nice is located in a deep bay, where the waves break continuously, generating a constant background noise, so that all the elements that transmit sound are subjected to this high-intensity bombardment of low frequencies".[260]

On a recent trip to Nice with my wife, we had the opportunity to spend an evening at the Opera House, a beautiful building that evoked times gone by. We noticed that the acoustics were not excellent, even though they had remodeled the stage, placing wooden panels that better reflected the sound.

That Tomatis quote reminds me of an article I read about the frogs of Huangshan in China, which live near deafening waterfalls. With that noise, the calls of the males would never reach the females, so they have adapted their hearing and croaking to the environment. They are a rarity among their kind, as they communicate by ultrasound.[261]

Meanwhile, the researcher Cecilia Pemberton discovered that the voices of Australian women had become deeper, by comparing recordings from 1945 and 1993. According to her, the explanation could have to do with psychological factors, since a deep voice is associated with greater authority.[262]

If we could analyze the phonetics of native Australian languages (which is impossible, as most of the over two hundred languages that

---

[260] See note 25

[261] **AFP/Reuters.** Frogs croacks in ultrasound. [Online] http://www.abc.net.au/science/articles/2006/03/16/1592962.htm.

[262] *Have women's voices lowered across time? A cross sectional study of Australian women's voices.* **Pemberton, C., McCormack, P. and Russell, A.** 2, 1998, Journal of Voice, Vol. 12, pp. 208-213.

used to be spoken have disappeared), we would surely see that Australian English is absorbing acoustic characteristics of the native languages, as happened in America, influenced by the environment where it is spoken. In fact, English vowel formants show a lower frequency when pronounced by Aboriginal people.[263] I am not claiming that the evolution of languages is merely a matter of acoustics, but it certainly has its influence.

Newborn babies' crying serves to identify the mother tongue. Researchers who have worked in this field can distinguish between English, French or German babies from their cries.[264] French babies show an ascending frequency curve, pitching their cries higher and higher, while German ones present a descending curve, in line with the prosody of their language.

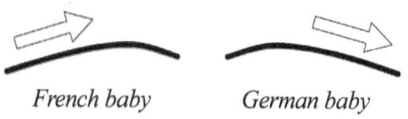

French baby   *German baby*

During gestation, the baby has been listening attentively and has adjusted his or her hearing to the mother's language. In a memorable experiment by Janet Werker, at the University of British Columbia in Canada, we see a newborn girl with a pacifier connected to a computer. When she hears a language she does not know, nothing happens, but with her mother tongue, she begins to suck avidly.

In a second experiment, one that is even more extraordinary as it implies a certain grammatical expertise, lists of words without specific content, such as prepositions and adverbs, were presented through the loudspeaker. No reaction. But when the baby heard nouns and verbs, the pacifier was brought back into action.[265]

Mothers talk to their children by playing with sounds, exaggerating prosody, and emphasizing language segments they want to highlight. Instinctively, they know how to capture the auditory attention of their babies by adapting their voice to each circumstance and the age of the growing child.[266]

---

[263] *The Vowels of Australian Aboriginal English.* **Butcher, A. and Anderson, V.** s.l. : Flinders University, 2008.

[264] *Newborns' Cry Melody Is Shaped by Their Native Language.* **Mampe, B. et al.,** 2009, Current Biology 19, 1994–1997, December 15, 2009, Vol. 19.

[265] *Newborn infants' sensitivity to perceptual cues to lexical and grammatical words.* **Shi, R., Werker, J.F. and Morgan, J.L.** 2, Sep 30, 1999, Cognition, Vol. 72.

[266] *Korean Mothers Attune the Frequency and Acoustic Saliency of Sound Symbolic Words to the Linguistic Maturity of Their Children.* **Jinyoung, J. and Eon-Suk, K.** 2225, Dec, 2018, Frontiers in Psychology, Vol. 9.

We should also consider selectivity, the capacity to discern fine frequency differences, in each language. We all know that the main problem with hearing aids is that, although they amplify sound perfectly, that is not enough to achieve proper understanding in adverse conditions. Other factors are involved.

We could re-educate hearing aid users by training them in fine discrimination of their language's passing band, using music. The percentage of customers dissatisfied with their devices would probably be reduced. This could also be used preventively, which would facilitate hearing-aid adjustment when needed.

Languages, furthermore, have their own rhythm. For example, the average duration of each syllable varies, instilling a characteristic cadence that can be appreciated in the popular music of each ethnic group.[267] Thus, for example, syllable length in English congregates in a range between 160 and 280 msec.[268]

Tomatis measured these times and incorporated them into the technology of his electronic ear: 0.15 sec. for French, 0.20 for English, etc. This is obtained by dividing the time a conversation takes by the number of syllables. It is a very similar concept to Caruso's timing delay when singing, which I mentioned in chapter 1.

To illustrate this internal rhythm, Tomatis would tell how during the Second World War, those in charge of intercepting the enemy's Morse messages often did not understand a word of what they were writing down, but they immediately recognized the language from the cadence of the sender's tapping.

Nina Kraus and her team at Northwestern University believe that the ability to follow rhythms is a reflection of neurological accuracy in auditory processing, and predicts which children may have future reading disorders.[269]

You cannot talk without singing at the same time, as the prosody of speech is made up of melody and rhythm,[270] and musical abilities favor the learning of a second language. In both cases we use similar

---

[267] *Comparing the rhythm and melody of speech and music: The case of British English and French.* **Patel, A.D., Iversen, J.R. and Rosenberg, J.C.** 5, 2006, J. Acoust. Soc. Am., Vol. 119.

[268] *La duración silábica y clasificación rítmica del inglés.* **Cuenca, M.H.** 1998, Philologia Hispalensis, Vol. 12, pp. 161-177.

[269] *Beat synchronization predicts neural speech encoding and reading readiness in preschoolers.* **Woodruff Carr, K. et al.** 40, 2014, PNAS, Vol. 111.

[270] *Music and speech prosody: a common rhythm.* **Hausen, M. et al.** 566, 2013, Frontiers in Psychology, Vol. 4.

hearing skills,[271,272] since music and language share neurological networks and structures.[273,274,275] Knowing this allows us to intervene therapeutically in advance, using music to develop skills that will later be necessary in the development of language.

Musical training structures auditory perception,[276,277] facilitating the immediate identification of tonal and rhythmic constructions and recognition of sounds: skills that are equally necessary for speaking.[278] Musicians often get better scores in verbal tests. They are faster and are better at spotting the important information.[279]

At the first Audio-psycho-phonology congress I attended, in 1995, the Eurocopter Company (the second largest helicopter manufacturer in the world at the time, which later became part of the Aerospatiale holding) presented a paper in the form of a short film. They had calculated the annual losses they suffered as a result of the lack of language proficiency of their aircraft maintenance staff worldwide. I do not remember the figures, but they were certainly high.

When a helicopter broke down, their mechanics would head off to repair it wherever necessary, transporting the tools and spare parts. They often paid the price for ineffective communication with the client: the repair job was not as expected, parts were missing, or the wrong staff had been sent out. To remedy this, they launched a project to learn English through Tomatis's techniques and in a short time they noticed the positive effects. In the presentation, the project's effectiveness was measured directly in French francs. The company was very happy with the results.

---

[271] *Relación entre la aptitud musical y el grado de comprensibilidad del habla en una segunda lengua.* **Osle, A.** 2012, Porta Linguarum, Vol. 17.

[272] **Toscano, C.M.** Estudio empírico de la relación existente entre el nivel de adquisición de una segunda lengua, la capacidad auditiva y la inteligencia musical del alumnado. [ed.] Dpto. Filología Inglesa University of Huelva. Huelva : s.n., 2011.

[273] *Speech and music shape the listening brain:evidence for shared domain-general mechanisms.* **Asaridou, S.S. and McQueen, J.M.** 321, 2013, Frontiers in Psychology, Vol. 4.

[274] *Shared and distinct neural correlates of singing and speaking.* **Özdemir, E., Norton, A. and Schlaug, G.** 2006, NeuroImage, Vol. 33, pp. 628-635.

[275] *Neural overlap in processing music.* **Peretz, I. et al.** March, 2015, The Royal Society Publishing.

[276] *Art and science: how musical training shapes the brain.* **Barrett, K.C. et al.** 713, 2013, Frontiers in Psychology, Vol. 4.

[277] *Musical intervention enhances infants' neural processing of temporal structure in music and speech.* **Zhao, T.C. and Kuhl, P.K.** April 25, 2016, PNAS.

[278] *Music Training Increases Phonological Awareness and Reading Skills in Developmental Dyslexia: A Randomized Control Trial.* **Flaugnacco, E. et al.** 2015, Plos One.

[279] *Coordinated plasticity in brainstem and auditory cortex contributes to enhanced categorical speech perception in musicians.* **Bidelman, G.M. et al.** 2014, European Journal of Neuroscience, pp. 1-12.

Subsequently, now as Aerospatiale, the language learning service was extended to the general public. The initiative even resonated with the European institutions, which financed the Audiolingua project that proved the usefulness of this methodology.[280] Several universities took part in it, among them a Spanish one, that of Zaragoza. Then other methods became fashionable and that knowledge was forgotten.

A great example of the application of Tomatis's techniques in working on the pronunciation of a language is the case of Mariana, a Brazilian actress living in Italy, who could not get rid of her native accent, which was a serious problem on stage.

She went to the Atlantis center in Belgium in search of a solution. My colleague Carmela Stillitano kept close track of the whole therapeutic process and published the results.[281] At the end of the therapy Mariana could speak at will in an Italian accent. It is almost impossible to recognize her Brazilian accent in the later recordings.

Convinced that language expresses a neurological substrate accumulated over millennia, Tomatis wondered if it was projected on to the written word in the same way. In order to do so, he sought the collaboration of a rabbi, so that he could read aloud the Hebrew alphabet with perfect diction, while a spectrum analyzer represented the sound visually.

The investigation soon came to an unexpected end, however. The rabbi stood in front of the microphone and pronounced the first letter: "Aleph". The graph plotted on the screen actually resembled the shape of the letter itself, and the rabbi took fright and refused to continue with the experiment.[282]

Years later, this work was taken up again by Carlo Soares, who published the book: *The Sonograms of the Hebrew Alphabet,*[283] in which he comments, letter by letter, on the similarities between the shape of the written letters and their spectral analysis. It is a work that will interest Kabbalah researchers more than audiologists, but this correspondence between sound pattern and written symbol is striking. It suggests that letters were not invented arbitrarily, but through their

---

[280] **Kanzer, U.A. and Gianni, F.** The Audio Language Project. [Online] https://isoraneurociencia.com/wp-content/uploads/2015/12/The_Audio-Language_Project_2c_Program_Socrates_UK.pdf.

[281] **Stillitano, C.** [Online] 2016. http://www.tomatisnew.com/biblioteca/EFECTO%20TOMATIS.pdf.

[282] See note 39

[283] **Suarès, C.** *Les spectrogrammes de l'alphabet hébraïque.* Genève : Editions Mont-Blanc, 1973.

acoustic perception, a type of synesthesia, which had an unconscious influence on their shape.

From time to time, the press calls our attention to an unusual way of learning languages. After severe trauma, some people wake up fluently speaking a language they barely had notions of before the accident. Several cases of this have been documented throughout history.

In 2016, for instance, a 16-year-old from Atlanta, Reuben Nsemoh, suffered a kick to the head during a football match, which left him in a coma for several days. When he woke up, he could speak correct Spanish.[284] Also, in that same year, in Australia, Ben McMahon, after a week in a coma from a car accident, discovered that he spoke perfect Mandarin Chinese.[285] He went so far as to present a TV program in that language.

These are extreme cases of the *foreign accent syndrome*, a rare dysfunction that causes some patients to speak with the characteristics of another language after a brain injury.[286]

AUDIOMETRY: A TEST OF DEVELOPMENT

Some traumatic childhood events leave their mark on the listening test. A complicated birth, for example, as osteopaths well know, can cause harmful torsions in the baby, especially in the dorsal and cervical areas. In these cases, scotomas usually appear on the audiometric graph in the bone conduction curve, both at 750 Hz (lumbar area) and 2,000 Hz (cervical area), which indicate the trauma suffered. This is seen in the left ear.

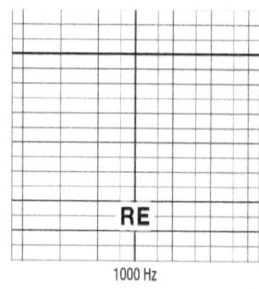

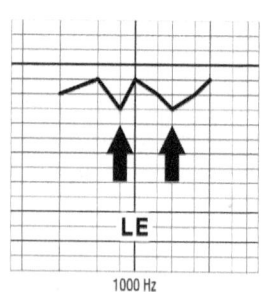

[284] **Redacción Barcelona.** Un joven de Atlanta se despierta de un coma hablando en perfecto español. *La Vanguardia.* Oct 25, 2016.

[285] **BBC.** Australiano despierta del coma hablando chino mandarín. *BBC Mundo.* March 22, 2016.

[286] *Transient foreign accent syndrome.* **Srinivas Bhandari, H.** 2011, BJM Case Reports.

If the air conduction curve also falls in the treble zone, it is very likely that there was anoxia during childbirth:

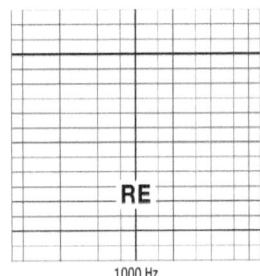
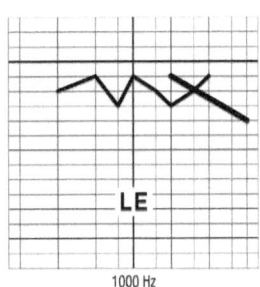

The selectivity test is also related to the person's life history. The ability to distinguish between two sounds evolves with age and can be truncated by a trauma. Hence, on analyzing this, along with other audiometric characteristics, we may suspect that something happened at a certain age. However, there are several factors that can be involved, and we must be cautious about interpretations.

In children up to 6–8 years of age, we usually find a lot of peaks and scotomas, selectivity errors and curve inversion, especially in the bass range. Little by little, the audiometric curves take on an adult pattern: smoothing themselves out and erasing errors, and showing parallel air and bone curves.

If an adult has a "child's" audiometric pattern, we know that something was not resolved correctly during childhood. In these cases, we usually discover psychological causes, such as an unhealthy environment or family circumstances.

The degree of maturation of the auditory system is currently evaluated by analyzing the brain waves obtained with evoked potentials. Their shape and latency change with age, so we can verify the level we are currently at. Auditory development has been shown to be affected by adverse psychological factors. A study conducted in Brazil, for example, tracked the auditory and psychological development of a group of children, up to their first birthday. The study presented these conclusions.

"Lesser maturation of the auditory pathway correlates with the presence of psychological risk. Problems in the mother–child relationship during the first 6 months of life harm not only cognitive development, but also hearing".[287]

[287] *Auditory maturation and psychological risk in the first year of life.* **Rechia, I.C. et al.** 4, 2018, CoDAS, Vol. 30.

The Case of Ingrid

This was Ingrid's test result at the age of five. She needed sleeping pills and her behavior was very irritating. She was so active that her parents were desperate and exhausted. They argued about how best to bring up their daughter, because they no longer knew what to do. As a result, the girl had adopted the habit of constantly provoking and challenging them.

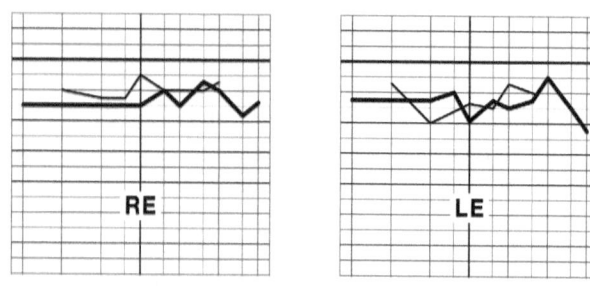

Initial test

It was not easy to rectify the situation, but after a few months we began to see results. She no longer needed medication to sleep. She stopped pestering and disobeying out of pure habit and they learned that they could do things together without shouting and arguing. In the final test the curves are more harmonious, the air and bone curves join together, and right and left ear are quite similar. As the audiometric pattern became smoother, the girl's behavior also improved, as if her brain had agreed to function with the harmony suggested by the new curve.

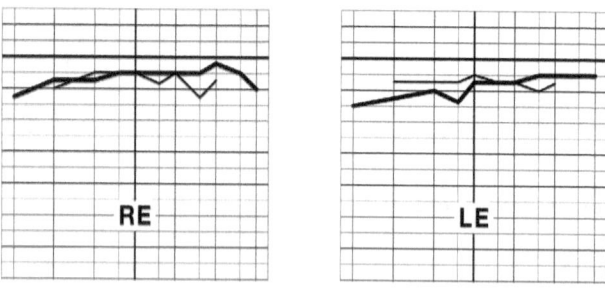

After therapy

AUDIOMETRY AND DYSLEXIA

The scientific literature regularly addresses the relationship between hearing and learning disorders, especially dyslexia. The studies almost always follow the same pattern: a group with difficulties is compared to a control group by means of various types of audiological tests, of central processing, evoked potentials, etc. And statistically significant differences do indeed tend to be found, though we do not understand why.

I am going to take the liberty of telling a story belonging to the Sufi tradition that reflects what I am trying to say:

A neighbor finds Nasrudin at night, looking for something on the ground by the light of a streetlamp.
-What are you looking for?, he asks.
-My keys; I have lost them.
-I'll help you.
They start searching together and after a while, more neighbors join in the search. Finally, tired of not finding them, one of the neighbors asks again:
-And you're sure you dropped them around here
-No, but this is where there is light.

Research on certain disorders such as dyslexia shows a close resemblance to this story. With every technical novelty at our disposal, with every new streetlamp, new studies are published, confirming that dyslexics are different, but we have still not found the underlying cause or causes.

Where are the keys to dyslexia? I would suggest they are in the results of therapies that have proved to be clearly successful, so we need to look in detail at these in order to find answers. Although we can sometimes see contradictory data, broadly speaking there seems to be no doubt that the hearing system works differently in children with learning difficulties. This sweeping statement does not mean, however, that hearing tests are robust and capable enough by themselves to identify dyslexia or other disorders. Many of the typical characteristics of "dyslexic hearing" are found in children without any learning problems, so they do not help us to diagnose accurately.

From the audio-psycho-phonological perspective, we have not identified an audiometric pattern specific to the dyslexic child either, but some patterns are repeated. The most common one is the fall we observe in Sector 2, that of language, with or without distortions.

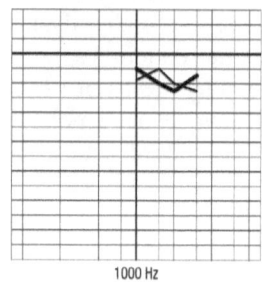
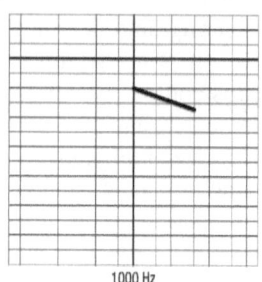

This descent is usually accompanied by alterations in Sector 1, often with curve inversion. According to Tomatis, it is to be interpreted as a deficient construction of language, a consequence of still immature motor skills.

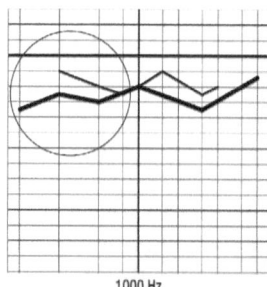

Tomatis wrote *Education and Dyslexia* in 1976, at the same time that Paula Tallal was publishing her first works on the topic in the United States.[288] Tallal is a world authority on dyslexia research and has always suspected that the auditory system is involved in the syndrome, while Tomatis, for his part, considered that in dyslexia the ear does not know how to synchronize with the visual captor and is not well lateralized to the right. The leading ear—always the right one for Tomatis—has not yet assumed its responsibilities. Certainly, in dichotic listening tests, there is no clear predominance of the right ear among dyslexic children, as there is in the general population.[289]

---

[288] *Auditory perception, phonics and reading disabilities in children.* **Tallal, P.** Miami Beach : s.n., 1977. 94th Meeting of the Acoustic Society of America.

[289] *Identificación de la lateralidad auditiva mediante una prueba dicótica nueva con dígitos en español, y de la lateralidad corporal y orientación espacial en niños con dislexia y en controles.* **García, F. et al.** 4, 2005, Revista de neurología, Vol. 41, pp. 198-204.

Tomatis also understood that the coordination of eye movements depended largely on the auditory system. For example, the reaction time of saccadic movements (the rapid eye movements we use when reading) is modified by auditory stimulation.[290]

Rivers of ink have been written about laterality and dyslexia and I will not dwell on the issue, but I will cite an article published in 2012 by the team at the Miguel Servet hospital in Zaragoza. They had found a high proportion of right-ear otitis in the histories of children with language disorders:[291] something that would prevent a proper lateralization process.

Are these otites just a health problem? Tomatis claimed that all otites are of psychological origin, unless proven otherwise, emphasizing the link between the skin (with its inner mucous lining) and the nervous system, which shares its ectodermal origin.

One of Tomatis's former dyslexic patients, psychologist Paul Madaule, runs an audio-psycho-phonology center in Canada. He wrote a book recounting his own experience[292] and over time has become an authority on this therapy. The famous psychiatrist Norman Doidge, author of the bestseller *The Brain Changes Itself*, explains his work in detail in his latest publication.[293]

The Case of Sara

Sara, a ten-year-old girl, came to our center for serious reading problems. She hated reading. Her teachers suspected dyslexia. She had thrown in the towel, not caring about anything. She did not

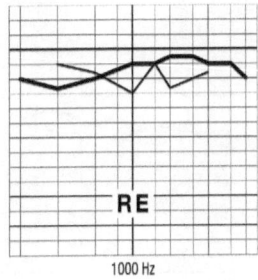
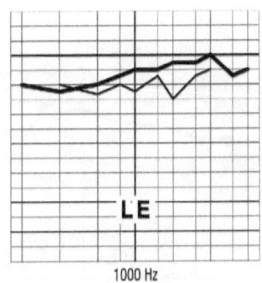

[290] *Visual-auditory interaction in saccadic reaction time: effects of auditory masker level.* **Steenken, R. et al.** Jul 18, 2008, Brain Res., Vol. 1220, pp. 150-6.

[291] *The Importance of Right OtitisMedia in Childhood Language Disorders.* **Uclés, P. et al.** International Journal of Otolaryngology : s.n., 2012.

[292] **Madaule, P.** *Escuchar despertar a la vida.* Mexico : Editorial Patria, 1994.

[293] **Doidge, N.** *The brain's way of healing.* New York : Vikin Penguin, 2015.

misbehave in class and went unnoticed. Her attitude was more concerning than her school difficulties. Her worst moment was when the teacher made her read aloud in front of everyone. That was a mirror in which she did not want to see herself. When I asked her to read me a few lines, she flatly refused. We can see in the right ear of her first test how the bone curve falls off around Sector 2.

Progress with Sara through auditory re-education was quick. Her attitude changed radically. After a short time, she surprised all of us by volunteering as a narrator at a school festival and began to read effortlessly in front of hundreds of people, microphone in hand, something unthinkable months before. A feat that corresponds to this test:

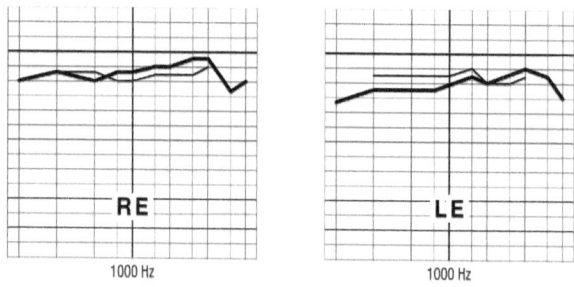

Both curves are approaching the ideal listening pattern, according to Tomatis, especially the right ear.

Sara's schooling continued normally from then on, but in one of the periodic checks we carried out, I found her curve to be somewhat disjointed again:

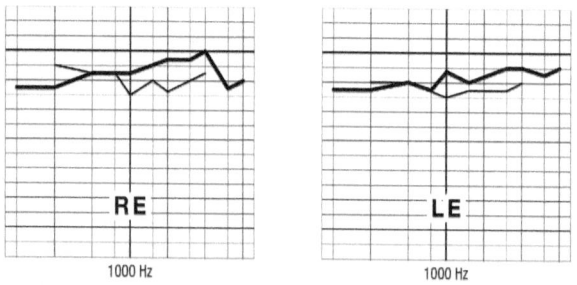

She had suffered a severe otitis, which had left her with a slight right facial hemiparesis. She had recovered fully, but the audiometry picked up the impact. Fortunately, this was a temporary setback, with no consequences.

THE EAR IN PSYCHIATRY

6

Tomatis took great interest in psychiatry. No doubt one of the reasons for this was a study in which he collaborated in 1962.[294] A medical team evaluated the hearing of 180 children diagnosed with mental disorders, at the Armentières Child Psychotherapy Center, in northern France. They were able to obtain reliable audiograms from 103 of them, with the following results:

- 42 cases of transmissive bilateral hearing loss,
- 31 cases of mixed bilateral hearing loss,
- 15 cases of undetermined bilateral hearing loss.

They also detected other types of pathologies. Only two audiograms were normal. The reader may assume that greater precautions are now taken before diagnosing a mental illness, and this is in fact the case, but these data show that hearing disorders and psychiatric disorders can be closely related and even share symptoms. In a 2008 article, Kendall and Rosenheck asked themselves why, in their veterans' hospital, hearing impaired people needed more psychiatric care than other patients.[295]

In the light of the studies already carried out, audiological diagnosis could become very useful in psychiatry[296] and auditory

---

[294] *Résultats de l'examen de l'audition chez 180 enfants hospitalisés au centre de psychothérapie infantile d'Armentiéres.* **Castets, B., et al.** June, 1962, Annales médico-psychologiques, Vol. 1.

[295] *Use of mental health services by veterans disabled by auditory disorders.* **Kendall, C. and Rosenheck, R.** 9, 2008, Journal of Rehabilitation Research & Development, Vol. 45, pp. 1349-1360.

[296] *Brain stem audiometry may supply markers for diagnostic and therapeutic control in psychiatry.* **Nielzén, S.et al.** 2016, Neuroscience Letters, Vol. 632, pp. 163-168.

therapy is deserving of in-depth study. Although I have hardly ever worked in clinical psychology, people with depression, bipolar disorder, paranoia and schizophrenia have come to my practice and I have been able to confirm that the audiometric test usually produces the profiles described by Tomatis. However, when the medication is massive, the hearing curves are not easily interpretable.

Once I shared a table with the Fromenteau, a married couple, both psychiatrists working in Bordeaux. They told me they had used Tomatis's therapy for fifteen years in a psychiatric hospital in Pau, in the south of France, until pharmacological methods were imposed. In their opinion, Tomatis's observations on mental illness were very much on target. For my part, I have found that auditory therapy, focused on improving listening, does help these patients. Their symptoms are eased and the audiometric curve becomes smoother, facilitating the work of psychiatrists.

The Case of Maria

One day a middle-aged woman, diagnosed with bipolar disorder, came to my consulting room. She had been on medication since she was 18. A very unfortunate childhood had had severe consequences.

Maria became a great teacher for me. At each visit she gave me a lesson in audiology and in humanity. She had an exquisite sensitivity. One day I mistakenly let her listen to an auditory training file that had been designed for another patient. They were very similar, no one else would have noticed, but she said: "I don't know what it is about that music, but I didn't like it at all."

After a year of auditory therapy, her psychiatrist withdrew her medication for good. She did not need it anymore. I asked her to come in from time to time for a check-up, so I saw her regularly for a few years. She did not relapse.

Mary managed to normalize a life marked by traumatic events in all respects. As she once explained to me, she had never enjoyed her conjugal life until she did Tomatis's therapy.

Schizophrenia is characterized by a high level of ideation. Deliriums and hallucinations appear; the patients live inside their fantasy. Depressives, on the other hand, manifest their apathy in a discourse that is poor and lackluster. They close in on themselves, showing total disinterest in the outside world. This is a very general description, but it will help us to understand the auditory dynamics involved in these pathologies.

In schizophrenia and depression, we often find opposite audiometric profiles, in line with Tomatis's observations. Let me clarify that the audiometric curve does not show anyone to be mentally ill. At most, it could be a risk factor. Some other factors to bear in mind are that medication can also modify auditory thresholds and that it is difficult to obtain reliable audiograms for a statistical study unless you work in a psychiatric hospital and have the necessary means.

THE EAR AND DEPRESSION

In depression, the curve often descends in the treble range: a shape that can also correspond to an incipient hearing loss. So how do we distinguish it?

This is a tough question to answer, especially as the two pathologies are often associated. In depression, we usually find the bone conduction curve to be better than the air curve:

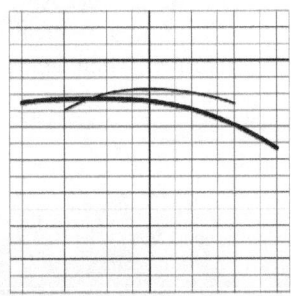

Auditory therapy hardly modifies the thresholds in the case of hearing loss, but it is effective in depression, with symptoms improving in parallel with the curves.

Another audiometric profile that we can obtain from a patient with depressive symptoms is a falling curve in the bass area. This is the curve of a vestibular-type person who has become sedentary. Sector 1 shows a fall due to lack of stimulation.

These patients tend to progress well with physical activity. Vestibular auditory therapy is a good initial aid.   As Tomatis described, a worsening of the audiometric curve has been observed in depressive patients, mainly in the higher frequencies and in the left ear.[297]

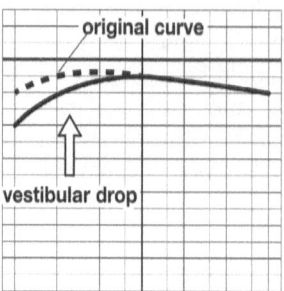

Whether hearing loss leads to depression due to the social isolation it causes or for neurological reasons[298] is under debate at present. Depression has indeed been considered to be an effect of deafness, a consequence of the social problems that hearing loss brings with it. The data tell us that the greater the hearing deficit, the greater the degree of depression[299,300,301,302] and although common sense leads us to think of deafness as the cause, because of its negative social effects, it may well be that shared neurological factors are behind the association.[303,304] Hearing improves when depression subsides.[305]

---

[297] *Hearing loss and asymmetry in major depression.* **Yovell, Y. et al.** 1, 1995, J Neuropsychiatry Clin Neurosci., Vol. 7, pp. 82-9.

[298] *Association Between Hearing Loss and Depressive Symptoms in Elderly.* **Ribeiro, A. et al.** 4, 2010, Intl. Arch. Otorhinolaryngol., Vol. 14, pp. 444-449.

[299] *Hearing Impairment Associated With Depression in US Adults, National Health and Nutrition Examination Survey 2005-2010.* **Li, C.M. et al.** March 6, 2014, JAMA Otolaryngology–Head & Neck Surgery.

[300] *Severe hearing impairment and risk of depression: A national cohort study.* **Kim, S.Y. et al.** 6, 2017, Plos One., Vol. 12.

[301] *Relación entre el déficit sensorial auditivo y depresión en personas mayores: revisión de la literatura.* **Millán-Calenti, J.C. et al.** 2011, Revista Española de Geriatría y Gerontología, Vol. 46(1), pp. 30-35.

[302] *Association of Audiometric Age-Related Hearing Loss With Depressive Symptoms Among Hispanic Individuals.* **Golub, J.S. et al.** 2, 2019, JAMA Otolaryngol Head Neck Surg., Vol. 145, pp. 132-139.

[303] *Pure-tone auditory thresholds are decreased in depressed people with post-traumatic stress disorder.* **Aubert-Khalfa, S. et al.** 2010, Journal of Affective Disorders. doi:10.1016/j.jad.2010.05.011.

[304] *Depressive Disorders in Relation to Neurootological Complaints.* **Nagy, E. et al.** 1, 2004, International Tinnitus Journal, Vol. 10, pp. 58-64.

[305] See note 183

Abnormalities have been found in the auditory processing of depressive patients, such as smaller waves with longer latencies in evoked potentials like MMN[306] or P300.[307]

In a recent study carried out in Holland on a sample of almost 3,000 people, it was found that the elderly who suffered from hearing loss had smaller brains, an atrophy that could be induced by receiving less stimulation. The loss of volume affected the whole brain, mostly in certain areas of the right hemisphere. The researchers were careful to isolate other variables in order not to contaminate the results: this reduction in size was not due to alcohol consumption, cardiovascular disease or cognitive level, but parallel to the degree of hearing loss.[308]

The severity of depressive symptoms goes up and down in parallel with the effectiveness of the left hemisphere in dichotic listening tests, which means these tests could be useful in the diagnosis of depression.[309] Cognitive impairment in old age is lower in people who maintain good hearing. They are even less at risk of falling[310].

These findings have initiated an incipient collaboration between ENT physicians and psychiatrists.[311] As Tomatis suggested, it seems that reduced activity of the auditory system can lead to atrophy in certain areas of the brain.

Tomatis claimed that deafness is not limited strictly to hearing, but should be considered in its energy dimension. The brain stops receiving much of the stimulation it needs to function correctly, falling into sensory deprivation. This effect is not immediate, but long-term, and activates compensation mechanisms. Persons who are hearing-impaired but with an active life (high vestibular activation) are able to find a balance. Two examples will serve to illustrate Tomatis's point of view.

---

[306] *Abnormality of Auditory Mismatch Negativity in Depression and Its Dependence on Stimulus Intensity.* **Restuccia, D.et al.** 2, 2016, Clin EEG Neurosci., Vol. 47, pp. 105-12

[307] *Auditory P300 study in patients with convalescent bipolar depression and bipolar depression.* **Fu, L. et al.** 11, 2018, Neuroreport., Vol. 29, pp. 968-973.

[308] *Hearing Impairment Is Associated Brain Volume in Aging.* **Rigters, S.C. et al.** Jan 20, 2017, Front. Aging Neurosci.

[309] *Dichotic listening asymmetry: A Potential Neuro-Behavioural Marker of Depression.* **Pandey, R. and Singh, I.L.** 2013, SIS J. Proj. Psy. & Ment. Health, Vol. 20, pp. 68-73.

[310] *Hearing Loss and Falls: A Systematic Review and Meta-analysis.* **Nicole Tin-Lok Jiam, N., Li, C. and Agrawal, Y.** Nov, 2016, Laryngoscope, Vol. 126.

[311] *Sensation and Psychiatry: Linking Age-Related Hearing Loss to Late-Life Depression and Cognitive Decline.* **Rutherford, B.R. et al.** 3, 2018, Am J Psychiatry., Vol. 175, pp. 215-224.

The first one is taken from my experience at the Tomatis center in Paris as a trainee student, when I accompanied a brilliant psychologist, Miss Cavé, on her daily visits. Once we received a newly retired lady who showed the typical symptoms of depression. Her audiometric curve was terrible, a consequence of damage suffered when a bomb fell on her home as a child, during the Second World War. In spite of this, she had worked as an interpreter, accompanying politicians on their travels. On retirement, her pace of life had undergone a radical change. She had begun to paint, her great hobby but, instead of feeling happy, she felt worse every day.

From the Tomatis perspective, this was a clear-cut case. A damaged but well-exercised ear fulfils its function of stimulating the nervous system perfectly. However, the lack of movement and conversation or, in other words, the absence of vestibular and cochlear stimulation that characterized her retirement had deprived her brain of the necessary energy. The therapy the psychologist prescribed was very simple: "Learn a new language and be active. Silence and stillness do not suit you."

To explain the above in neurophysiological terms: if the ear is deprived of stimuli, so will the reticular formation be, rendering it unable to perform its functions well, including activation of the hippocampus and maintenance of cortical arousal. This is an ideal terrain for depression to appear.

The second example arises from an observation by Tomatis which I have been able to confirm several times. Some people are terribly tired after their holidays. These are usually people whose auditory curves fall slightly in the treble range, but who compensate for this perfectly through their daily activity, with movement and vestibular energy. When resting, however, they become exhausted. A few days of total relaxation are enough to defeat them. They soon show signs of restlessness: looking for something to keep them busy, which is really an attempt to recover their vestibular energy recharge. This is a similar case to that of the retired interpreter.

THE EAR AND SCHIZOPHRENIA

In schizophrenic patients we usually see a noticeable upward slope, starting from low down in the bass range and reaching high into the trebles. This is the *artist's* profile, in its pathological version:

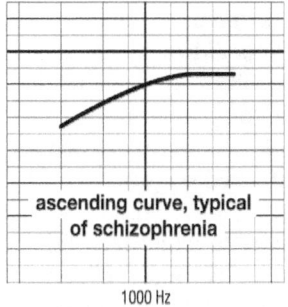

In fact, it is not usually as harmonious as we have drawn it here, but very distorted, something unusual in an adult. If the patient is medicated, the profile is smoother, mainly in the right ear. The bass area may even look normal, although high sensitivity will persist in the treble area. This is a real curve of a schizophrenic patient:

Three elements stand out:

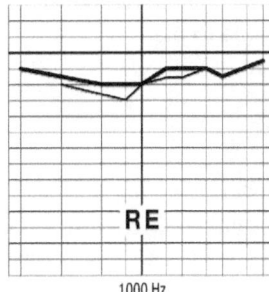
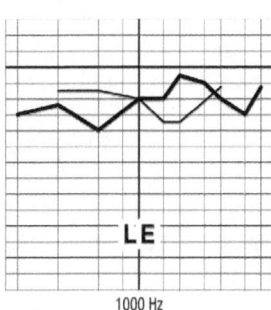

- A left ear with erratic lines, without any parallelism between air and bone. I have already mentioned that, in adults, we seldom see this and it suggests a disruption to personality structure.
- The curves rise in the treble range.
- In the vestibular area of the left ear the bone conduction curve is above the air curve.

The patient was stable, on medication. The curves of the right ear are much more harmonious. During a psychotic break, they would present more irregularities.

The relatively low sensitivity in the bass range (air curve, left ear) indicates poor body control, which is confirmed by the behavior of schizophrenics: they care little about their appearance and reject sport and any kind of physical effort. If we can get them to go to the gym for a few hours, their symptoms improve quickly, but it does not usually happen. Discipline and regularity are not their strong points. They isolate themselves from external reality and build their own inner world, centered on themselves. In the discourse of a schizophrenic, the word "I" appears at a rate of 8.4%, practically twice that seen in non-affected subjects.[312]

Auditory hallucinations are common, so their hearing has been thoroughly studied in order to understand the mechanism that triggers them. At first, the hearing impairments observed in schizophrenia were thought to result from a dysfunction of the whole brain, mainly the left hemisphere. Under this hypothesis, audiological diagnosis is an indirect way of assessing brain function. Tomatis's position, however, was almost diametrically opposed to this, pointing to the ear as a cause and not as an effect. From his perspective, auditory therapy takes on another meaning: we are dealing with a cochlea that has lost its ability to regulate and recharges too much, flooding the nervous system with high frequencies, the most energizing ones. The brain is overwhelmed by a great number of stimuli that it is unable to manage.

The energy of a sound wave, measured in joules is:

$$E = 2\pi^2 \rho St A^2 v f^2$$

The formula indicates that energy depends on the medium in which it is propagated, the transversal surface covered by the wave, its temporal duration, its amplitude and its speed. The final f represents the frequency. If this is 100 Hz the last factor of the formula will be 10,000. If the frequency is 10,000 Hz, we multiply by 100 million. Treble sounds carry much more energy than bass ones.

Auditory processing in psychiatric disorders is, to say the least, peculiar. Among schizophrenics there are disruptions to otoacoustic emissions, to dichotic listening tests,[313] to the efferent system,[314] to the P300 wave[315] and a wide range of neurological

---

[312] See note 118

[313] *Aplicaciones de la escucha dicótica verbal a la clínica neurológica y neuropsiquiátrica.* **Gadea-Doménech, M. y Espert-Tortajada, R.** 1, 2004, Revista de Neurología, Vol. 39, pp. 74-80.

[314] *Abnormal peripheral auditory asymmetry in schizophrenia.* **Veuillet, E. et al.** 2001, J Neurol Neurosurg Psychiatry, Vol. 70, pp. 88-94.

[315] *Confirmation of a relationship between reduced auditory P300 amplitude and thought disorder in schizophrenia.* **Kirihara, K. et al.** 80(2-3), 2005 : s.n., Dec 15, 2005, Schizophrenia Research, Vol. 15, pp. 197-201.

measurements of the auditory system[316,317]. A literature review conducted in 2003 found 564 articles linking hearing to some type of mental disorder, mostly (31%) to schizophrenia.[318]

The latest research tells us that these patients do not regulate sound entry properly, as Tomatis himself stated. Impairments have been found in the third auditory cortex layer, an important area in efferent regulation. The pyramidal cells are thinner and the axonal density is lower.[319] These findings fit in with other data that indicate low inhibitory capacity in these patients. Also, distinctive anatomical features appear in certain areas, such as Heschl's gyrus[320,321], a language processing area in which greater reactivity to variations in pitch or duration of sounds has been observed.[322] Post-mortem studies in schizophrenics have revealed shrinking of the auditory cortex: the smaller its size, the more auditory hallucinations they suffered.[323] Another singularity that can identify and predict schizophrenia is alteration of the tonotopic organization that characterizes the entire auditory pathway, from the cochlea to the cortex. A disordered frequency distribution could be the origin of these patients' hallucinations.[324]

Several studies confirm that psychotic patients have a greater record of auditory pathology than in general population. Of these, I

[316] *Auditory dysfunction in schizophrenia: integrating clinical and basic features.* **Javitt, D.C. and Sweet, R.A.** Sept, 2015, Nat Rev Neurosci., Vol. 16(9), pp. 535–550.

[317] *Preliminary Evidence for Reduced Auditory Lateral Suppression in Schizophrenia.* **Ramage, E.M. et al.** March, 2015, Schizophr Res., Vol. 162(0), pp. 269–275.

[318] *Contribution of psychoacoustics and neuroaudiology in revealing correlation of mental disorders with central auditory processing disorders.* **Iliadou, V. and Iakovides, S.** May, 2003, Annals of General Hospital Psychiatry 2003, 2, Vol. 2.

[319] *The Auditory Cortex in Schizophrenia.* **Shi, W.X.** 7, 2007, Biol Psychiatry., Vol. 61, pp. 829-830.

[320] *Hemispheric asymmetry of primary auditory cortex and Heschl's gyrus in schizophrenia and nonpsychiatric brains.* **Smiley, J.F. et al.** 3, 2013, Psychiatry Res., Vol. 214.

[321] *Auditory cortex asymmetry, altered minicolumn spacing and absence of ageing effects in schizophrenia.* **Chance, S.A. et al.** 2008, Brain, Vol. 131, pp. 3178-3192.

[322] *Auditory processing abnormalities in schizotypal personality disorder: An fMRI experiment using tones of deviant pitch and duration.* **Dickey, C.C. et al.** 1-3, Aug, 2008, Schizophr Res., Vol. 103, pp. 26-39.

[323] *Neuroanatomy of 'Hearing Voices': A Frontotemporal Brain Structural Abnormality Associated with Auditory Hallucinations in Schizophrenia.* **Gaser, C. et al.** 2004, Cerebral Cortex, Vol. 14, pp. 91-96.

[324] *Abnormal auditory tonotopy in patients with schizophrenia.* **Doucet, G.E. et al.** 16, 2019, NPJ Schizophrenia, Vol. 5.

would highlight the work of M. Van der Werf and her team in the Netherlands, analyzing a sample of over 3,000 German teenagers. Their figures suggest that the greater the hearing impairment, the more severe are the psychotic symptoms.[325] A Greek study of 3,500 children for whom medical data had been available since birth yielded similar results[326] and, in the UK, Mason and colleagues reported a higher incidence of middle-ear pathology among schizophrenic patients: a link that was even closer when the affected ear was the left one.[327] Their findings coincide with those of Tomatis himself.

On receiving two equal consecutive acoustic stimuli, the second one has less impact on us. This can be seen in wave P50, which shows a smoother profile during the second stimulus. A filtering takes place which avoids oversaturation of the system. We could say that we get over our initial "surprise" and our reaction diminishes. However, a characteristic of patients with schizophrenia is a lack or noticeable decrease in this sensory filtering (auditory gating), something that we also find in bipolar disorder[328] and, surprisingly, in dyslexic adults.[329] Consecutive P50 waves are similar.[330] It is as if they are always open to receiving any stimulus. The results on some cognitive tests are also worse in subjects with a decreased auditory gating.[331]

Other waves also show disparities, such as MMN and P300, which appear reduced and constitute a robust specific feature of the disorder.[332] The typical hearing patterns found in healthy people fade away.

---

[325] *Adolescent development of psychosis as an outcome of hearing impairment: a 10-year longitudinal study.* **van der Werf, M. et al.** [ed.] Cambridge University Press. April, 2010, Psychological Medicine, pp. 1-9.

[326] *Hearing impairment and psychosis: A replication in a cohort of young adults.* **Stefanis, N. et al.** 1-3, July, 2006, Squizophrenia Research, Vol. 85, pp. 266-272.

[327] *Middle-ear disease and squizophrenia: case-control study.* **Mason, P. et al.** 3, Sept, 2008, Br J Psyquiatry, Vol. 193, pp. 192-6.

[328] *Auditory sensory gating in patients with bipolar disorders: A meta-analysis.* **Cheng, C.H. et al.** 2016, J Affect Disord., Vol. 203, pp. 199-203.

[329] *Auditory gating in adults with dyslexia: An ERP account of diminished rapid neural adaptation.* **Peter, B. et al.** July, 2019, Clinical Neurophysiology.

[330] *Sensory Gating Deficits and their Clinical Correlates in Drug-Free/Drug-Naive Patients with Schizophrenia.* **Ravichandra, K. et al.** 3, May-June, 2018, Indian J Psychol Med., Vol. 40, pp. 247-256.

[331] *Cognitive mechanisms associated with auditory sensory gating.* **Jones, L.A. et al.** 2016, Brain and Cognition, Vol. 102, pp. 33-45.

[332] *Mismatch Negativity (MMN) y esquizofreniz: una revisión.* **Mondragón-Maya, A.et al.** 6, 2011, Actas Esp Psiquiatr, Vol. 39, pp. 363-73.

We observe further alterations that we are not yet able to understand. For instance, efferent inhibitory action increases at certain points in the system, while in others it diminishes.[333,334] Those who say they hear voices show bilateral activations in brain areas where they should not be found.[335] The M100 wave, linked to the temporal gyrus, is more symmetrical than usual in both schizophrenia and bipolar disorders .[336,337] It is strange but, yet again, the same happens with dyslexics.

People at risk of schizophrenia, without symptoms, may show pathological indicators in hearing tests.[338] Some have been found among the relatives of schizophrenics.[339] The same thing seems to occur in depression[340] which suggests that auditory dysfunction precedes mental dysfunction.

Tomatis was the first to notice that the audiometric curve is closely related to these pathologies, opening up a new field of research. The possibilities of brainstem audiometry in the diagnosis of bipolar disorder and schizophrenia are currently being explored.[341] A team from the University Hospital of Northern Norway has been working for years on the development of an algorithm to assist psychiatrists, based on audiometric assessment. Although it is still under development, preliminary results are promising.[342] The evaluation of

---

[333] See note 314

[334] *The Hyperactivity of Efferent Auditory System in Patients with Schizophrenia: A Transient Evoked Otoacoustic Emissions Study.* **Wahab, N.A. et al.** 1, 2016, Psychiatry Investig, Vol. 13, pp. 82-88.

[335] *Relationship of auditory verbal hallucinations with cerebral asymmetry in patients with schizophrenia: an event-related fMRI study.* **Zhang, Z. et al.** 6, 2008, J Psychiatr Res., Vol. 42, pp. 477-86.

[336] *Reduced auditory M100 asymmetry in schizophrenia and dyslexia: applying a developmental instability approach to assess atypical brain asymmetry.* **Edgar, J.C. et al.** 2, 2006, Neuropsychologia, Vol. 44, pp. 289-99.

[337] *Absence of Auditory M100 Source Asymmetry in Schizophrenia and Bipolar Disorder: A MEG Study.* **Wang, Y. et al.** 12, 2013, Plos One, Vol. 8.

[338] *Language Lateralization and Auditory Attention Impairment in Young Adults at Ultra-High Risk for Psychosis: A Dichotic Listening Study.* **Aase, I. et al.** 608, 2018, Frontiers in Psychology, Vol. 9.

[339] *Auditory Steady State Response in the Schizophrenia, First-Degree Relatives, and Schizotypal Personality Disorder.* **Rass, O. et al.** 1-3, Apr, 2012, Schizophr Res., Vol. 136, pp. 143-149.

[340] *Risk of depression enhances auditory Pitch discrimination in the brain as indexed by the mismatch negativity.* **Bonetti, L. et al.** 10, 2017, Clin Neurophysiol., Vol. 128, pp. 1923-1936.

[341] *Brainstem audiometry as a diagnostic tool in psychiatry: Preliminary results from a blinded study.* **Wahlström, V. and Wynn, R.** Apr, 2017, European Psychiatry, Vol. 41.

[342] *Auditory Brainstem Response as a Diagnostic Tool for Patients Suffering From Schizophrenia, Attention Deficit Hyperactivity Disorder, and Bipolar Disorder: Protocol.* **Wahlström, V. et al.** 2015, JMIR Research Protocols, Vol. 4.

vestibular activity is also a powerful tool for identifying mental disorders, as we will see in the following pages.

Based on the data, it can be concluded that hearing disorders are a risk factor to be taken into account in psychiatry.[343] There is still no robust theory to explain this relationship between hearing and psychosis, but Tomatis's energy hypothesis is certainly a good approach.

As I mentioned earlier, in schizophrenia the lowest level of the audiometric curve lies in Sector 1, the vestibular sector, which matches schizophrenics' way of life: they do not like playing sports, DIY or any work that involves physical effort. If we succeed in overcoming this rejection, positive effects appear. I have seen remarkable improvements in patients who agreed to exercise regularly, and positive developments have been reported in psychoses treated with rhythmic movement therapy, which is a great vestibular activator.[344]

DEMENTIA

Yet again we come across the auditory connection in dementia, as it takes a greater toll on the deaf, to the extent that the degree of hearing impairment is considered a marker of cognitive dysfunction.[345,346]

Lin and his team from the Department of Otolaryngology at Johns Hopkins School of Medicine in Baltimore, USA, found that cognitive impairment in deaf patients was three years (in a period of ten) ahead of those without hearing problems. This was reflected equally in both verbal and non-verbal tests, which suggests that hearing impairment causes generic effects, not restricted to the specific brain areas concerned with hearing and language.[347]

---

[343] *Increased risk of psychosis in patients with hearing impairment: Review and meta-analyses.* **Mascha, M.J. et al.** March, 2016, Neuroscience & Biobehavioral Reviews, Vol. 62, pp. 1-20.

[344] **Bolmberg, H.** *Terapia de movimiento rítmico, movimientos que curan.* 2011.

[345] *Hearing Loss and Incident Dementia.* **Lin, R.F. et al.** 2, Arch Neurol, Vol. 68, pp. 214-220.

[346] *Relationship of Hearing loss and Dementia: a Prospective, Population-based Study.* **Gurgel, R.K. et al.** 5, June, 2014, Otol Neurotol, Vol. 35, pp. 775-781.

[347] *Hearing Loss and Cognitive Decline Among Older Adults.* **Lin, F.R. et al.** 4, Feb 25, 2013, JAMA Intern Med, Vol. 173.

Additionally, a longitudinal study carried out in Germany, evaluating more than 150,000 subjects over the age of 65, has confirmed that the risk of dementia is higher among people with hearing loss.[348] The lower degree of social interaction of deaf people is suggested as a possible explanation. From the Tomatis perspective, they are in a state of continuous sensory deprivation: their auditory dynamo does not recharge sufficiently.

Adapted hearing aids improve the quality of life of these persons, but do not reverse the progression of the dementia.[349] Music therapy is of great help in alleviating the symptoms.[350]

STRESS

The stress of our hectic Western life is behind most of the illnesses we suffer. Our body was not designed to live under constant strain. The immune system works poorly in these conditions and eventually our health suffers.

The hearing system is very sensitive and we have already seen that stress can hurt it. Together with the olfactory system, it is the most closely connected system to the amygdala, in the limbic lobe,[351] a structure directly involved in regulating mood and the development of depressive states. Stress has always been regarded as one of the possible triggers of mental illness.

A team of Chilean researchers has investigated how the auditory system could be involved in this process.[352] Neural damage caused by stress on the amygdala could prevent proper sound processing, both emotional and cognitive, placing the patient in functional sensory deprivation. They remind us that the limbic and the auditory systems have evolved together since ancient times, in application of concepts that are very close to those of Tomatis described above.

---

[348] *Hearing Impairment Affects Dementia Incidence. An Analysis Based on Longitudinal Health Claims Data in Germany.* **Fritze, T. et al.** 7, Jul 8, de 2016, Plos One, Vol. 11.

[349] *The effects of improving hearing in dementia.* **Allen, N.H. et al.** 2, 2003, Age and Ageing, Vol. 32, pp. 189-193.

[350] *Impact of Music Therapy on Dementia Behaviors: A Literature Review.* **Fakhoury, N. et al.** Oct 10, 2017, Consult Pharm, Vol. 32.

[351] See note 183

[352] *Effects of stress on the auditory system: an approach to study a common origin for mood disorders and dementia.* **Pérez-Valenzuela, C. et al.**: s.n., Sept, 2018, Reviews in the neurosciences.

The amygdala assesses the emotional importance of events in collaboration with the limbic system. If this is high and generates sensations of great intensity, it will cause the hypothalamus to react, triggering activation of the whole autonomic nervous system. A specific nerve pathway connects the auditory centers to the amygdala. Crying and, above all, laughter, activate it immediately.[353] This is the neurological mechanism of laughter therapy.

The vestibular system links to our emotional and cognitive areas.[354] From the vestibular nuclei, fibers extend out to the limbic system and the hypothalamus. Others, supplied by the facial, glossopharyngeal and vagus nerves, reach the nucleus of the solitary tract, where auditory, gustatory and visceral afferences converge. The information they provide is used to process various autonomic reflex reactions such as coughing or nausea.

The vestibule also embraces the endocrine system, and indeed it is hard to find a hormone not under its influence. Its links to the hypothalamus-pituitary-adrenal axis, the pancreas, the thyroid, etc. have been described.[355] It plays a decisive role in our psychic and physical balance.

V.S. Ramachandran, a professor at the University of California, in San Diego, USA, has described a strange clinical case that illustrates the consequences of a neurological disconnection between the sensory and emotional systems. One of his patients was unable to recognize his mother visually. When he saw her, he thought she was someone else posing as her (Capgras syndrome), but showed no symptoms when talking to her on the telephone. The auditory pathway had kept its emotional nexus intact.[356]

AUTISM

"One of his most remarkable feats was the performance of three musical pieces at the same time. He played Fisher's Hornpipe with one hand and Yankee Doodle with the other while simultaneously singing Dixie". Oliver Sacks, 2006[357]

---

[353] *Audition of laughing and crying leads to right amygdala activation in a low-noise fMRI setting.* **Sander, K. et al.** 2, 2003, Brain Res Protoc., Vol. 11, pp. 81-91.

[354] *Interactions between stress and vestibular compensation - a review.* **Saman, Y. et al.** 116, 2012, Frontiers in Neurology, Vol. 3.

[355] See note 89

[356] **Ramachandran, V.S.** *Lo que el cerebro nos dice.* Barcelona : Espasa Libros, 2012.

[357] **Sacks, O.** *Un antropólogo en Marte.* Barcelona : Anagrama, 2006.

Almost 10% of autistic people have an outstanding talent: for music, calculation, drawing, etc. This percentage is a thousand times greater than that of the general population.[358] The singular features of their hearing system are still being debated, such as hyper- and hypo-sensitivity, phonophobia, etc.; but it is not known to what extent these peculiarities could be the cause of their symptoms.[359] One recent study has found a lower neural density in the superior olivary complex, in the brainstem, accompanied by dysmorphia.[360] We will have to wait for further research to learn how important this finding is.

Auditory therapy in relation to autism is a delicate matter to deal with. Even when we try to be extremely rigorous, information can be misinterpreted.

When I met Tomatis, his center in Paris welcomed autistic children from all over the world. There had been notable improvements in some cases and the news had spread like wildfire. The advances were seen primarily in desire to communicate and language development. However, in a document published in 1983, Tomatis acknowledged that his therapy did not achieve progress in 50% of the cases treated. He did not know why.[361]

The baton has now been picked up by Jozef Vervoort's team at their center in Sint-Truiden, where they conduct brain mappings on their patients, with the collaboration of a neurologist, Van den Bergh..[362] This technique allows them to objectively assess the changes taking place in the course of auditory therapy, and verify the extent to which brain activity is normalized at the same time as the audiometric curves.[363] This work is achieving successes that can hardly be put down to chance or the placebo effect.

Both favorable[364,365] and unfavorable[366] studies have been published on Tomatis's therapy for autistic people, but none yet that

---

[358] Ibid.

[359] *Auditory abnormalities in children with autism.* **Tan, Y.H. et al.** 33-37, 2012, Open Journal of Psychiatry, Vol. 2.

[360] *Malformation of the human superior olive in autistic spectrum disorders.* **Kulesza, R., Lukose, R. and Stevens, L.** 2011, Brain Research, Vol. 1367, pp. 360-371.

[361] **Tomatis, A.** Communication sur l' autism. París : s.n., 1983.

[362] *The Improvement of Severe Psychomotor and Neurological Dysfunctions Treated with the Tomatis Audio-Psycho-Phonology Method Measured with EEG Brain Map and Auditory Evoked Potentials.* **Vervoort, J. et al.** Sept 4, 2008, Journal of Neurotherapy: Investigations in Neuromodulation, Neurofeedback and Applied Neuroscience, Vol. 11, pp. 37-49.

[363] See note 5

[364] *The Effect of Tomatis Therapy on Children: with Autism: Eleven Case Studies.* **Garritsen, J.** 2010, International Journal of Listening.

display sufficient scientific rigor. There is a serious methodological obstacle. Two groups are usually compared: one that receives the therapy (the same therapy for each individual) and another that does not (control group), to see whether there is any significant difference between both in statistical terms. These comparisons yield misleading results, however, as they do not reflect reality. Auditory therapy is always individually adjusted in accordance with the diagnosis and subsequent progression, so no two subjects receive the same auditory training. This complicates the protocol needed to carry out valid and reliable research, and raises its costs.

In short, not all autistic people improve with Tomatis's therapy and there are no rigorous studies to endorse or rule out its application to this disorder; but if I had had an autistic child, I would certainly have done my best to seek the help of the professionals at Sint-Truiden.

I have had the opportunity to meet Dan Copes several times at the biannual conferences organized in this city. Dan is a physician and runs a center in Houston that specializes in autism. He is the father of two autistic twins, something that made his professional life take a new turn. Dan integrates Tomatis's techniques in his treatments and has always insisted on the importance of nutrition in these children. Recent findings on the role of bacterial flora in the syndrome are a major step forward towards understanding it better.[367,368]

The role of the hypothalamus in the regulation of microbiota is being investigated.[369] The hypothalamus is very sensitive to sound and modulates the hormonal system and stress:[370] something to take very much into account in premature births.[371] I would also like to emphasize that our current diet is contaminated with endocrine disruptors capable of altering hypothalamic function. It is suspected,

---

[365] *Sound Therapy: an Experimental Study with Autistic Children.* **AbediKoupaei, M. et al.** 2013, Procedia - Social and Behavioral Sciences, Vol. 84, pp. 626-630.

[366] *Brief report: the effects of Tomatis sound therapy on language in children with autism.* **Corbett, B.A., Shickman, K. and Ferrer, E.** 3, 2008, J Autism Dev Disord., Vol. 38, pp. 562-6.

[367] *New evidences on the altered gut microbiota in autism spectrum disorders.* **Strati, F. et al.** 24, 2017, Microbiome, Vol. 5.

[368] *Altered composition and function of intestinal microbiota in autism spectrum disorders: a systematic review.* **Liu, F. et al.** 43, 2019, Translational Psychiatry, Vol. 9.

[369] *Hypothalamic Control of Systemic Glucose Homeostasis: The Pancreas Connection.* **Pozo, M. and Claret, M.** 1329, 2019, Trends in Endocrinology & Metabolism.

[370] *Effect of sound on the hypothalamic-pituitary-adrenal axis.* **Henkin, R.I. and Knigge, K.M.** 1963, Am J Physiol., Vol. 204, pp. 701-4.

[371] *Prenatal noise stress impairs HPA axis and cognitive performance in mice.* **Jafari, Z. et al.** 10560, 2017, Nature Scientific Reports, Vol. 7.

for example, that mercury is one of the causes of ADHD.[372] My colleague, Monica Cuenca, a psychologist and mother of an autistic child, has become my guiding light on the syndrome. A tireless fighter, she knows all about the disorder and has achieved notable improvements in her son's development. She applies Tomatis's techniques in Madrid.

VESTIBULAR KEYS

In medicine, the vestibule is often referred to in pathological terms, mostly in relation to vertigo and balance disorders. As I mentioned in Chapter 3, Tomatis considered it to be the main source of stimulation of the nervous system:

"The human ear secures a great deal of cortical energy. It intervenes in a proportion of 60% in relation to the other sensory organs. If we add to this the responses of the skin, whose sensory function is phylogenetically linked to the auditory function and if we also consider the sensory-muscular and sensory-articulatory responses, which arise from differentiated sensors that share their auditory origin, we reach a percentage of 90% as regards the energy attributed to the cochleo-vestibular apparatus, which is a considerable amount".[373]

Many people turn to reading aloud, while walking, for better memorization. This activates cochlear and vestibular stimulation. Have you seen any Koranic or Jewish schools, with children sitting on the floor, rhythmically moving their trunk back and forth, while reciting the sacred scriptures aloud? Although their teachers probably do not know mnemonic physiology, in practice they know that it works best that way.

The vestibular stimulation from swaying and the cochlear stimulation from reading activate the brain and facilitate a cognitive process, in this case, memory. For Carla Hannaford, an expert in education, vestibular involvement in learning is so capital that she claims:

"If we do not move and activate the vestibular system, we are not assimilating environmental information". [374]

---

[372] **Medina, M.A.** La recomendación de que los niños no coman atún llega 20 años tarde. *El País.* Nov 19, 2019.

[373] See note 42

[374] See note 184

My generation learned the multiplication tables by singing, songs being more easily remembered than texts. Psychologist J.A. Sloboda points out that music is undoubtedly the best tool for memorization in non-literate cultures,[375] and the great musical pedagogue Edgar Willems tells us: *"The fact that sensory hearing and rhythm are tributaries of the same physiological, dynamic or agogic laws explains why certain sounds are best imprinted in memory when they are rhythmic".*[376]

An experiment carried out at the University Hospital in Zurich[377] shows how vestibular stimulation conditions our mental activity. The participants had two tasks to perform: the first, about spatial location (associated with the right hemisphere) and the second, a language test (associated with the left).

Vestibular activity can be modified by irrigating the ear with cold or hot water. This generates currents in the intralabyrinthine liquids that activate the macules of hair cells. In this case, cold water was used, with the intention of increasing the activity of the brain hemisphere on the opposite side, through vestibular stimulation.

The subjects irrigated in the corresponding ear performed the tasks better than the control group. Something similar was raised by A. Gopinath in his psychology thesis.[378] In a typical orientation task in a maze, the mice irrigated with hot water remembered better where the prize was, evidencing a positive effect on their memory.

Several researchers have described a vestibular system related to the attention, mood and behavior processes, hormonal processes and processes of self-image perception, including anorexia, phantom limb syndrome and pain. The suspicion of a relationship between vestibular system and mind goes a long way back,[379] as disorders of balance and muscle tone appear in a large number of mentally ill people. Paul Ferdinand Schilder, in the early 20th century, was one of the first psychiatrists to notice this link.

---

[375] **Sloboda, J.A.** *La mente musical: La psicología cognitiva de la música.* Madrid : Machado Grupo de Distribución, 2012.

[376] See note 92

[377] *Spatial and verbal-memory improvement by cold-water caloric stimulation in healthy subjects.* **Bächtold, D. et al.** 2001, Exp Brain Res, Vol. 136, pp. 128-132.

[378] **Gopinath, A.** Effect of caloric vestibular stimulation on memory. s.l. : Kerala University of Health Sciences, 2016.

[379] *The moving history of vestibular stimulation as a therapeutic intervention.* **Grabherr, L., Lenggenhager, B. and Macauda, G.** 5-6, 2015, Multisensory Research, Vol. 28, pp. 653-687.

Schilder was a disciple of Freud and husband of the famous psychologist Lauretta Bender. In 1933 he wrote an article entitled *The vestibular apparatus in neurosis and psychosis,*[380] describing the muscle tone disorders among these patients. His work was truncated when he was hit by a car and killed after visiting his wife in hospital when their daughter was born. Mats Niklasson, quoting Schilder, writes this:

"Organic changes in the vestibular apparatus will be reflected in the psychic structures. Not only will they influence tone, the vegetative system and the attitudes of the body, but they will also change our entire perceptual apparatus and even our consciousness. These general considerations make it possible that the study of the vestibular apparatus can have great importance for the understanding of psychotic and neurotic states ". Schilder, P. (1942). *Mind: Perception and thought in their constructive aspects. Freeport, NY.*[381]

Several researchers confirmed this mind–vestibule connection in the laboratory almost eighty years ago, by comparing schizophrenics with control groups.[382,383] Around 1940, A. Angyal described the atypical reactions of these patients in vestibular caloric stimulation tests and their muscle tone disorders.

In the same vein, psychiatrist E.M. Ornitz confirmed that in both schizophrenia and autism, reactions to vestibular stimulation (such as ocular nystagmus) were not as expected and hypothesized that vestibule dysfunctions could be the cause of these pathologies.[384]

Despite these discoveries, the vestibular hypothesis for mental disorders has remained forgotten for decades, with a few exceptions, [385,386] but now there does seem to be a renewed interest, thanks in part

---

[380] *The vestibular apparatus in neurosis and psychosis.* **Schilder, P.** 1933, Journal of Nervous and Mental Disease, Vol. 78

[381] **Niklasson, M.** Could Motor Development Be an Emergent Property of Vestibular Stimulation and Primary Reflex Inhibition?... [book author] Wichian Sittiprapaporn. *Learning disabilities.* 2012.

[382] *Vestibular reactivity in schizophrenia.* **Angyal, A. and Blackman, N.** 1940, Arch. Neurol. Psychiat., Vol. 44, pp. 611-620.

[383] *Postural reactions to vestibular stimulation in schizophrenic and normal subjects.* **Angyal, A. and Sherman, M.** 1942, Amer. J. Psychiat., Vol. 98, pp. 857-862.

[384] *Vestibular dysfunction in schizophrenia and childhood.* **Ornitz, E.M.** 2, 1970, Comprehensive Psychiatry, Vol. 11.

[385] *Otolith Formation and Trace Elements: A Theory of Schizophrenic Behavior.* **Erway, L.C.** 1, 1975, Orthomolecular Psychiatry, Vol. 4, pp. 16-26.

to modern neuroimaging techniques. At Monash University in Australia, they have been able to establish the correlation between vestibular activity and psychiatric illnesses, such as depression, by analyzing electrovestibulographic records using a new device: the EVestG. Distorted patterns in vestibular activity become visible before symptoms of mental illness occur, the researchers say,[387] allowing early diagnosis. In a recent paper, they also report being able to detect post-concussion syndrome, with and without depression.[388]

Diagnosis of schizophrenia has also been achieved, with almost 100% accuracy, by examining ocular motility,[389] which largely depends on the vestibular system.

Activating the vestibule

When we dance to the beat of a song we activate the vestibule.[390] Acoustic rhythmic stimulation has been used for years in gait rehabilitation programs.[391] It excites motor neurons in both brainstem and spinal cord. In the laboratory we can trigger vestibular responses in controlled situations. Caloric stimulation, with water irrigation in the auditory canal, and galvanic stimulation, through electromagnetic fields, are commonly used. Both cause endolymph currents within the vestibular apparatus, modifying its activity. Unequivocal and sometimes almost instantaneous recoveries have been reported in patients with psychiatric or neurological pathology following vestibular caloric stimulation. Dudson, from New Zealand, recounts the case of a 29-year-old patient with a history of bipolar disorder since she was 19, who was admitted to the hospital in the middle of a

---

[386] *High Thresholds for Movement Perception in Schizophrenia may indicate Abnormal Extraneous Noise Levels of Central Vestibular Activity.* **Wertheim, A.H. et al.** 1985, Biol Psyquiatry, Vol. 20, pp. 1197-1210.

[387] *Separating mental disorders using vestibular field potentials.* **Maller, J.J. et al.** 1, 2015, Arch Neurosci., Vol. 2.

[388] *Investigating the validity reliability of Electrovestibulography (EVestG) for detecting post-concussion syndrome (PCS) with and without comorbid depression.* **Suleiman, A. et al.** 2018, Scientific Reports, Vol. 8, pág. 14495.

[389] *Simple Viewing Tests Can Detect Eye Movement Abnormalities That Distinguish Schizophrenia Cases from Controls with Exceptional Accuracy.* **Benson, P.J. et al.** 9, 2012, Biological Psychiatry, Vol. 72, pp. 716-724.

[390] *Why Movement Is Captured by Music, but Less by Speech: Role of Temporal Regularity.* **Dalla Bella, S., Białuńska, A. and Sowiński, J.** 8, 2013, Plos One, Vol. 8.

[391] *Effects of gait training with rhythmic auditory stimulation on gait ability in stroke patients.* **Song, G. and Ryu, H.G.** 2016, J. Phys. Ther. Sci., Vol. 28, pp. 1403-6.

manic phase, with great excitement and irritability. She did not respond to pharmacological treatment, even at high doses.

They tried vestibular caloric stimulation: cold in this case as they irrigated her ear with 50 ml of water at 4 degrees Celsius. Using the YMRS scale to determine the severity of the manic episode, her progression was checked at 20 minutes, one hour, 6, 24 and 48 hours. She calmed down after only a few minutes and remained that way for several hours. Next day, however, her symptoms started to get worse again. At 72 hours her condition had returned to the initial situation. They repeated the vestibular stimulation process with cold water and once more she regained the state of calm, which she gradually lost.[392]

We do not know how such a quick and beneficial reaction is possible, but there is no doubt that the vestibule has a wide network of connections with the limbic system, our emotion manager.[393] The psychiatrist J. Levine describes a similar progression in three cases of schizophrenia, noting that the effectiveness was greater when the irrigated ear was the left one,[394] which, from the Tomatis's perspective, is the most important one in personality disorders.

Doing magic

One experiment shows us strikingly how the vestibule is involved in the perception of our body image.[395] André and his collaborators applied vestibular caloric stimulation to subjects with amputated limbs, some of whom had phantom limb syndrome (perception of the severed part, usually accompanied by pain). During the procedure, they discovered two spectacular phenomena:

- In patients with phantom limbs, the pain disappeared.
- Those who did not have the syndrome began to feel the amputated part again.

---

[392] *Vestibular stimulation in mania: a case report.* **Dodson, M.J.** 2004, J Neurol Neurosurg Psychiatry, Vol. 75, pp. 163-171.

[393] *Understanding the links between vestibular and limbic systems regulating emotions.* **Rajagopalan, A. et al.** 1, 2017, Journal of Natural Science, Biology and Medicine, Vol. 8.

[394] *Beneficial effects of caloric vestibular stimulation on denial of illness and manic delusions in schizoaffective disorder: a case report.* **Levine, J. et al.** 3, 2012, Brain Stimul., Vol. 5, pp. 267-273.

[395] *Temporary phantom limbs evoked by vestibular caloric stimulation in amputees.* **André, J.M. et al.** 3, 2001, Neuropsychiatry Neuropsychol Behav Neurol., Vol. 14, pp. 190-6.

This experiment is the auditory version of the work of Ramachandran, who wrote one of the most beautiful pages in the history of neurology by discovering how to eliminate phantom limb pain with the sole help of a mirror.[396]

N. D. Schiff and M. Pulver, from the New York Hospital - Cornell Medical Center, describe the case of an 81-year-old patient who suffered a stroke in the left hemisphere.[397] MRI indicated multiple cortical infarctions around the middle cerebral artery. She presented the concomitant symptoms: blindness in the right visual field, aphasia, she was not aware of her right hand and the muscle tone of all that side was weak.

After vestibular caloric stimulation, all of her symptoms improved within thirty seconds and she was able to recognize visual and auditory stimuli presented on her right side. The examiner showed her her right hand and asked: "Whose hand is this?" She clearly answered: "It's my hand!" Just a minute before, she did not know. Then, after four minutes, the positive effects gradually faded, and she returned to her initial state.

What had happened? What alternative neural pathway had allowed that sudden change and what triggered it? The authors' own hypothesis is that there was temporary cortical activation, resulting from the participation of thalamic structures, in which all sensations integrate with the emotions.

Tomatis used to say that sometimes the thalamus was full of "emotional garbage" that we had to clean up, because the accumulation of negative emotions prevented it from functioning correctly which, in turn, affected the auditory system. As he was coming to the end of one of his lectures, a neurologist asked him to briefly summarize the effect mechanism of his therapy. Tomatis looked up and replied: *"One word is enough: thalamus!"*

A recent paper describes a case of neurorehabilitation involving the application of Tomatis's principles in a patient who had suffered a subarachnoid hemorrhage. The patient was made to listen to music with rapid changes in equalization, from low- to high-pass filtering. Her balance and audiometric curve improved quickly, as did her

---

[396] *The use of visual feedback, in particular mirror visual feedback, in restoring brain function.* **Ramachandran, V.S. and Altschuler, E.L.** 2009, Brain, Vol. 132, pp. 1693–1710.

[397] *Does vestibular stimulation activate thalamocortical mechanisms that reintegrate impaired cortical regions?* **Schiff, D. and Pulver, M.** 1999, Proc. R. Soc. Lond., Vol. 266, pp. 421-423.

motor and cognitive functions.[398] In the same vein, a Chinese university team has also reported ongoing improvement of memory in stroke patients, after an intervention with techniques similar to those of Tomatis.[399]

The above examples open up a new dimension in the treatment of brain disorders and rehabilitation.[400] They show us that the human body is able to find alternative ways to compensate for seemingly irreversible injuries, and that a therapeutic intervention focused on auditory stimulation can be very beneficial.

Continuing to look at this area of work, we could also consider vestibular therapies based on rhythm, such as the Ronnie Gardiner method, [401] which seems to be of great help in the recovery of patients with neurological damage. Rhythmic stimulation with music, for instance, has been shown to be effective in stroke rehabilitation.[402,403] At 87, Gardiner is still active, giving seminars all over the world.

Tomatis therapy contains a specific protocol for vestibular stimulation, which is based on the specific use of frequencies below 1,000 Hz. Other approaches using music with a large proportion of low frequencies are also reported to have had beneficial effects on the vestibular function. For example, a study in Japan revealed better performance in balance tests among young people who had previously listened to music that was boosted in the 100 Hz region.[404]

Vestibule and rhythm are so intertwined that, experimentally, a perception of rhythm can be induced by activating the vestibule through

---

[398] *Restoration of Balance and Unilateral Hearing Using Alternating and Filtering Auditory Training in Shunt-Treated Hydrocephalus Following Subarachnoid Hemorrhage: A Case Report.* **Milantoni, N., Di Bella, N. and Chahbazian, K.** 2018, Am J Case Rep., Vol. 19, pp. 935-940.

[399] **Jingjing, A. and Changxiang, C.** Tomatis® Audio Training on Memory Disorder of Patients with Stroke. *Australian Tomatis® Method.* [Online] 2017. www.tomatis.com.au.

[400] *Studies of caloric vestibular stimulation: implications for the cognitive neurosciences, the clinical neurosciences and neurophilosophy.* **Miller, S.M. and Ngo, T.T.** 2007, Acta Neuropsychiatrica, Vol. 19, pp. 183-203.

[401] *The Ronnie Gardiner Method: An Innovative Music-Based Intervention for Neurological Rehabilitation.* **Pohl, P.** 1, 2018, Neurophysiology and Rehabilitation, Vol. 1.

[402] *Rhythmic Auditory Stimulation Improves Gait More Than NDT/Bobath Training in Near-Ambulatory Patients Early Poststroke: A Single-Blind, Randomized Trial.* **Thaut, M.H. et al.** 5, 2007, Neurorehabilitation and Neural Repair, Vol. 21.

[403] *Effects of (music-based) rhythmic auditory cueing training on gait and posture post-stroke: A systematic review & dose-response meta-analysis.* **Ghai, S. and Ghai, I.** 2183, 2019, Scientific Reports, Vol. 9

[404] *Improvement of balance in young adults by a sound component at 100 Hz in music.* **Xu, H. et al.** 16894, 2018, Scientific Report, Vol. 8.

galvanic stimulation.[405] This effect has proved useful, for example, in the recovery of gaze control after a stroke.[406]

MENTAL HEALTH AND CANCER

In a lecture he gave in Barcelona around 1991, Tomatis commented that cancer and schizophrenia were quite incompatible, alluding to the low rates of cancer he had found in psychiatric hospitals. This assertion is still disputed today in the scientific community, because the research results are sometimes contradictory.[407] However, large-scale data do seem to back up his claim.

In one of the largest studies exploring the cancer–schizophrenia nexus,[408] the entire Swedish population was analyzed from 1965 to 2008. On comparing the 60,000 psychiatric patients and their relatives to the rest of the population, lower rates of cancer were observed, but only in men. A detailed analysis showed that the rates were different for each type of cancer, but overall, it seems that there is some protective factor, perhaps genetic, in families of schizophrenics. The results are even more significant considering that these patients do not usually lead a healthy life (regular physical exercise, balanced diet, moderate or zero consumption of alcohol, tobacco, etc.), so their cancer rate, a priori, should be higher.

In Israel, a group of 3,226 mentally ill patients (1,247 women and 1,979 men) were followed up for 10 years.[409] For the total population, a 6,5% incidence of cancer was estimated, while among the mentally ill it was only 3,7%. 1.8% of the women developed breast cancer, compared to 3% of the general population.

In another study, conducted in 2008, these same researchers found even lower rates of breast cancer in women diagnosed with severe

---

[405] *The primal role of the vestibular system in determining musical rhythm.* **Trainor, L.J.** et al. 2009, cortex, Vol. 45, pp. 35-43.

[406] **Hassanein, A., Arafa, M. and Ahmed, A.** *Effect of Galvanic Vestibular Stimulation on Recovery from Gaze Palsy.* Neurology and Faculty of Physical Therapy, Cairo University. El Cairo : s.n., 2012.

[407] *Cancer in schizophrenia: is the risk higher or lower?* **Grinshpoon, A. et al.** 2-3, 2005, Schizophr Res., Vol. 73, pp. 333-41.

[408] *Incidence of Cancer in Patients With Schizophrenia and Their First-Degree Relatives: A Population-Based Study in Sweden.* **Ji, J. et al.** 3, 2013, Schizophrenia Bulletin, Vol. 39, pp. 527-536.

[409] *Reduced Cancer Incidence among Patients with Schizophrenia.* **Barak, Y. et al.** 12, 2005, Cancer, Vol. 104.

mentally illness.[410] An inverse correspondence between Alzheimer's and cancer has also been observed.[411] We still do not know what causes this strange relationship.

Certain genes linked to deafness may also be involved in some types of cancer, such as DFNA5,[412] which is inactivated in half of gastric cancers. A clinical case of this disease has been described whose only symptomatology was sudden bilateral deafness.[413]

---

[410] *Breast cancer in women suffering from serious mental illness.* **Barak, Y. et al.** 1-3, 2008, Schizophr Res., Vol. 102, pp. 249-53.

[411] *Inverse occurrence of cancer and Alzheimer disease.* **Musicco, M. et al.** 4, 2013, Neurology, Vol. 81.

[412] *DFNA5, a Gene Involved in Hearing Loss and Cancer: A Review.* **De Beeck, K.O., Van Laer, L. and Van Camp, G.** 3, Annals of Otology, Rhinology & Laryngology, Vol. 121, pp. 197-207.

[413] *Sudden bilateral hearing loss in gastric cancer asthe only symptom of disease.* **Rakusic, Z. et al.** 2015, OncoTargets and Therapy, Vol. 8, pp. 1285-1289.

EAR AND HEALTH: SOME OTHER LINKS   7

"Singing is a dynamic activity essential to the balance of a being. Therefore, we will never be able to treat it with the seriousness and attention it truly deserves. "

A. Tomatis[414]

We have seen the close relationship between ear and voice, the mirror of our state of mind. Tomatis liked to say that "we sing with our ears". Some scientists have tried to go further and measure which voice parameters vary according to our emotions or health, and they have made extraordinary findings.

What do we measure in the voice? Mainly the fundamental tone, or pitch; jitter and shimmer, which are small oscillations in frequency and intensity, respectively, in a given time; silences; the rhythm of pauses, etc.; and even grammatical and lexical parameters. Gathering all this data, we obtain characteristic profiles that reveal our emotions [415] or help to detect pathologies. It is a promising line of work which, due to its technical complexity, is closer to the field of informatics than to audiology itself.

Certain voice alterations allow the detection of diseases, such as depression or Alzheimer's,[416] or even assessment of the effects of

---

[414] See note 27

[415] *When voices get emotional: A corpus of nonverbal vocalizations for research on emotion processing.* **Lima, C.F., Castro, S.L. and Scott, S.K.** Feb 27, 2013, Behav Res.

[416] *Advances on Automatic Speech Analysis for Early Detection of Alzheimer Disease: A Non-linear Multi-task Approach.* **López de Ipiña, K.** 2, 2018, Curr Alzheimer Res, Vol. 15, pp. 139-148.

psychotropic drugs.[417] A team of researchers coordinated from New York's Mount Sinai School of Medicine has developed automated speech analysis software capable of diagnosing psychosis with an accuracy of close to 80%.

Psychiatrist Charles Marmar applies similar software to identify people affected by post-traumatic stress. In a study published in 2015, he selected a group of war veterans, with and without post-traumatic stress disorder. The computational analysis correctly classified 70% of the subjects.[418] In an interview published in January 2019, he claims to have already achieved an accuracy of 90%.[419] Even the voice of people with suicidal tendencies is examined to find out when they need to be hospitalized.[420] MIT scientists are attempting to diagnose Covid-19 from acoustic analysis of coughing.[421]

Audiologist Dorinne Davis states that there is a total correlation between voice and otoacoustic emissions, so that, in the presence of a disease, the acoustic spectrums of both are modified in parallel. According to Davis, this phenomenon can be useful in diagnosis and in therapy.[422]

EAR, KIDNEY AND HEART

A study conducted on a sample of 2,564 people over 49 years of age determined that most patients with asymptomatic kidney disease presented hearing loss (54%). Among the subjects without kidney disease, the percentage of those affected by hearing loss was approximately half (28%). It was observed that the greater the degree of renal pathology, the greater the hearing impairment. This relationship was established independently of other variables such as age, sex,

[417] *A Window into the Intoxicated Mind? Speech as an Index of Psychoactive Drug Effects.* **Bedi, G. et al.** 2014, Neuropsychopharmacology, Vol. 39, pp. 2340-2348.

[418] *Speech-Based Assessment of PTSD in a Military Population using Diverse Feature Classes.* **Vergyri, D. et al.** 10, Dresden : s.n., 2015, Intersepeech, Vol. 6.

[419] **Marmar, C.** [interview] A. Brown. *NYU langone Health.* Jan de 2019. https://nyulangone.org/news/harnessing-voice-recognition-software-screen-post-traumatic-stress-disorder.

[420] **Hasan, W.A.** Acoustic analysis of speech based on power spectral density features in detecting suicidal risk among female patients. *Doctoral Thesis.* Nashville : Vanderbilt University, May, 2011.

[421] **EFE.** Científicos catalanes del MIT ensayan con una app que detectará quién tiene coronavirus por la tos. *La Vanguardia.* April 17, 2020.

[422] *The Davis addendum to the Tomatis effect.* **Davis, D.** 4, 2004, The Journal of the Acoustical Society of America, Vol. 116.

medication or other health factors.[423] Several explanations have been proposed, but the question remains open.[424,425]

In Chinese medicine the ear is the sensory organ of the kidney and the size and shape of the auricle is examined to assess the quality of renal function. A study carried out in Thailand addressed this special relationship.[426] The researchers wanted to know whether it had any basis, so they took precise measurements of the ears of kidney donors, before and after the transplants. At the same time, data were taken on other variables, such as the glomerular filtration rate (GFR), a good index of kidney function. The results showed a significant correlation between the observed variation in ear length and donor's GFR.

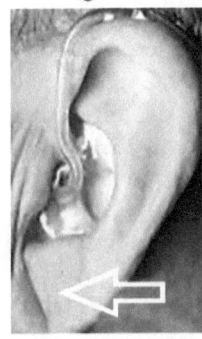

The heart can also give warnings by leaving marks on the ear. A diagonal fold in the lobe is a serious sign of imminent heart attack or stroke. It is known as Frank's sign, for the doctor who first described it in 1973.

Nose and ear grow throughout life. If we suffer from vascular problems, uneven tissue will be generated, which we will see in the form of a fold.[427,428]

SUDDEN INFANT DEATH

A few years ago, Daniel Rubens, an American anesthesiologist, decided to occupy his time on quiet on-call days by investigating sudden infant death syndrome. The cause of this syndrome is still

[423] *The Association Between Reduced GFR and Hearing Loss: A Cross-sectional Population-Based Study.* **Vilayur, E. et al.** 4, American Journal of Kidney Diseases, Vol. 56.

[424] *Ear and kidney syndromes: Molecular versus clinical approach.* **Izzedine, H. et al.** 2004, Kidney International, Vol. 65, pp. 369-385.

[425] *Kidney Disease and Inner Ear Sufferance of Non-Familial Origin: A Review of the Literature and a Proposal of Explanation.* **Pirodda, A. et al.** 1, 2012, The Journal of International Advanced Otology, Vol. 8, pp. 118-122.

[426] *Ear length and kidney function decline after kidney donation.* **Katavetin, P. et al.** 11, Nov, 2016, Nephrology, Vol. 21, pp. 975-978.

[427] *Asociación entre el pliegue diagonal del lóbulo de la oreja y enfermedad cardiovascular.* **Rodríguez-López, C. et al.** Santiago de Compostela : s.n., 2014. Congreso de Enfermedades Cardiovasculares.

[428] *Ear lobe crease as a marker of coronary artery disease: A meta-analysis.* **Lucenteforte, E. et al.** Dec, 2010, European Journal of Integrative Medicine.

unclear, despite medical efforts to find the reason why some newborns die suddenly, without any apparent illness.

He began by reviewing their medical records, hoping to find some common link. The only thing that caught his attention was an auditory characteristic. Even though it did not seem related to the pathology, he decided to check it. He published his article in 2008.[429] Compared to healthy children, those who died of this syndrome presented decreased signals in their TEOAE (otoacoustic emissions) at 2,000, 3,000 and 4,000 Hz, in the right ear.

Since then, in successive articles published with other collaborators, he has explored the origin of this relationship.[430,431] The ear is apparently involved in our response to asphyxia. When we are not breathing in enough oxygen, we change our breathing rate and move, trying to place ourselves in a position with better ventilation. This is what all mammals do. However, when the researchers experimentally damaged the hearing of a group of mice, their respiratory rate remained the same with hypoxia and they barely moved. The typical ventilatory response of the control group did not appear.

It was already known that abnormal respiratory responses were related to sudden death syndrome[432] but not that the ear was involved. It has been suggested that their delicate hair cells could act as alarms, immediately detecting a shortage of oxygen in the blood.

Vestibular cells are also very demanding and trigger sympathetic reactions when they detect a lack of blood supply during hypotension.[433] The vestibular system has a role in regulating the autonomic nervous system and breathing [434] and it modulates blood

[429] *Newborn oto-acoustic emission hearing screening tests: preliminary evidence for a marker of susceptibility to SIDS.* **Rubens, D.D. et al.** Apr, 2008, Early Hum Dev, pp. 225-9.

[430] *Inner ear insult ablates the arousal response to hypoxia and hypercarbia.* **Allen, T et al.** Dic, 2013, Neuroscience, pp. 283-91.

[431] *Inner ear lesion and the differential roles of hypoxia and hypercarbia in triggering active movements: Potential implication for the Sudden Infant Death Syndrome.* **Ramirez, S et al.** 19, Nov, 2016, Neuroscience, pp. 337-9.

[432] **Nathanielsz, P.W.** *Life Before Birth.* New York : W.H. Freeman and Co., 1992.

[433] *Role of peripheral vestibular receptors in the control of blood pressure following hypotension.* **Jin, G.S. et al.** 4, 2018, Korean J Physiol Pharmacol, Vol. 22, pp. 363-368.

[434] *Physiological evidence that the vestibular system participates in autonomic and respiratory control.* **Yates, B.J. and Miller, A.D.** 1, 1998, Journal of Vestibular Research., Vol. 8, pp. 17-25.

flow probably through stimulation of the otoliths in an upright position,[435] which brings us back to Tomatis's concept of *energy*.

An exhaustive review, covering the last forty years, of the literature relating to autopsies of children who had died from the syndrome, revealed a high incidence of otolaryngologic abnormalities, which lends consistency to Rubens' observations.[436]

PRESBYCUSIS

One third of the population over the age of 65 suffers from significant hearing loss associated with other ailments. Deafness is 54% more common in people with cardiovascular disease [437] and lower sensitivity to high frequencies accompanies diabetes.[438] Hair cells are thought to be so sensitive that hearing loss may be the first sign of the onset of some diseases.

We are so accustomed to the elderly becoming deaf that we accept it as inevitable. The hair cells gradually die off and, as they are not replaced, hearing is lost. This is a reasonable explanation, but it does not appear to be well grounded in science. Prolonged accumulation of aggressions such as noise and poor nutrition can pave the way for deafness, but not aging on its own.

In 1960, two ENT physicians, Samuel Rosen and Pekka Olin, embarked on the adventure of travelling to Sudan to evaluate the hearing of the Mabbans, a tribe that lived in harmony with nature, without noise, and with a healthy diet. As a result, their cholesterol levels were 160 mg % on average, compared to 250 mg % in the USA and there was no hypertension. In these healthy conditions, hearing loss in the elderly was mild: they could hear better than young Americans.[439]

Other investigations have produced similar results. In 2008, for instance, 35 researchers from various countries took part in an international study. They analyzed data from over 4,000 people between the ages of 53 and 67, and concluded that the most important

---

[435] *Vestibular effects on cerebral blood flow.* **Serrador, J.M. et al.** 2009, BMC Neuroscience, Vol. 10.

[436] *Otolaryngological aspects of sudden infant death syndrome.* **Marom, T. et al.** 2012, International Journal of Pediatric Otorhinolaryngology, Vol. 76, pp. 311–318.

[437] *Study finds higher cardiovascular fitness associated with greater hearing acuity.* **Alessio, H.M. et al.,** 8, 2002, The Hearing Journal, Vol. 55.

[438] *Impairment of extra-high frequency auditory thresholds in subjects with elevated levels of fasting blood glucose.* **Das, A. et al.** 2018, Journal of Otology, Vol. 13, pp. 29-35.

[439] *Hearing loss and coronary heart disease.* **Rosen, S. Olin, P.** 10, New York : s.n., Oct, 1965, Bull. N. Y. Acad. Med., Vol. 41.

risk factors for presbycusis were exposure to continuous noise, smoking and obesity, while moderate alcohol consumption was beneficial.[440]

Recent research on a sample of 1,500 teenagers reported worse hearing among the obese.[441] Another study found analogous results in a sample of women.[442] In Spain, childhood obesity is an alarming problem, according to the preliminary results of a study carried out by the Gasol Foundation. In children between the ages of 8 and 16, over 60% do not get the recommended amount of daily physical exercise and a third are overweight.[443]

Children with recurrent episodes of otitis have been observed to tend to be obese.[444] Hearing impairments occur before we reach old age if we do not take care of ourselves. There were no fat people among the Mabbans.

Landegger, Psaltis and Stankovic[445] compared the auditory tissue of 131 deceased people with their last audiometric data. They expected to find a correspondence between the main damaged areas and the audiometric curves, since the frequency distribution in the cochlea is tonotopic (trebles at the base and basses at the apex). However, they failed to establish such a relationship. Audiograms with very similar profiles belonged to cochleas with dissimilar lesions. The title of their article summarizes the results well: Human audiometric thresholds do not predict specific cell damage in the inner ear.

Viana et al. reached similar conclusions.[446] They suggest that the cochlear nerve degenerates before damage to hair cells appears, and that this would be the case in hearing loss between the ages of 50 and 60.

---

[440] *Occupational Noise, Smoking, and a High Body Mass Index are Risk Factors for Age-related Hearing Impairment...* **Fransen, E. et al.** 2008, Journal of the Association for research in Otolaringology, Vol. 9, pp. 264-276.

[441] *Obesity Is Associated with Sensorineural Hearing Loss in Adolescents.* **Lalwani, A.K. et al.** 2013, The Laryngoscope.

[442] *Visceral adipose tissue is significantly associated with hearing thresholds in adult women.* **Kim, T.S., et al.** 3, 2014, Clin Endocrinol (Oxf)., Vol. 80, pp. 368-75.

[443] **Fundación Gasol.** *Resultados preliminares del estudio Pasos.* Sant Boi de Llobregat, Barcelona : s.n., 2019.

[444] *Relationship Between Pediatric Obesity and Otitis Media With Effusion.* **Kim, J.B. et al.** 2007, Arch Otolaryngol Head Neck Surg, Vol. 133.

[445] *Human audiometric thresholds do not predict specific cellular damage in the inner ear.* **Landegger, L.D., Psaltis, D. and Stankovic, K.** 2016, Hearing Research, Vol. 335, pp. 83-93.

[446] *Cochlear neuropathy in human presbycusis: confocal analysis of hidden hearing loss in post-mortem tissue.* **Viana, L.M. et al.** Sept, 2015, Hearing Research, Vol. 327, pp. 78-88.

We can prevent presbycusis by staying in good physical condition [447] and learning music.[448] Patients following a Tomatis's program often report better hearing in noisy environments, regardless of their hearing thresholds. There is probably a training of the efferent system, which facilitates discrimination. Hopefully, in future, hearing will be restored through stem cell transplants in the Corti organ or other techniques,[449] but in the meantime, we will have to keep protecting our hair cells.

Cavinato and her team from Padua University, in Italy, pose another question to add to our special collection of enigmas. They report on the case of a patient who became totally deaf after an extensive injury to both temporo-parietal lobes. As expected, they found no brainstem potentials but did record cortical evoked potentials, indicating a reaction to acoustic stimuli: something that was impossible in view of the damage suffered. Obviously, the patient was unaware of her brain's responses. Since we cannot obtain cortical potentials unless there is a functional nerve pathway from the ear to the cortex, it is difficult to understand the phenomenon from a conventional perspective.[450]

We must revise that old dogma about the irreversibility of hair-cell loss. We have known for more than twenty years that it is possible to regenerate them in mammals.[451,452] Even the role of the support cells is being reconsidered, with a view to using them in therapy.[453]

The best way to maintain a functional nerve is to keep it active. I do not think that Tomatis's therapy can resurrect hair cells, but it is likely to help preserve the functionality of the neurons of the auditory system.

---

[447] *Study finds higher cardiovascular fitness associated with greater hearing acuity.* **Alessio, H.M. et al.** 8, Aug, 2002, The Hearing Journal, Vol. 55.

[448] *Music training: lifelong investment to protect the brain from aging and hearing loss.* **Kraus, N. and White-Schwoch1, T.** 2, Aug, 2014, Acoustics Auistralia, Vol. 42, pp. 2014-117.

[449] *Recent Advancements in the Regeneration of Auditory Hair Cells and Hearing Restoration.* **Mittal, R. et al.** 236, July, 2017, Frontiers in Molecular Neuroscience, Vol. 10.

[450] *Preservation of Auditory P300-Like Potentials in Cortical Deafness.* **Cavinato, M. et al.** 1, 2012, Plos One, Vol. 7.

[451] *Ultrastructural evidence for hair cell regeneration in the mammalian inner.* **Forge, A. et al.** 5101, 1993, Science.

[452] *Regeneration in the mammalian inner ear: A glimpse into the future.* **Ciorba, A. and Martini, A.** 2014, Hearing, Balance and Communication, Vol. 12.

[453] *Inner ear supporting cells: Rethinking the silent majority.* **Wan G., Corfas G., Stone J.F.** Washington : s.n., 2013, Semin Cell Dev Biol Author manuscript.

TINNITUS

Tinnitus is one of the most widely studied disorders, and yet it is reluctant to reveal its secrets to us. In broad terms, we know neither its causes nor the treatment to follow. Even a cochlear implant does not guarantee a solution to tinnitus, indicating that the cause can be located anywhere along the auditory pathway and involve other brain structures.[454]

In tinnitus, the tonotopic representation of sound (by frequencies) traveling through the auditory pathways is restructured and we do not understand these changes well. Some neurons pulsate uncontrollably, over and over again, and we do not know how to deactivate them.

It is a multi-causal pathology that is often associated with hearing loss, but can also occur after an episode of otitis, or trauma, or for no apparent reason. High percentages (71%) of sleep breathing disorders, such as apneas, have been found in tinnitus patients: pointing to another link between oxygen and the ear? The connections of the auditory system with the limbic lobe would explain why stress aggravates the symptoms.[455] Tinnitus triggers the dopaminergic pathways and the activity observed in the limbic lobe is greater than in the auditory cortex itself.[456]

Therapies for the treatment of tinnitus can be divided into two groups: medical interventions, which try to reduce or suppress tinnitus, and therapies focused on optimizing the patient's attitude towards these annoying noises. The latter tend to be psychological in nature, such as EMDR.

Among the medical therapies, none has stood the test of time for now. No drug is really effective. Nor have listening to filtered music, white noise training, Swedish herbs, magnetic stimulation, neurofeedback, or hypnosis proven to be convincing remedies. Only a few improvements and remissions have been achieved in isolated cases. In severe cases, surgery has been attempted, severing the auditory nerve: a drastic intervention that still does not improve the

---

[454] *The dorsal cochlear nucleus as a participant in the auditory, attentional and emotional components of tinnitus.* **Kaltenbach, J.A.** 2006, Hearing Research , 224–234, Vols. 216-217.

[455] *Neuronal connectivity and interactions between the auditory and limbic systems. Effects of noise and tinnitus.* **Kraus, K.S. and Canlon, B.** 1-2, Jun, 2012, Hearing Research, Vol. 288, pp. 34-46.

[456] *Dopamina. Vía común final de acúfenos.* **López González, M.A.** [ed.] Hospital Universitario Virgen del Rocío. Granada : s.n., 2010. XXIV Congreso de la Sociedad Andaluza de Otorrinolaringología y Patología Cérvico-Facial. p. 61-81.

symptoms in half of the patients; and when the nerve is severed on removing a tumor, tinnitus appears in half the subjects affected![457]

Additionally, many users of frequency transposition hearing aids have reportedly seen their tinnitus improve: to the point of disappearing in some cases.[458] As we know, frequency transposition is used in patients with major hearing loss – so great that using a conventional hearing aid to amplify sounds in the damaged area proves to be unviable. In such cases, special hearing aids are used, which transfer the sound that is inaudible to the patient to the area where it is audible.

This involves great acoustic distortion, but after a period of learning these patients usually improve their language comprehension through this system. It is surprising that the total sensory deprivation they are thus subjected to in their area of hearing loss should reduce their tinnitus, since favorable results are also obtained through the opposite therapy: hyperstimulation of the same area. The only possible explanation is that the term "tinnitus" encompasses widely differing neurological processes, for all that these present with the same symptoms.

I have seen improvements in some patients who followed a program of auditory training, but the success rate is low, partly because it is a long-term therapy and the dropout rate is high. With disciplined patients, it is worth a try, at least in my own experience. My colleague Carmela Stillitano has published about it.[459]

Every so often inventions are announced that awaken new hope: Oto-313® project, Ototech®, and so on. In addition, some partial studies have obtained promising results with oxytocin, gingko biloba, acupuncture and music therapy.[460,461] I hope one of these takes hold and turns out to be the definitive solution.

A few years ago, I heard about the device invented by Martin L. Lenhardt, the Ultraquiet®.[462,463] I contacted him and he told me its

[457] *Plasticity in Tinnitus Patients: A Role for the Efferent Auditory Systems.* **Geven, L.I. et al.** 2014, Otol Neurotol, Vol. 35, pp. 796-802

[458] *Long-Term Tinnitus Suppression with Linear Octave Frequency Transposition Hearing Aids.* **Peltier, E. et al.** 12, 2012, Plos One, Vol. 7.

[459] *The effects of the Tomatis Method on Tinnitus.* **Stillitano, C. et al.** 2, June, 2014, International Journal of Research In Medical and Health Sciences, Vol. 4.

[460] *Music therapy as an early intervention to prevent chronification of tinnitus.* **Grapp, M. et al.** 7, 2013, Int J Clin Exp Med, Vol. 6, pp. 589-593.

[461] *Listening to Filtered Music as a Treatment Option for Tinnitus: A review.* **Courtenay Wilson, E. and Schlaug, G.** 4, 2010, Music Percept., Vol. 27, pp. 327-330.

[462] *Long-term Inhibition of Tinnitus by UltraQuiet™ Therapy Preliminary Report.* **Goldstein, B.A.** 2002, International Tinnitus Journal.

development had come to a halt. I did not ask him why. Months later I heard he had passed away. Unfortunately, his prototype was never marketed. It used music whose frequencies had been artificially shifted to the 10,000–20,000 Hz range at an intensity of 6 dB above the auditory threshold, transmitted via bone conduction. Preliminary tests documented positive results with only two one-hour sessions per week. Hopefully someone will take up the baton and continue these investigations.

Around 75% of tinnitus patients improve when listening to white noise, at least temporarily.[464] This is the phenomenon of residual inhibition, the basis for sequential sound therapy[465], a line of research that could still come up with new discoveries.

Tinnitus and psychiatric disorders have a high degree of comorbidity. Approximately half of those suffering from tinnitus also suffer from mental illness (according to some researchers, over 80%).[466] The reasonable explanation could be that anxiety and depression develop as a result of living under insistent, out-of-control noise. That constant stress, accompanied by insomnia on many occasions, would take its toll.

Of course, this is a valid argument, but we have to take other factors into account: for example, that both tinnitus and mental disorders seem to generate neurological changes in the same brain structures,[467] as if they were two sides of the same coin. Tinnitus can be a warning of the appearance of a psychotic break, and can respond positively to psychiatric treatment, even when this is non-pharmacological.[468] Once more, we find mental health linked to hearing.

The terms "social epigenetics of the ear" and "otosociology" have been coined. ENT specialists have realized that tinnitus does not appear by itself but tends to be accompanied by anxiety, resulting from tense work or family situations that modulate the

[463] *Tinnitus Improvement with Ultra-High-Frequency Vibration Therapy.* **Goldstein, B.A.** 1, 2005, International Tinnitus Journal, Vol. 11.

[464] Geven, op.cit. 457

[465] *Terapia Sonora Secuencial en Acúfenos.* **López, M.A. y López, R.** 2004, Acta Otorrinolaringol, Vol. 55, págs. 2-8.

[466] *A Brain Centred View of Psychiatric Comorbidity in Tinnitus: From Otology to Hodology.* **Salviati, M. et al.** 2014, Neural Plasticity, Vol. 2014.

[467] *Tinnitus como síntoma de psicosis de inicio reciente. A propósito de un caso.* **Alberdi-Páramo, I., Jesús Enrique Ibáñez-Vizoso, J.E. and Saiz-González, M.D.** 2, 2018, Psiquiatría Biológica, Vol. 25, pp. 68-71

[468] *Tinnitus as a Symptom of Psychotic Depression Successfully Treated With Electroconvulsive Therapy.* **Popeo, D.M. et al.** 1, 2011, Journal of ECT, Vol. 27.

intensity of the symptoms. The cochlea is very vulnerable to stress and this could be the origin of many auditory pathologies.

ACOUSTIC DRUGS

Frequencies between 20 and 20,000 Hz make up the conscious audible band, but the effects of sound on our organism span a much wider range.[469]

High-intensity infrasounds, such as seismic waves, cause headaches, dizziness and vision problems, and can damage internal organs. However, we actually live with them, as brain waves pulsate in this frequency range. The alpha waves, which correspond to the state of relaxed wakefulness, oscillate between 8 and 14 Hz and the delta waves, characteristic of deep sleep, between 1 and 4 Hz.

If we send two different frequencies to the ears, an unexpected phenomenon occurs: the brain waves begin to align with the mathematical difference between the two. For example, if I send the frequency 104 Hz to one ear and 100 Hz to the other, a 4 Hz pulse is produced, inducing sleep.[470]

This discovery led the Monroe Institute to develop the Hemi Sync®, a device to promote relaxation and other mental states through binaural waves.[471] However, this kind of acoustic stimulation is not always of benefit to the patient and is being used to provoke altered states of consciousness. We can find websites that offer "acoustic drugs" based on this mechanism: a very unfortunate idea.

Auditory brain areas are especially sensitive to increased gamma waves, which is achieved when the difference between the sounds presented is 40 Hz.[472]

---

[469] **Advisory group on non-ionising radiation.** *Health effects of exposure to ultrasound and infrasound.* s.l. : Health Protection Agency, 2010.

[470] **Llancafil, N.F.** Efectos de los infrasonidos en la conducta humana. *Tesis doctoral.* Valdivia, Chile : s.n., 2013.

[471] *Auditory driving of the autonomic nervous system:Listening to theta-frequency binaural beats post-exercise increases parasympathetic activation and sympathetic withdrawal.* **McConnell, P.A. et al.** 1248, Nov, 2014, Frontiers in Psychologie, Vol. 5.

[472] *Brain responses to 40-Hz binaural beat and effects on emotion and memory.* **Jirakittayakorn, N. and Wongsawat, Y.** 2017, International Journal of Psychophysiology, Vol. 120, págs. 96-107.

MOTHER'S VOICE AND NEWBORNS 8

Tomatis began his research on intrauterine listening around 1950, influenced by the works of Negus, Lorenz and Thomas. He had great admiration for Victor Negus, an English zoologist, who had written a monumental work about the larynx.[473] He met him at a conference in Barcelona in 1949.

In his book, Negus mentioned a surprising fact: when a songbird's egg is incubated by another bird of a different species, the chick's song is more like that of its adoptive parents than the biological ones. And if some songbird eggs are incubated by a non-singing bird the chicks do not sing.

Later, Tomatis learned about Konrad Lorenz's famous experiment in which he began to talk regularly to some goose eggs in incubation. When hatching, the little geese followed Lorenz's voice, even preferring him over their own mother. For his work in ethology, Lorenz received the Nobel Prize in Medicine in 1973.

The third and definitive clue came to him from the hand of André Thomas, a famous neuro-pediatrician, whom he met while working at the Trousseau Hospital in Paris. Thomas was an expert in the neurological assessment of newborns. One of the tests he performed was the so-called *name sign* which we can perform before the baby is 10 days old.[474] If we stand behind the newborn, who is in a seated position, and call him by his

---

[473] **Negus, V.** *The mechanism of the larynx.* London : C.V. Mosby Co., 1929. p. 528.

[474] *Spontaneous audibility of the maternal voice; conditioned audibility of every other voice.* **Thomas, A. and Autgaerden, S.** 1963, Presse Med., Vol. 71.

name, nothing happens, but if it is the mother who calls him, he turns around towards the side he was called from.

Determined to find out what the fetus heard, Tomatis built a rudimentary device that recreated the conditions of the mother's womb. He concluded that intrauterine listening consisted of treble sounds, mostly from 8,000 Hz. This result was actually due to a failure in one of the devices he was using. If it had worked well, he would have established the exact opposite: that it was the bass sounds that were reaching the fetus. Paradoxically, however, this error led him to discover the positive effect that filtered sounds caused in people and used it therapeutically. Two amazing experiences subsequently led him to understand the power of filtered sounds.

THE END OF THE TUNNEL!

The first one occurred during the visit of a friend, who came accompanied by his little daughter. While explaining his research on intrauterine listening, he switched on a tape recorder to let him listen to the filtered voice. After a few minutes, the little girl started talking. She said she saw a tunnel, and at the end of it a lot of light and two angels. Then she said she saw her mom. When her father asked her what she looked like, she placed herself in the usual gynecological delivery position at the time. She was remembering her own birth.[475]

The second experience was shared with Françoise Dolto, the famous pediatrician and psychoanalyst. She had a schizophrenic patient, a twelve-year-old boy with highly disruptive behavior. She and Tomatis decided to try out the effect filtered sounds could produce in such a case.

Everyone gathered in Tomatis's laboratory: the child and his mother, F. Dolto and her assistant Bernard This, as well as Tomatis himself, equipped with a loudspeaker. He began to direct the filtered maternal voice towards the child.

The boy's reaction stunned them. When he heard the sounds, he went to the light switch, turned off the light and lay on his mother's lap, something unusual because he permanently rejected her. Hugging his mother, he began to suck his thumb, until the tape ended. Then, he got up and turned on the light.[476]

---

[475] See note 32
[476] See note 3

There was a second session—also successful—but not a third, as the boy manifested serious episodes of aggression towards his mother and against himself. At this, F. Dolto decided to abandon this line of work. Tomatis continued it. He realized he had gone too fast. He had to perfect the method.

He returned to university and studied psychology at the Sorbonne, where professors with psychoanalytic training taught. Although Tomatis did not follow this current, its influence is noticeable in his work: always emphasizing the relationship with the mother regarding the structuring of personality and the importance of the intra-uterine experience to the child's subsequent development. He believed that the origin of many pathologies lay in gestation and that filtered sounds could give patients a sort of second chance. He said that the mother's voice had the ability to "reset" the system, as when we restart a computer.

The maternal voice is not systematically applied in Tomatis's therapy. Mozart's music and Gregorian chants work very well in most cases.

A FORTUNATE MISTAKE

Tomatis's work did not go unnoticed and other researchers replicated his experiments, but obtained conflicting results. Within the acoustic universe of the mother's womb, low-frequency sounds reign: breathing, intestinal movements, the heartbeat and also noises coming from outside that cross the uterine wall, which are mainly bass sounds.

At first, Tomatis attached little importance to these criticisms, but since they came from prestigious experts, he rebuilt his device fifteen years later. In doing so, he noticed the technical glitch: one of the sound analyzers he used was acting as a filter, eliminating the bass sounds. This affected his reputation in the scientific community, but by then the therapeutic power of treble sounds was obvious. Bass sounds do not produce the same effects.

This apparent contradiction could only have one explanation: immersed in the chaotic sound environment of the womb, the fetus is already listening, deliberately selecting the sounds it wants to capture: in particular the mother's voice. The fetus listens by bone transmission.[477] The sound runs down the mother's spine, to be amplified by the pelvis acting as a soundboard.

In ontogenetic development, the appearance of hair cells does not occur in the entire cochlea at once, but begins at the base, its widest part, where high-pitched sounds are analyzed. This process is common to all animal species and is therefore considered a law of evolution. Internal hair cells mature earlier than external ones and vestibular ones earlier than cochlear ones.[478] Therefore, it is quite likely that the first sounds the fetus hears are high frequencies. Hair cells are theoretically functional at 20 weeks of gestation.[479] After birth, the amniotic fluid remains in the newborn's ear and Eustachian tube for a few days, as protection, facilitating a progressive transition from aquatic to aerial hearing.

Adults feel that children listen differently. We tend to speak to them in a higher pitch and exaggerate the intonation. Do we do this to facilitate understanding? What are the advantages of talking to them in this way? It is hard to answer these questions. Studies on sound discrimination in childhood are sometimes contradictory. In any case, bearing in mind that the 2,000–4,000 Hz frequency range provides 90% of the intelligibility of the word, it would be almost impossible for children to learn to speak if they could not discriminate enough in this range of sounds.[480]

SPEAKING ENGLISH

In his book *The Conscious Ear*, Tomatis refers to one of the many cases in which prenatal listening manifested itself:

"Not long ago I treated a four-and-a-half-year-old girl who was brought to me for a total verbal blockage. The treatment was quick to take effect: the little one began to speak. She came to the sessions in the company of her mother, as I had asked, and also her father, who

---

[477] *The pathway enabling external sounds to reach and excite the fetal inner ear.* **Somher, H. et al.** May-Jun, 2001, Audiol Neurootol, Vol. 6(3), pp. 109-16.

[478] *Anatomical and physiological development of the human inner ear.* **Lim, R. and Brichta, A.M.** 2016, Hearing Research, Vol. 338, pp. 9-21.

[479] *Temporal bone study of development of the organ of Corti: correlation between auditory function and anatomical structure.* **Bibas, A.G. et al.** 122(4), Apr, 2008, J Laryngol Otol., pp. 336-42.

[480] **McCracken, W. and Mulla, I.** *What are children hearing?* s.l. : University of Manchester, 2012.

served as the family chauffeur [...] The girl had started talking when one day her father said:

-Listen, doctor, I don't know what's going on, but something seems strange to me. We have four children, my wife and I. That makes it difficult for us to isolate ourselves at home to tell each other things they shouldn't hear. So, we solved the problem: when we need to say something about those sorts of things, we use English, which we both speak fluently. Our daughter being treated at your center gives the impression that she understands English better than French. Naturally the girl has never taken English classes in her life...
-Perhaps your wife spoke English during the pregnancy...
-During the pregnancy? Oh no! Not at all! Out of the question.
And that is how we left it. Busy with my work, I forgot about this story. Eight days later, the girl came for a routine check-up, accompanied by her father.
-Ah!" said the father when he saw me, "I must apologize!
-Apologize?
-Yes, last week I was wrong. I was very sure of myself but after making inquiries, it seems I was wrong. I asked my wife and she reminded me that while she was pregnant with the child, she was employed as an English translator in an import–export company.
-May I ask at what stage of the pregnancy?"
-Only the first three months.

I believe that this anecdote will enlighten us better than a long theoretical argument. And I hasten to point out that it is just one of many that I could tell. I hear testimonies like this every week, if not every day, and without asking! I have cited this case because it is one of the most recent and therefore fresher in my memory.
The elaboration of listening is done in the deepest uterine night: I place its beginnings in the first days of conception. And I maintain this. I do not go even further back, like others, to a hypothetical previous life".[481]

Personally, I had never seen anything like that until, a few years ago, I found myself in an almost identical situation. A boy was brought into my consulting room who hardly spoke at all, and least of all the languages of his environment, Spanish and Catalan. However,

---

[481] See note 3

he showed a special predilection for English. He asked for cartoons and stories in that language and when he addressed his parents, the few words he used were English. Indeed, his mother had spoken that language during pregnancy, but he had not been exposed to it again since then.

After the therapy, the child showed a greater desire to communicate, which led him to increase his use of his mother tongue, Spanish. From then on, everything was simpler. I must confess that I have never gotten used to situations like this. They still amaze me.

SURPRISING VOICE

With his studies on the maternal voice, Tomatis opened up an important research path, which has captivated other professionals. Inside the uterus, the fetus has a predilection for its mother's voice and language,[482,483] just like the newborn. Other people's voices, including the father's, do not generate the same reactions.[484] Its brain responds differently, as shown by tests using evoked potentials,[485] ultrasounds,[486] magnetic resonance[487] and electrophysiology.[488]

Baby dolphins behave similarly to humans. Their mothers "talk" to them during pregnancy and, after birth, the babies recognize those sounds.[489]

The maternal voice may produce effects on the hippocampus and the amygdala, thus configuring the limbic lobe: the emotion manager.[490] A recent study, using MRI, found that children whose

[482] **Purhonen, M. et al.** Cerebral processing of mother's voice compared to unfamiliar voice in 4-month-old infants. *Int J Psychophysiol.* May, 2004. 52(3), pp. 257-66.

[483] **Kisilevsky BS, et al.** Effects of experience on fetal voice recognition. *Psychol Sci.* 2003 May. May, 2003. 14(3), pp. 220-4.

[484] *Fetuses respond to father's voice but prefer mother's voice after birth.* **Lee, G.Y. y Kisilevsky, B.S.** 1, 2014, Dev Psychobiol., Vol. 56, pp. 1-11.

[485] *Cerebral processing of mother's voice compared to unfamiliar voice in 4-month-old infants.* **Purhonen, M. et al.** 3, 2004, Int J Psychophysiol., Vol. 52, pp. 257-66.

[486] *Ultrasonographic Investigation of Human Fetus Responses to Maternal Communicative and Non-communicative Stimuli.* **Ferrari, G.A. et al.** 354, 2016, Front Psychol., Vol. 7.

[487] *Young children's neural processing of their mother's voice: An fMRI study.* **Liu, P. et al.** 2019, Neuropsychologia, Vol. 122, pp. 11-19.

[488] *Mother and stranger: an electrophysiological study of voice processing in newborns.* **Beauchemin, M. et al.** 8, 2011, Cereb Cortex., Vol. 21, pp. 1705-11.

[489] **Pappas, S.** LiveScience. [Online] Aug 9, 2016. [Cited: Oct, 2019.] https://www.livescience.com/55699-mother-dolphins-teach-babies-signature-whistle.html.

[490] *Separation-induced receptor changes in the hippocampus and amygdala of Octodon degus: influence of maternal vocalizations.* **Ziabreva, I. et al.** 12, 2003, J Neurosci., Vol. 23, pp. 5329-36.

mother's voice had a strong impact on their auditory and emotional areas later developed better social skills.[491]

According to Tomatis, the mother's voice is the first sound the fetus would hear, and this would explain its therapeutic efficacy. At the beginning of gestation, acoustic stimulation circulates freely towards the nervous system, without any mechanism regulating its entry, as neither the efferent pathways nor the middle ear have yet been constructed. The maternal voice is, therefore, a sound that has free access and it may maintain that property even after birth, throughout adult life. Some areas of the brainstem have neuromodulatory effects on the rest of the brain, allowing or blocking the changes we know as plasticity.[492] The mother's voice could be able to activate those areas.

A clinical case displays the extent to which the bond with the mother is maintained through her voice. An eight-year-old boy who had been in a vegetative state for four years due to an accident (drowning) had his brain waves monitored while listening to his mother's or an unknown woman's voice. The records were conclusive. Somehow, his brain was still able to identify the mother, generating totally different brain waves when he heard her.[493]

PRE- AND PERINATAL HEARING

Hormones are closely related to auditory perception. Women's voices are higher pitched during ovulation[494,495] and their audiograms change throughout pregnancy.[496] The resonance frequency of the ear is modified and sensitivity to bass sounds decreases.[497] However, menopause does not seem to affect the hearing threshold directly[498]

---

[491] *Neural circuits underlying mother's voice perception predict social communication abilities in children.* **Abrams, D.A. et al.** 22, 2016, Proc Natl Acad Sci U S A., Vol. 113, pp. 6295-300.

[492] **Barry, S.R.** *Ver en estéreo.* Madrid : BGA Asesores, 2012.

[493] *Recognizing a mother's voice in the persistent vegetative state.* **Machado, C. et al.** 3, 2007, Clin EEG Neurosci., Vol. 38, pp. 124-6.

[494] *Vocal cues of ovulation in human females.* **Bryant, G.A. and Haselton, M.G.** Oct, 2009, Biol. Lett., Vol. 5, pp. 12-15.

[495] *Women's voices become more high-pitched during ovulation.* **Gregory, A.B. et al.** Dec, 2008, Biology Letters.

[496] See note 242

[497] *Decrease in middle ear resonance frequency during pregnancy.* **Dag, E.M., Gulumser, C. and Erbek, S.** 147, 2016, Audiology Research, Vol. 6.

[498] *Comparative audiometric evaluation of hearing loss between the premenopausal and postmenopausal period in young women.* **Oghan, F. and Coksuer, H.** 3, 2012, Am J Otolaryngol., Vol. 33, pp. 322-5.

except in some cases, such as menopausal women suffering from sarcopenia.[499]

The hearing system learns fast in the prenatal stage—much more quickly than the other senses—so we can hear before the fifth month of gestation.[500] And the vestibular apparatus starts functioning even before that, to capture gravity.[501] However, when Tomatis claimed in the 1960s that the ear was functional from the fourth and a half month of gestation, no one took him seriously until 1994, when Peter G. Hepper and B. Sara Shahidullah confirmed fetal responses to sound at 19 weeks, which coincides in time with the opening of the Corti tunnel in the fetus.[502]

The physiological response of the fetus to the maternal voice has been proven beyond doubt[503] The mother's voice acts on the neurovegetative system, regulating blood cortisol levels, respiratory rate and brain waves.[504]

An investigation by the Marqués Institute in Barcelona[505] places hearing at 16 weeks and has given rise to a device that emits music from the vagina or abdominal wall. Although it has been approved by health-care institutions, I have serious doubts as to whether it will be of any benefit. Rather, I suspect the opposite. The fetus is very sensitive to sound, so we should be very careful with the acoustic stimulation it receives. The uterine acoustic environment offered by nature is probably the most suitable one for fetal development and, in my opinion, we should not alter it. We must exercise extreme caution in the care of hearing during pregnancy.

In 1997, the American Academy of Pediatrics issued a series of recommendations regarding newborns' exposure to noise,[506] in recognition of the fact that in their incubators they can close their

---

[499] *Association between sarcopenia and hearing thresholds in postmenopausal women.* **Hui Kang, S. et al.** 5, 2017, International Journal of Medical Sciences, Vol. 14, pp. 470-476.

[500] *Fetal facial expression in response to intravaginal mussic emission.* **López-Teijón, M. et al.** 2015, Ultrasound. https://www.institutomarques.com/pdf/ultrasound.pdf

[501] *Early embryogenesis of the vestibular apparatus in mammals with different ecologies.* **Solntseva, G.N.** 2, Moscú : s.n., 2002, Aquatic mammals, Vol. 28.

[502] See note 474

[503] **Beauchemin Maude, et al.** Mother and Stranger: An Electrophysiological Study of Voice Processing in Newborns. *Cerebral cortex.* Montreal : s.n., Aug, 2011. https://www.ncbi.nlm.nih.gov/pubmed/21149849.

[504] *Effect of mother's voice on neonatal respiratory activity and EEG delta amplitude.* **Uchida, M.O. et al.** 2018, Developmental Psychobiology, Vol. 60, pp. 140-149.

[505] See note 500

[506] *Noise: A Hazard for the Fetus and Newborn.* **Committee on Environmental Health.** s.l. : American Academy of Pediatrics, 1997.

eyes, but not their ears. Their hearing system is largely formed, with the exception of certain listening skills, such as knowing how to protect themselves from noise. For this, they need their olivo-cochlear system to mature, which will be achieved by the sixth month of postnatal life.[507] Hearing disorders have been observed in children whose mothers were exposed to high noise levels during pregnancy even though the uterus is well protected acoustically.[508]

The correct neurological development of the brain areas involved in hearing depends to a large extent on a favorable acoustic environment.[509] In neonatal intensive care units, the sound level of the room is constantly monitored, as noise is harmful to the babies,[510] but those exposed to soft music spend less time in incubators. That means considerable savings for the hospital.[511,512]

Thanks to magnetic resonance techniques, a Swiss team has been able to visualize and accurately determine the positive effect of music on premature babies: it accelerates maturation of brain structures and increases connectivity between them.[513] Babies bring their cortisol levels into balance when their mothers sing to them.[514] Sound has the ability to alter our metabolism, for better or worse.

Tomatis is not alone in using the mother's voice.[515] Some hospitals have introduced it in incubators, with excellent results. It has a relaxing effect on the autonomic nervous system,[516] slowing down the

[507] *The human auditory system: A timeline of development.* **Moore, J.K. and Linthicum, F.H.** 2007, International Journal of Audiology, Vol. 46, pp. 460-478.

[508] *Maternal Occupational Exposure to Noise during Pregnancy and Hearing Dysfunction in Children: A Nationwide Prospective Cohort Study in Sweden.* **Selander, J. et al.** 6, 2016, Environmental Health Perspectives, Vol. 124.

[509] *Auditory brain development in premature infants: the importance of early experience.* **McMahon, E., Wintermark, P. and Lahav, A.** 2012, Annals of the New York Academy of Sciences, Vol. 1252.

[510] *The effects of noise on preterm infants in the NICU.* **Wachman, E.M. and Lahav, A.** 2010, Arch Dis Child Fetal Neonatal.

[511] **Schwartz, F.J. and Ritchie, R.** *Music listening in neonatal intensive care.* 2007.

[512] *A meta-analysis of the efficacy of music therapy for premature infants.* **Standley, J.M.** 2, 2002, Journal of pediatric nursing, Vol. 17.

[513] *Music in premature infants enhances high-level cognitive bran networks.* **Lordier, L. et al.** 24, Washington : s.n., Jun 11, 2018, PNAS, Vol. 116, p. 2019.

[514] *Maternal singing modulates infant arousal.* **Shenfield, T., Trehubta, S.E. and Nakata, T.** 4, 2003, Psychology of Music, Vol. 31.

[515] *Therapeutic effects of music and mother's voice on premature infants.* **Standley, JM and Moore, RS.** 21(6), Nov-Dec, 1995, Pediatr Nurs., pp. 509-12.

[516] *The role of mother's voice in the organization of brain function in the newborn.* **Fifer, WP and Moon, CM.** 397, June, 1994, Acta Paediatr Suppl, pp. 86-93.

heartbeat,[517] and its anti-stress benefits (measured by the oxytocin it generates) are comparable to those of physical contact.[518]

The maternal voice also helps children recover from the effects of anesthesia after surgery[519] and is capable of reducing pain[520] which is of great importance in newborns.[521] When exposed to it, they present more highly developed auditory areas,[522,523,524] they increase their food intake and suffer fewer food intolerances,[525] they gain weight faster, they improve blood oxygen saturation,[526] etc. In short, they make better progress.[527,528]

Its effect is even visible in anatomical studies. Auditory brain areas are larger in children stimulated with maternal voice.[529] Prenatal experience has a strong influence on shaping auditory structures and subsequent musical preferences.[530] Some medical conditions in pregnancy, such as diabetes, can alter the fetus' response to the

---

[517] *Maternal sounds elicit lower heart rate in preterm newborns in the first month of life.* **Rand, K. and Lahav, A.** 10, 2014, Early Hum Dev., Vol. 90, pp. 679-83.

[518] *Social vocalizations can release oxytocin in humans.* **Seltzer, L.J., Ziegler, T.E. and Pollak, S.D.** 277, 2010, Proc Biol Sci., Vol. 7, pp. 2661-6.

[519] *Mother's recorded voice on emergence can decrease postoperative emergence delirium from general anaesthesia in paediatric patients: a prospective randomised controlled trial.* **Byun, S. et al.** 2, 2018, Br J Anaesth., Vol. 121, pp. 483-489.

[520] *Randomised study showed that recorded maternal voices reduced pain in preterm infants undergoing heel lance procedures in a neonatal intensive care unit.* **Chirico, G. et al.** 10, 2017, Acta Paediatr., Vol. 106, pp. 1564-1568.

[521] *The Effect of Mother's Voice on Arterial Blood Sampling Induced Pain in Neonates Hospitalized in Neonate Intensive Care Unit.* **Azarmnejad, E. et al.** 6, 2015, Glob J Health Sci., Vol. 7, pp. 198-204.

[522] See note 515

[523] *A pacifier-activated music player with mother's voice improves oral feeding in preterm infants.* **Chorna, O.D. et al.** 3, 2014, Pediatrics, Vol. 133, pp. 462-8.

[524] *Mother's voice and heartbeat sounds elicit auditory plasticity in the human brain before full gestation.* **Webb, A.R. et al.** Feb, 2015, Proceedings of the National Academy of Sciences.

[525] *Maternal Voice and Short-Term Outcomes in Preterm Infants.* **Krueger, C. et al.** 2, 2010, Dev Psychobiol., Vol. 52, pp. 205-212.

[526] *Positive effects of low intensity recorded maternal voice on physiologic reactions in premature infants.* **Saijadian, N. et al.** 2017, Infant Behav Dev., Vol. 46, pp. 59-66.

[527] *Exposure to Maternal Voice in Preterm Infants: A Review.* **Krueger, C.** 1, 2010, Adv Neonatal Care., Vol. 10, pp. 13-20.

[528] *Do mothers sound good? A systematic review of the effects of maternal voice exposure on preterm infants' development.* **Provenzi, L. et al.** 2018, Neurosci Biobehav Rev., Vol. 88, pp. 42-50.

[529] See note 524

[530] *Linking prenatal experience to the emerging musical mind.* **Ullal-Gupta, S. et al.** 48, 2013, Frontiers in Systems Neuroscience, Vol. 7.

mother's voice.[531,532] In such cases the protocol designed by Tomatis for pregnant women could be of great help, facilitating this mother–child dialogue.

As I have mentioned, the fetus perceives its mother's voice via bone conduction,[533] through contact with the pelvis: something that needs to be taken into account when this is used for therapeutic purposes. Sound reaches the fetus differently depending on how it is positioned.

Near my practice is that of a well-known osteopath, María Ángeles Paredes, who, among other things, is known for her ability to reposition the fetus when it is wrongly placed for delivery.[534] One day I asked her how she did it, thinking she would describe some complicated osteopathic maneuver. However, her answer was much simpler:

"I teach mothers to communicate with their babies. I tell them to talk to them and ask them to turn around."

She left me speechless.

FEMININE AND MASCULINE

Men and women do not hear the same way, there being appreciable differences in otoacoustic emissions from birth. In girls they show greater amplitude. Males tolerate background noise better and are faster in some temporal and spatial location hearing tests.[535] Most probably, as hunters, they developed certain skills that were not so important to the female sex.

Women, on the other hand, are better at discriminating sounds and their academic advantage in the area of language, mainly before adolescence, is well known. However, they are less able to withstand loud noises, with discomfort thresholds about 6 dB lower than men.

---

[531] *Atypical fetal voice processing in preeclamptic pregnancy.* **Kisilevsky, B.S. et al.** 1, 2011, J Dev Behav Pediatr., Vol. 32, pp. 34-40.

[532] *Atypical fetal response to the mother's voice in diabetic compared with overweight pregnancies.* **Kisilevsky, B.S. et al.** 1, 2012, J Dev Behav Pediatr., Vol. 33, pp. 55-61.

[533] See note 477

[534] **Paredes, M.A.** *El primer regalo de vida: terapia craneosacral.* Barcelona : Ediciones Obelisco, 2015.

[535] *Sex Differences in Hearing. Implications for best practice in the classroom.* **Sax, L.** 2010, Advances in Gender and Education, Vol. 2.

Dennis McFadden, who was a professor of Psychology at the University of Texas, published a series of papers in which he linked hearing not to gender, but to sexual orientation,[536] suggesting that both the ear and future sexual orientation could be conditioned by a greater or lesser circulation of androgens during pregnancy. Recent studies seem to support his theory.[537,538] This is a controversial topic, with ethical and even religious implications.

McFadden found that otoacoustic emissions (both spontaneous and evoked) were more abundant and of greater amplitude in women, but varied depending on whether they were homosexual or heterosexual. In homosexual women, both number and amplitude decreased significantly. Something similar occurred among males, but to a lesser extent.

Furthermore, McFadden stated that otoemission patterns remain stable over time. The results obtained in a baby hardly vary thirty years later. Therefore, this appears to be a biological marker that could be determined at birth.

FULL SPEED VESTIBULE

Why is Nature in such a hurry to complete the hearing system before birth?[539] This cannot be a whim, but a necessity or a biological advantage. The developing nervous system may need this stimulation to mature: the *nervous energy* to which Tomatis referred. In an article published by Swedish psychologist Mats Niklasson, we can read:

"Appearing nine weeks after conception, the vestibular nuclei are functional by the eleventh week (Humphrey, 1965). At about the 21st week (Robbins, 1977; Larsen, 1993), aside from the interoceptive sensory receptors (sensory receptors in the walls of the thoracic, abdominal, and pelvic viscera), the vestibular system is the only sensory system which is mature. Although it develops this early, some

---

[536] *Sexual Orientation and the Auditory System.* **McFadden, D.** 2, 2011, Front Neuroendocrinol., Vol. 32.

[537] *Otoacoustic Emissions, Auditory Evoked Potentials and Self-Reported Gender in People Affected by Disorders of Sex Development (DSD).* **Wisniewski, A.B. et al.** 3, 2014, Horm Behav., Vol. 66, pp. 467-474.

[538] *Prenatal masculinization of the auditory system in infants: The MIREC-ID study.* **Nguyen, T.V. et al.** 2019, Psychoneuroendocrinology, Vol. 104, pp. 33-41.

[539] *Time course of axonal myelination in the human brainstem auditory pathway.* **Moore, Jean K., Perazzob, L. M. and Brau, A.** 91(1-2), Nov, 1995, Hear Res, pp. 208-9.

authors (Windle, 1971; Prechtl, 1984) believe that the system is inhibited during prenatal life.

Others like Odent (1986) and Restak (1979) claim that the floating fetus is constantly stimulated by the mother's movements and registers its first perceptions through the vestibular system. **It is because of this early maturation that the vestibular system is so important for brain development and a disturbance of its function by any factor will be reflected in the formation of the whole nervous system"** [bold type added]. Klosovskii, 1963, p. 116.[540]

I have previously cited an experiment (see p. 49) in which pregnant rats were sent to space to check the effects of weightlessness.[541] Once born, the offspring were returned to Earth. They were clumsy and did not have the typical reflexes of rodents at birth.

Thousands of jellyfish have also been sent into space to observe their development. As adults, their motility was that of any jellyfish, but it became chaotic when they returned to Earth.[542] I believe this is something to keep in mind when working with rhythmic movement training (RMT) to integrate the primary reflexes.[543] The circumstances of gestation affect the development of the vestibular captors.[544]

The vestibule manages everything related to the struggle against gravity, including the bones. Rats with damaged vestibules have been observed to lose bone mass compared to those who keep them intact, regardless of the physical exercise they perform.[545] However, the application of a moderate vibration can help in the prevention and treatment of osteoporosis.[546]

VESTIBULAR MUSIC

Some expectant women have to rest during pregnancy. I have seen children with motor disorders coming from such a background. They

---

[540] See note 381

[541] See note 56

[542] *Development Studies of Aurelia (Jellyfish) Ephyrae Which Developed During The SLS-1 Mission.* **Spangenberg, D., et al.**, 1994, Advanced Space Research, V14N87

[543] See note 344

[544] See note 58

[545]*Bone remodeling is regulated by inner ear vestibular signals.* **Vignaux, G. et al.** 10, Oct, 2013, J Bone Miner Res, Vol. 28, pp. 2136-44.

[546] *The Potential Benefits and Inherent Risks of Vibration as a Non-Drug Therapy for the Prevention and Treatment of Osteoporosis.* **Ete Chan, M., Uzer, G. and Rubin, C.T.** 1, 2013, Curr Osteoporos Rep. March, 2013, Vol. 11, pp 36-44

did not suffer from weightlessness but did receive less vestibular stimulation due to lack of movement.

I have always suspected that there is a link between rest time during gestation and later motor development, especially if it is from the third month of pregnancy, when the vestibule is already functional. I have observed frequent manifestations of vestibular hyperreactivity, just like the rat pups gestated in space, but I do not have statistical data to confirm this.

I usually ask children I am treating, and even adults, to dance to a musical beat or just follow it with their hands. When their timing is all wrong, I know where to start working. The vestibular system, together with its annex, the cerebellum, plays a prominent role in rhythm, one of the manifestations of something more generic: temporal perception.[547]

I consider the lack of a sense of rhythm, which can sometimes be absolute (rhythmic deafness), a good indicator of the maturation level of these two structures: an important point to take into account in the diagnosis of learning disorders.[548]

For Tomatis, Sector I of the audiometric curve, up to 1,000 Hz, is influenced by vestibular activity, as the vestibule can analyze bass sounds. When distortions appear in that sector, along with problems of balance, posture, etc., we suggest vestibular stimulation therapy through music with low pass filters.

This works very well when applied in combination with other motor therapies, such as Harald Blomberg's RMT, or Padovan, an interesting method of neurofunctional reorganization that also incorporates the cochlea into the exercises, each of which is accompanied by a poem or a song.[549] Here in Spain, the pedagogue and speech therapist Teresa Feliu has been able to effectively integrate this therapy with the Tomatis approach.

Both Padovan and RMT work on the vestibular system, integrating the primary reflexes that are still active, adapting muscle tone to the situation and organizing motor coordination. Learning difficulties often have their origin and solution here.[550]

---

[547] See note 405

[548] *The cerebellum's contribution to beat interval discrimination.* **Paquette, S. et al.** 2017, Neuroimage, Vol. 163, pp. 177-182.

[549] **Feliu, T.** La reorganització neurofuncional segons el mètode de Beatriz Padovan. [Online] https://sincroniayoga.com/wp-content/uploads/2018/10/Teresa-Feliu-article-Padovan.pdf.

[550] *Effects of replicating primary-reflex movements on specific reading difficulties in children: a randomised, double-blind, controlled trial.* **McPhillips, M., Hepper, P.G. and Mulhem, G.** 9203, London : s.n., 2000, The Lancet, Vol. 355, pp. 537-541.

I'M CRYING FOR YOU TO UNDERSTAND ME

A baby's nervous system is expressed through its cries and acoustic analysis of crying can be used to make extremely precise diagnoses.[551] In some countries, such as Cuba, scientists have been accumulating research on this for thirty years.

Although the computational analysis used includes several indicators, variation in the fundamental tone or pitch alone provides valuable information and can be used as a screening tool. In a study carried out in India, they analyzed the fundamental frequency of pain-induced crying in babies less than one month old, which is around 400 Hz. Unlike the adult voice, it was higher pitched in boys (420 Hz versus 370 Hz in girls).[552]

Crying is the result of intense activity of the autonomic nervous system (ANS). The sound emitted depends on the manner of breathing and muscle tone, regulated by an ANS that is very attentive to primary sensations, such as hunger or pain.[553]

Informatics allows multiple variables of the acoustic spectrum to be analyzed, and mobile phone apps have already appeared, to tell us why the baby is crying. The crying of autistic children has been seen to present certain differential elements, such as a rise and oscillation in pitch.[554]

WHAT THE EAR SAYS ABOUT YOU

Modern thermometers measure the temperature in the ear canal almost instantaneously. What is less known is that this instrument can be used as a personality test.

At 91, Jerome Kagan is still one of the world's leading figures in child psychology. I was thrilled to see his name on an original work

---

[551] **Escobedo Beceiro, D.I.** Análisis acústico del llanto del niño recién nacido orientado al diagnóstico de patología en su neurodesarrollo debido a hipoxia. Santiago de Cuba : s.n., 2006. Doctoral thesis.

[552] **Daga, Raina P. and Panditrao, Anagha M.** Acoustical Analysis of Pain Cries' in Neonates: Fundamental Frequency. *Special Issue of International Journal of Computer Applications (0975 – 8887) on Electronics, Information and Communication Engineering - ICEICE.* Dec, 2011. 3.

[553] **Newman, J.D.** Neural circuits underlying crying and cry responding in mammals. *Behavioural Brain Research.* 2007. 182, pp. 155-165.

[554] *Atypical cry acoustics in 6-month-old infants at risk for autism spectrum disorder.* **Sheinkopf, S.J. et al.** 5,Oct, 2012, Autism Research, Vol.5.

that closely intertwines hearing and the psyche once again.[555] According to the research team, a left ear with a higher temperature is an indicator of calmness whereas, when it is the right ear, babies tend to be more restless. This seems to be related to an asymmetry in the activation of certain zones of the cerebral hemispheres. The study recalls Yair Bar-Haim's paper on the stapedial reflex of introverts and extroverts, which I mentioned earlier (see Chapter 5).

---

[555] *Temperament, tympanum and temperature: four provisional studies of the biiobehavioural...* **Boyce, W.T. et al.** 3, 2002, Child Development, Vol. 73.

THE THERAPY OF A. TOMATIS 9

The ear, in addition to providing us with diagnostic data, is an excellent therapeutic tool. Through the techniques of audio-psycho-phonology we are always aiming for better listening. We follow the same procedures with patients as with singers, trying to achieve a more balanced audiometric profile, free of obstacles, and what we find is that symptoms are relieved as the curves gradually improve.

Our body behaves as if it were always looking for coherence, a phenomenon not restricted to the ear. Acupuncture, foot reflexology and other techniques act on the same principle: if we are able to improve certain symptoms, there is a positive effect on overall health.[556] I would suggest that some medications work in the same way. Why does an antipyretic relieve us so much, if all it does is lower the fever? As its temperature is normalized, the body acts as if it has regained its health.

Likewise, if we are able to enhance listening, the positive effects are reflected not only in hearing but in general health. The body tries to fit in with the new situation: "If the audiometric curve is a good one, I should behave accordingly".

We still do not properly understand the processes that connect certain disorders with the hearing system, so we can never say—or at least for the moment—that auditory therapy can be used to cure diseases. However, little by little, scientific studies are accumulating

---

[556] See note 91

in support of what we therapists have been observing in clinical practice for decades.

USES OF THERAPY

Undoubtedly, the most controversial thing about Tomatis is his therapy. It has been used to treat the voice, learning problems, psychiatric disorders and so on: "Too many things", detractors say. However, I have already said that his therapy only pursues one objective: to obtain better listening. All other benefits that may appear are positive side effects of this.

The listening test is a good indicator of the therapeutic possibilities. If there are many irregularities, our patient is very likely to make progress after we intervene. If the initial curve is already good, our technique may not be the most suitable one. The information gathered in the intake interview will be crucial in deciding whether to intervene or not.

In fact, three factors are taken into account: the patient's goals, the intake interview and the tests. If these three match up, we will surely make progress just by exercising listening. Let's take an example: a patient comes in and asks us to solve his gastritis problem, because a friend of his did Tomatis and it went away. He has a long history of stomach pain and the test confirms this, showing a disturbance in the 1,000 Hz region, in both ears. What do we do? Very simple: refer him to a gastroenterologist. He is not a candidate for the therapy.

However, if the objective of this same patient was to refine his musical ear, we might hear him say in his sessions that he has changed his way of eating, that he now prefers healthier, lighter meals, that he no longer gets irritated so easily at work, etc., and his gastritis could well improve, indirectly.

WHAT USUALLY HAPPENS

What can we expect after the therapy?

In relation to hearing tests, a better audiometric curve, with smoothed out peaks and scotomas and a more harmonious structure: getting closer to the ideal curve. Blockages (distortions and errors of spatialization, selectivity or left-ear laterality) gradually disappear. I should emphasize here that the therapy will not be able to cure hearing loss except in very special cases. We will see changes in the audiometric profile, but HAIC levels will hardly vary.

In terms of patient experience, the following positive changes tend to be observed.

- Desire to communicate and enjoy socializing
- Enjoyment of music
- Oral expression: ability to find the right words, and control prosody.
- Voice quality, tunefulness and an ear for music or languages
- Posture: walking more upright without realizing it.
- Feeling energetic, eager to work and take on challenges.
- Alertness, rapid reasoning and effective memory.

Patients also report sleeping better and feeling calmer, not so overwhelmed by small daily problems, which are signs of progressive vagal activation.

The autonomic nervous system conditions the audiometric profile. It makes sense for damage caused by stress in the structure of the neurons of the auditory system to be reflected in the audiometric test.[557] Stressed people who live most of the time in sympathicotonia show curves full of distortions, while those who face the ups and downs of life calmly, exhibit uniform ones. The therapy developed by Tomatis addresses this sympathetic–parasympathetic dynamic, favoring an equilibrium, which explains the multiple benefits observed.

In childhood, the parasympathetic is activated by our mothers. Both their voice and being rocked in their arms relax us.[558,559] When we are adults, we look for the same thing: therapies to activate the vagus nerve, to calm down and feel better. Analgesics and tranquilizers are the best-selling drugs and Spain is a world leader in per capita consumption of these: an unequivocal sign that we are failing to maintain good health.

Tomatis's techniques access the parasympathetic system through the ear, where the vagus nerve spreads out wide. On the basis of other theories, the same effect is being explored. Vagal stimulation from the external ear has been proposed as a therapy for heart conditions: modulating blood pressure and heartbeat.[560,561] The device developed

---

[557] See note 183

[558] See note 514

[559] *Impact of cocooning and maternal voice on the autonomic nervous system activity in the premature newborn infant.* **Alexandre, C. et al.** 9, 2013, Arch Pediatr., Vol. 20, pp. 963-8.

[560] *Messages from the auricle: Limiting progression of heart failure with preserved ejection fraction through transcutaneous nerve stimulation of nerves in the external ear.* **Deuchars, S.A. and Deuchars, J.** 2019, Experimental Physiology, Vol. 104, pp. 11-12.

by Porges works in a similar way. He has also found the entrance
door to be in the ear.

THE THERAPY: HOW IT WORKS

Tomatis therapy aims to lead the patient towards more efficient
listening through auditory conditioning. A device called the electronic
ear insistently offers a better listening option. After many repetitions,
the audiometric curve looks more and more like that proposed by the
device.

The hearing system has great plasticity. Musicians are studied by
neurologists due to their ability to generate changes in the brain in a
very short time, for example, increasing the size of the corpus
callosum.[562] This plasticity also encompasses subcortical areas.
Brainstem response can be shaped through acoustic experience.[563]

Tomatis used to say that his therapy was nothing more than
gymnastics for the musculature of the middle ear. The muscles of the
hammer and stirrup behave like flexors and extensors. Changes in the
acoustic signal produced by the electronic ear can favor these auditory
exercises. As seen before (see Chapter 1), he had observed that the
best singers had audiograms approaching that of Caruso, while the
least gifted ones remained far from that model.

Tomatis's first intervention in his opera-singing patients consisted
of equalizing the sound, allowing them to compensate for the
frequency regions with scotomas in their audiometric curve.
Technically, this was quite a feat before 1950, when electronics was
taking its first steps.

The procedure proved to be effective in the consulting room. The
singers recovered the harmonics in their voices on listening to
themselves better but, once the headphones were removed, it was
back to square one. Obviously, they could not go on stage with
headphones on. Tomatis had to find a way to get permanent results, so
he designed a conditioning method.

The singers alternated between two listening modes: normal
(channel 1) and equalized with the appropriate corrections (channel

---

[561] *The strange case of the ear and the heart: the auricular vagus nerve and its influence
on cardiac control.* **Murray, A. et al.** Autonomic Neuroscience: Basic and Clinical, Vol.
199, pp. 48-53.

[562] *Musicians and music making as a model for the study of brain plasticity.* **Schlaug, G.**
2015, Prog Brain Res., Vol. 217, pp. 37-55.

[563] *The scalp-recorded brainstem response to speech: Neural origins and plasticity.*
Chandrasekaran, B. and Kraus, N. 2010, Psychophysiology, Vol. 47, pp. 236-246.

2), by means of a manually operated switch. Just before singing a long, sustained note, they went from channel 1 to channel 2. From that moment, Tomatis began to observe an effect of remanence. In this way, the ear accepted the new way of listening proposed by channel 2.

Advances in technology later allowed the construction of the first electronic ear, in which this alternation from channel 1 to channel 2 took place automatically, thanks to the diode. Electronic ears continued to develop until bone conduction was added in the 1970s. This was a major step which reduced the time needed for therapy. The headphones have a vibrator on the top, plus side speakers.

The incorporation of bone conduction derives from Tomatis's theoretical conception of the mechanisms of hearing. To recap, according to him, sound travels to the inner ear through bone, from the tympanic ring, not through the ossicular chain. He bases his therapy on this: first sending the signal via bone conduction, and then by air.

The therapy consists of a passive phase of listening, and then an active one of reading and singing, in order to incorporate everything assimilated in the auditory re-education into the audio-vocal circuit. I attach great importance to this final stage, in which the patient's own voice is worked on by means of the electronic ear. I do not limit it to just reading exercises. My patients are surprised when I ask them to sing and move rhythmically. The positive psychological effects that occur after an excellent active phase are tremendous. The change is radical.

One of my colleagues, Mari Cruz Domínguez, a hearing and language specialist, has contributed new elements to the design of the active phase of the therapy developed by Tomatis, thanks to the years she has spent studying singing technique in depth. She works with her daughter Alba, a psychologist, in her center in Madrid.

The channels

The electronic ear is equipped with two filters, a low pass in channel 1 and a high pass in channel 2, both of 6 dB/octave slope and cut-off frequency at 1,000 Hz:

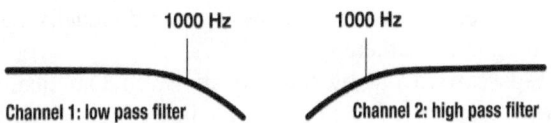

1000 Hz   1000 Hz

Channel 1: low pass filter   Channel 2: high pass filter

We listen through channel 1 and, starting from a certain volume, on channel 2:

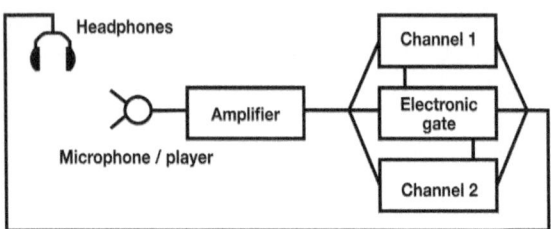

In the electronic ear, the switch from channel 1 to 2 is not immediate. It happens first via bone conduction and, after a set time (precession), via air conduction, following this sequence:

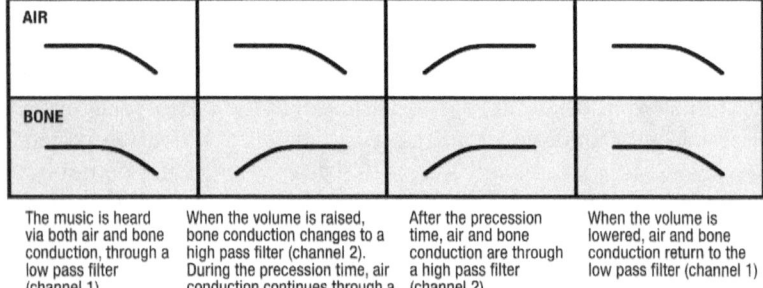

| The music is heard via both air and bone conduction, through a low pass filter (channel 1) | When the volume is raised, bone conduction changes to a high pass filter (channel 2). During the precession time, air conduction continues through a low pass filter (channel 1) | After the precession time, air and bone conduction are through a high pass filter (channel 2) | When the volume is lowered, air and bone conduction return to the low pass filter (channel 1) |

The equipment has also a set of high pass filters with different cut-off frequencies and a slope of 48 dB per octave, to work on specific areas of the auditory spectrum. They act on both channels in a stable fashion.

Precession

The most commonly used precession time is 250 msec, but this has varied as we have gained more experience with the therapy. In general, the more difficulties our patient presents, the longer the precession will be, but each case is assessed individually and is also modified throughout the therapy.

Brain maps carried out by the Mozart Brain Lab Institute have shown that precession is linked to the latency of the P300, the brain wave that indicates that the sound has already reached our level of consciousness and which, as its name suggests, appears around 300 msec after the stimulus. In my opinion, the value of precession is also related to the reaction time of the stirrup muscle, the stapedial reflex, whose latency is approximately the same.

Mozart is unique

The music that patients listen to during therapy is mainly Mozart. Gregorian chants are also used. Mozart has ideal characteristics due to its unpredictability and rich harmonies. Tomatis was questioned so much about this topic that he finally wrote a book exclusively dedicated to the great composer.[564] Much has been written about the possible benefits of Mozart's music. For example, some of his works reduce epileptic seizures in children.[565]

Copying nature

Tomatis therapy tries to reproduce the same sequence that children follow in their auditory development. In the first phase, the patient is gradually led towards exposure to treble sounds, eliminating the bass notes in the Mozart piece through the 48 dB/octave high-pass filters of the electronic ear. This phase is called *musical sonic feedback* (RSM in its French initials).

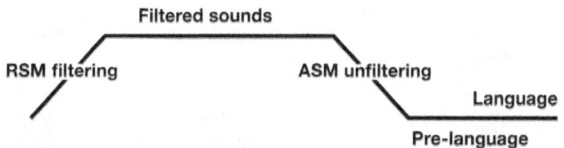

The second phase involves working with music by Mozart again or with the maternal voice, with high pass filters, emulating intrauterine listening. The third phase, contrary to the first, takes the patient back to unfiltered listening (*ASM phase,* from its initials in French, or *sonic birth*). Finally, there are sessions focused on language: the *pre-language* and *language* phases.

All this constitutes a recapitulation in a few weeks of the maturation process of the ear, according to Tomatis. In the future we may find new ways to sequence the therapy but when structured in this way it is very effective.

---

[564] **Tomatis, A.** *Pourquoi Mozart.* Paris : Fixot, 1991.

[565] *Mozart's music in children with epilepsy.* **Lin, Lung-Chang and Yang, Rei-Cheng.** 4, 2015, Translational Pediatrics, Vol. 4.

From the patient's perspective, the music they listen to is increasingly distorted (RSM phase), to a point that it is hard to identify it (filtered sound phase). Then it is heard better and better (ASM phase) until it is heard normally (pre-language and language phases).

The electronic ears developed in Belgium, can regulate the slope of the high pass filters of channels 1 and 2. If it was previously set at 6 dB/octave, it can now be applied at 12 and 18 dB/octave. This is a way of adjusting the intensity of auditory training.

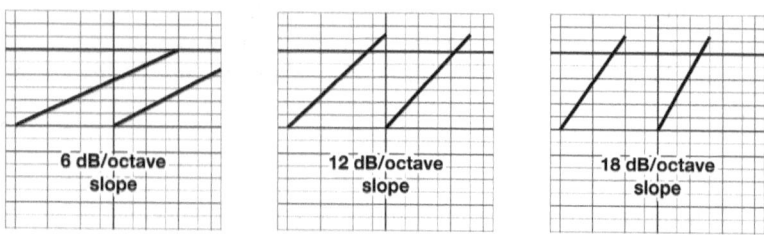

It is also possible to change the rotation point, previously always fixed at 1,000 Hz, by moving it to other frequencies, which allows the therapy to be adjusted precisely:

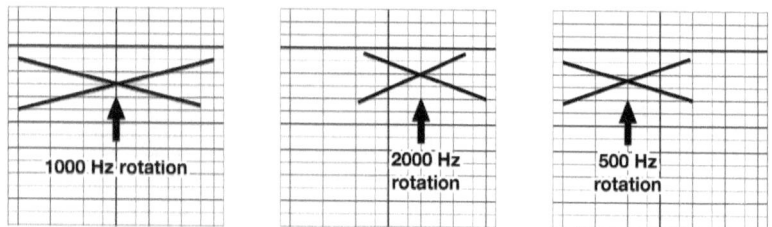

THE PRESENT AND FUTURE OF THE THERAPY

Since Tomatis passed away, several companies have started marketing devices based on his ideas. There is a wide variety of designs and prices. Which one should we choose? The therapist should know how to measure the acoustic parameters and verify the quality, and this needs to be repeated every so often to make sure the material being used with patients is fit for purpose: emitting the correct audio signal.

With the advent of music informatics and digital sound editing, the technical possibilities have become virtually infinite. It is like having an electronic ear with all imaginable settings, while costs have fallen substantially. Pandora's Box has been opened. Sound editing is allowing us to fine-tune therapy more and more, adapting it completely to the characteristics of the patient.

Among my colleagues, opinions are divided on these new possibilities. Some centers prefer to remain faithful to the original model. They distrust technical advances, such as the miniaturization of equipment, which offer great advantages, but can subvert the therapy and turn it into something that does not even come close to a proper therapeutic process. Others are committed to seizing the opportunities that today's technology makes available to them. The debate is still on.

I have spent many hours in the recording studio, conducting all sorts of tests with the help of a sound technician, thanks to which I have made minor changes to the therapy, trying to imagine what Tomatis would have done with today's technical marvels. Some of these innovations have worked very well and I have shared them with other colleagues, who have achieved similar results.

I respect all ideas that focus primarily on how best to help our patients. Technological progress is unstoppable, but we do need to steer it in the right direction, taking cautious steps, but always forward. Whatever the case, we must never lose sight of the fact that our job is more than just connecting the patient to a machine. Electronics is not the therapy: it is just one more tool in the hands of the therapist, who continues to be the decisive factor. Our training, our passion, our desire to help will be crucial to the final result.

Tomatis had sound knowledge of music, audiology and psychology. We need therapists capable of integrating these subjects with new technologies, within the framework of audio-psycho-phonology. Not everybody is willing to make such a great effort, so "express" training courses are more popular. Due to commercial pressure, it is very easy to acquire an electronic ear or a similar device and turn into a therapist in a few days, which is worrying, as it undermines the good reputation of our work. Fortunately, there are still many responsible professionals who seek training of high quality. In both Belgium and Spain this can be found.[566]

---

[566] De Voigt, op.cit. 5

OTHER HEARING THERAPIES

Tomatis immediately had to face competition. There are several hearing therapies based on his work, the best known of which is the Bérard method. Bérard was a physician who, having worked in Cambodia, returned to France in search of a solution to his tinnitus at the hands of Tomatis. He then went back to university and specialized in otolaryngology, developing a device very similar to Tomatis's: the earducator®. This device follows the same principles as the electronic ear, with channel switching, although technically it is much simpler. It has no bone conduction.

Bérard's technique (AIT: auditory integration training) was very successful in the USA and then in Europe. An eleven-year-old girl, Georgianna Stehli, came out of her autism after undergoing it and her mother published a book in appreciation that became a bestseller in the USA,[567] and made him famous. He recently passed away, but there is still an international association of practitioners of this therapy. There is an inaccurate article on internet stating that Bérard ended his working relationship with Tomatis because the latter accused the mothers of autistic children of being responsible for their condition. I believe this to be absolutely false. I never heard Tomatis say any such thing.

Although other hearing therapies have had less impact in Spain, the list is a long one: Johansen, Hemi-Sync, Interactive metronome, Samonas, Bioacoustics, Earobics, and many more. I am struck by the fact that most of them only take air conduction into account, whereas my own and my colleagues' experience constantly reveals the importance of bone conduction. There is a lack of scientific studies to support these therapies. They are patented by private companies, which usually operate as franchises and do not share their knowledge easily, to avoid plagiarism. Actually, it is common to find therapists applying these techniques who are almost totally unaware of their mechanism of action. They have received general training in the use of the equipment and little more. We have already seen that the connection between the nervous and auditory systems is a profound one. Any such therapy should be used by qualified personnel.

As the physicist Michio Kaku states: *"If you do not share knowledge, it is useless"*.[568] I would like information to flow freely, in

[567] **Stehli, A.** *Sound of a Miracle.* New York : Beaufort books, 1995.
[568] **Kaku, M.** Si no compartes el conocimiento, no sirva para nada. *BBVA, Aprendemos Juntos.* s.l. : https://www.youtube.com/watch?v=6rDxlolYUQw, 2019.

the public domain and available to universities for research purposes. I am convinced that, in this way, some of these techniques could be brought into the scientific fold, which would, in turn, help their practitioners to be given proper training.

THE POWER OF MUSIC

Kraus and her team have demonstrated the benefits that come with musical learning.[569] It is the great power of music, which activates our whole brain. One of my patients showed me how powerful a tool music really is. In this case, it was during a session of EMDR, a technique widely used to treat post-traumatic stress.[570] It is a therapy based on bilateral stimulation of both brain hemispheres, which is generally achieved through the visual pathway. However, it is also possible to apply EMDR by means of auditory or tactile stimuli.

The case of Natalia

When I met Natalia, she was 35. A woman who was full of curiosity, enterprising, likeable... but with a problem: she was unable to write. As soon as she tried, a tremor took hold of her hand and the handwriting was illegible. However, she could type on the computer perfectly well.

Natalia enjoyed a pleasant life, but suffered the consequences of a troubled past: living with her first husband, an obsessive, jealous man who watched over her every move, had taken an emotional toll on her. She had to endure his demeaning comments until the very day of their divorce. When she went to sign, she noticed that her hand was shaking and from then on, every time she tried to write, all she could manage was a scrawl. The years passed and she happily renewed her life with a wonderful new partner, but her hand kept remembering, every time she held a pen.

In the first EMDR session, she described to me a sad scene that she immediately related to a song she used to listen to at that time in her life, the lyrics of which portrayed her own feelings quite well.

For the next appointment, based on the clues she had given me, I prepared a somewhat atypical EMDR protocol, alternating auditory

---

[569] *Auditory Training: Evidence for Neural Plasticity in older adults.* **Anderson, S. and Kraus, N.** 1, May, 2013, Perspectives on Hearing and Hearing Disorders Research and Diagnostics, Vol. 17, pp. 37-57.

[570] **Shapiro, F.** *Emdr: Desensibilización y Reprocesamiento por medio de Movimiento Ocular.* Mexico : Editorial Pax Mexico, 2004.

stimulation with that special song. She soon entered a state of total abreaction, shedding tears and sobbing for a long time. At that moment, Natalia emptied herself of grief, literally.
She finally calmed down. We exchanged a few words. She took a pen and a piece of paper and started writing. She did it normally, as if nothing had ever happened. That moment was a great gift for both of us, an indescribable experience. From then on, her tremors ceased. Sometimes, on meeting again, she would say: "Look at my hand,", and write something with a smile on her face.

According to the great researcher Gottfried Schlaug, there is no human activity capable of involving as many brain areas at once as playing a musical instrument.[571] Similarly, Zatorre states: "The regions of the cortex that are activated when we listen to music are the same as when we imagine something".[572]

Audio-psycho-phonology also tells us that the auditory curves are plastic and modifiable by conditioning (within certain limits). This could have immediate applications, for example, in hearing-aid adjustment or prevention of deafness.

Hearing aids are a great help and contribute to brain plasticity,[573] but they are not always the definitive solution. Listening often remains difficult, requiring further assistance from an audiologist trained in auditory rehabilitation, a discipline that does not yet formally exist, but whose implementation should be considered.[574]

MUSIC AND HEALTH

All known cultures sing and dance. Even the Bible emphasizes the power of sound, when it says that "…in the beginning was the Word, and the Word was with God, and the Word was God" (John 1:1). Throughout history, music has accompanied humankind in all its solemn ceremonies, including rituals to regain health. It is the great anthropological common denominator, along with language. Our Western civilization, however, is displacing music and dance from

---

[571] *Keeping brains young with making music.* **Rogenmoser, L. et al.** Aug, 2017, Brain Struct Funct.

[572] **Estapé, N.** http://www.madrimasd.org/canales/salud-biomedicina /tendencias/la-musica-es-el-lenguaje-del-cerebro. [Online] 2013.

[573] *Acoustic Experience Alters the Aged Auditory System.* **Turner, J.G. et al.** 2, 2013, Ear Hear., Vol. 34, pp. 151-159.

[574] *The Ear–Brain Connection:Older Ears and Older Brains.* **Tremblay, K.L.** June, 2015, American Journal of Audiology, Vol. 24, pp. 117-120.

everyday life, turning them into mere spectacles. We are depriving the ear of much of its natural training. Could that have anything to do with the rise in learning and behavior problems we are seeing?

The combination of music and science has become popular. A few years ago, National Geographic published a wonderful report entitled *My Musical Brain*, in which the singer Sting collaborates with Levitin, one of the most renowned scientists in this field and who, in his youth, was a musician and producer.

Music, apart from offering undeniable aesthetic pleasure, is very beneficial to health. The Greeks themselves used it for medical purposes. It is universal: there are peoples who lack writing or mathematics, but singing and dancing are always present. Sound and motor skills, cochlea and vestibule together. Popular culture reflects the power of music and the therapeutic effects of sound in legends like the Pied Piper of Hamelin and sayings like "Sing your troubles away".

Samuel A. Mehr and his team try to understand what music is and provide some answers. They have found transcultural patterns, both rhythmic and melodic, adapted to specific social contexts. All human groups share common musical structures.[575]

Until the advent of psychotropic drugs, music therapy was the main tool for treating mental illness. Then, it was relegated by chemistry. However, recent research techniques have rediscovered its great therapeutic value. Hundreds of works on music therapy are published every year. Its beneficial effect on the nervous system is extraordinary. Stefan Mainka says: "*Music stimulates muscles, mind and feelings in one go.*" [576]

Singing has remarkable positive effects. It has been shown to be useful in rehabilitation of brain injuries, Parkinson's disease, autism, palliative care, etc. It generates changes in the neural networks, in the pulmonary system and in the cardiovascular system by modulating the heartbeat.[577] Professional singers show these benefits when compared to amateurs.[578]

---

[575] *Universality and diversity in human song.* **Mehr, S.A. et al.** 970, Nov 22, 2019, Science, Vol. 366.

[576] *Music stimulates muscles,mind,and feelings in one go.* **Mainka, S.** 1547, 2015, Frontiers in psychology, Vol. 6.

[577] *Music structure determines heart rate variability of singers.* **Vickhoff, B. et al.** 334, 2013, Frontiers in psychology, Vol. 4.

[578] *The terapeutic effects of singing in neurological disorders.* **Wan, C.Y. et al.** 4, 2010, Music Perception, Vol. 27, pp. 287-295.

Music lowers blood pressure in hypertensive patients and decreases anxiety before and after entering the operating theater,[579] reducing blood cortisol levels even better than tranquilizers and alleviating postoperative pain.[580]

Today, music and medicine come together in one of the most promising lines of research: brain plasticity. Neuroscientists have discovered in music a true experimental treasure. It activates the whole brain and, its learning, causes visible changes in a short time. The cerebellum grows, as do the auditory areas and the corpus callosum. Connections multiply. In the words of Koelsch, a music researcher at the Free University of Berlin: "Music can profoundly change the brain".[581] The pianist James Rhodes is a good example, as he explains in his autobiography.[582] Music saved his life.

This plasticity does not only occur in childhood. Adults who attend music classes also do well. Gottfried Schlaug believes that learning an instrument acts as brain gymnastics; it is ideal for rehabilitation and for keeping us functionally young.[583,584] In cognitive tests, musicians tend to outperform non-musicians almost always[585] obtaining results that correspond to younger people.[586]

Music shares its neural circuits with other functions, hence its broad influence.[587] The following quotation, from Fukui and Toyoshima, citing Abbott (2002), sums up the effect of music on our neurons very well:

"The most important finding has been that music improves synaptic changes in the brain. In other words, studies comparing musicians and non-musicians and music students and novices have made it clear that music causes brain plasticity. Music affects neural

---

[579] *The effects of music on the cardiovascular system and cardiovascular health.* **Trappe, H.J.** 2010, Heart, Vol. 96, pp. 1868-1871.

[580] *Effect of Music on Postoperative Pain in Patients Under Open Heart Surgery.* **Mirbagher Ajorpaz, N. et al.,** 3, 2014, Nurs Midwifery Stud., Vol. 3.

[581] **Sanchís, I.** La música puede variar profundamente el cerebro. *La Vanguardia.* Aug 17, 2011.

[582] **Rhodes, J.** *Instrumental.* s.l. : Titivillus, 2018.

[583] See note 480

[584] *Music Making as a Tool for Promoting Brain Plasticity across the Life Span.* **Wan, C.Y. and Schlaug, G.** 5, 2010, The Neuroscientist, Vol. 16.

[585] *The Relation Between Instrumental Musical Activity and Cognitive Aging.* **Hanna-Pladdy, B. and MacKay, A.** 3, 2011, Neuropsychology, Vol. 25.

[586] See note 571

[587] See note 275

learning and readjustment (response of brain cells to sound and musical stimuli, and changes in cell counts), and this effect lasts".[588]

The neural networks involved in music are widely shared with those of language.[589] Musical networks encompass the linguistic ones, so musicians have certain advantages when acquiring a new language.[590]

The changes caused by musical learning mitigate cognitive decline.[591] Such is its might, that it even raises some fears. Levitin, for example, makes this confession:

"Wagner has always disturbed me profoundly, and not just his music, but also the idea of listening to it. I feel reluctant to give in to the seduction of music created by so disturbed a mind and so dangerous (or impenetrably hard) a heart as his, for fear that I might develop some of the same ugly thoughts".[592]

In a scene in the documentary The Musical Brain, Sting also feels uncomfortable. He tells Levitin he does not want to hear any more about his brain in relation to music. He fears the magic will vanish and inspiration will abandon him.

Music has even been found to affect our genome. We do not know what research in this field will bring, but it could be a genuine revolution. When we listen to it, we trigger the activation of certain genes. The action of sound goes deep.[593]

Plants also react to sounds.[594] It is an exciting field of study. I have always wondered what the objective is, what evolutionary advantage this acoustic sensitivity gives them. Part of the explanation (though I suspect the best is yet to be discovered) is that the leaves respond to vibration, like our skin. When an insect eats

---

[588] **Fukui, H. and Toyoshima, K.** *Music and Steroids – Music Facilitates Steroid–Induced Synaptic Plasticity.* s.l. : Nara University of Education.

[589] *Modularity of music processing.* **Peretz, I. and Coltheart, M.** 7, 2003, Nature Neuroscience, Vol. 6.

[590] *Musical expertise and foreign speech perception.* **Martínez-Montes, E. et al.** 84, 2013, Frontiers in Systems Neuroscience, Vol. 7.

[591] See note 448

[592] **Levitin, D.J.** *Tu cerebro y la música.* s.l. : RBA, 2015.

[593] *The effect of listening to music on human transcriptome.* **Kanduri, C. et al.** 830, PeerJ, Vol. 3.

[594] *Effect of Music on Plants – An Overview.* **Roy Chowdhury, A. and Gupta, A.** 6, 2015, International Journal of Integrative Sciences, Innovation and Technology (IJIIT), Vol. 4, pp. 30-34.

them, they pick up the vibration produced and secrete defensive chemicals in response.[595]

In Tel-Aviv, Israel, they have managed to record the "cries" of plants such as tobacco or tomato, under different environmental conditions. They "cry out" in the ultrasonic band (around 55,000 Hz) at considerable intensity (over 66 dB at a distance of 10 cm). The research identified some patterns in the sounds emitted: plants did not cry out in the same way when they lacked water as when they were cut. It is thought to be a form of communication with their fellows.[596]

Kraus recorded the brain waves of people listening to music, filtered out noise and passed them through an amplifier and a loudspeaker. We can recognize the original music on listening to the recording. It is awe-inspiring. See the experiment here:

Every time someone hears words, music or noise, their brain waves are modified, literally reflecting what they have heard. This is why sound is so important: it permanently shapes brain activity.

I wonder why we do not take advantage of music in hearing-aid clinics. Users are taught to sharpen their discrimination with hearing aids, using language, but no use is made of singing and movement, which would multiply the therapeutic possibilities. Of course, there is no need to turn our intervention into a spectacle, but we should capitalize on the knowledge that science is making available to us. If we want access to brain plasticity, we have to respect its rules.

Sudden onset of musical abilities after a stroke or severe trauma has been documented. It is something that baffles me because it implies they were there all the time, hidden behind a curtain of inhibitory processes blocking access to them. Oliver Sacks, the recently deceased popular psychiatrist, recounts some of these experiences: a doctor who suddenly developed excellent musical

---

[595] *Plants respond to leaf vibrations caused by insect herbivore chewing.* **Appel, H. M. and Cocroft, R.B.** 2014, Oecologia, Vol. 175, pp. 1257-1266.

[596] *Plants emit informative airborne sounds under stress.* **Khait, I. et al.** Tel-Aviv : s.n., Dec 2, 2019, BioRxiv. peer reviewed.

skills as a result of trauma, or the case of Rolf Silber, who after suffering a cerebral hemorrhage began to understand and enjoy music as never before. However, as he recovered and regained language, he lost his new faculties.[597]

Another amazing phenomenon is the sudden onset of synesthesia, associated with vision loss. Some patients tell of seeing music in color. Listening to an orchestra becomes a pictorial work. Those hearing–vision connections were already there, in the brain. They could not have formed that quickly. The trauma was just the trigger.

The great musical pedagogue Paulo Lameiro affirms that our greatest auditory capacity appears at birth and on our death.[598] Children's songs are the last thing people with neurodegenerative disorders forget. For some reason, they leave an indelible mark. Parkinson's patients who are unable to start walking are able to do so if we mark time for them or the beat of a familiar song. Sacks speaks of a pianist who was no longer able to hold a fork to eat and whose fingers, incredibly, still flitted precisely over the keyboard.

Neurons love music—at least according to Neysa Navarro's doctoral thesis.[599] She studied embryonic neural stem cells to find out if music had any effect on them. She left the cultures in three different situations: Mozart, noise and silence. After 24 hours, the cells that had reproduced the most were those that listened to Mozart. After three days, 65% of the cells kept in silence and 70% of those subjected to noise had survived, compared to over 80% among the Mozartians.

Many years before, Tomatis had also experimented with the effects of sound on cells:

"I noticed in the Aeronautical Arsenals that the employees who worked in horrifying hygienic conditions (the machines on which they worked continually spewed oil and dust straight into their faces) never had suppurations.

This phenomenon had intrigued me for some time when it occurred to me that environmental noise could have a destructive effect on microbes. Eager to verify this hypothesis, I bought some boxes of Petri tubes and exposed them in my laboratory to sounds sent by small speakers.

---

[597] **Sacks, O.** *Musicofilia.* Barcelona : Editorial Anagrama, 2009.

[598] **Sanchís, I.** Pañales, amor y música. *La Vanguardia.* Nov 15, 2019.

[599] **Navarro, N.** Caracterización y cuantificación de la influencia de la música como agente físico sobre el comportamiento de células madre neurales embrionarias en cultivo. [ed.] Universidad de Valladolid. *Doctoral thesis.* 2010.

The microbes all died as from 2,000 Hz, except for one: the Koch bacillus. It survived, but I soon realized that by sending it low-frequency emissions, it was prevented from reproducing. The sound was enough to disrupt their lives profoundly. Thus, sound was capable, either of killing microbes once and for all, or at least of preventing their proliferation". [600]

Ultrasounds are now a common method of sterilization. The original idea of using sound to kill microbes seems to be attributed to Royal Rife, a controversial American inventor whose life was plagued by strange circumstances.

---

[600] See note 3

EAR AND LEARNING

10

Processing speed is a fundamental parameter in the assessment of hearing. In a well-known experiment, Paula Tallal presented pairs of sounds, asking two groups of children to indicate which was the highest-pitched one: a similar test to the Tomatis selectivity test, but taking into account the time interval between the two stimuli (ISI: inter stimulus interval). She observed that dyslexic children performed the task as well as the others if the ISI was greater than 150 milliseconds.[601] If the sounds were presented too close together in time, they could not distinguish between them. She then adapted the experiment so that it could be performed on babies and, after monitoring them for several years, found that the test predicted which children might have language disorders in the future.

Several experiments, measuring the latency of brain waves, also coincide in highlighting the slow processing of acoustic signals in developmental language disorders,[602,603] specifically dyslexia. For example, a longer response time on wave P100[604] or on P300.[605]

[601] *Neural Mechanisms of Language-Based Learning Impairments: Insights From Human Populations and Animal Models.* **Fitch, R.H. and Tallal, P.** 3, 2003, Behavioral and Cognitive Neuroscience Reviews, Vol. 2

[602] *Early auditory evoked potentials in children with language development disorders.* **von Suchodoletz, W. and Wolfram, I.** 5, 1996, Klin Padiatr., Vol. 208, pp. 290-3.

[603] *Auditory Brainstem Responses of Children with Developmental Language Disorders.* **Roncagliolo, M. et al.** 1, 1994, Child Neurology, Vol. 36.

[604] *Auditory processing in the dyslexic brain.* **Reid, M. et al.** 2010. Proceedings of the 9th Conference of the Australasian Society for Cognitive Science.

[605] *Auditory evoked potentials: predicting speech therapy outcomes in children with phonological disorders.* **Leite, R.A. et al.** 12, 2014, /clinics/2014, Vol. 3.

These are indicators that can help us to monitor the progress of a therapy.

In the laboratory run by Nina Kraus they have come to the same conclusions. Dyslexic children react to sound a little later: a tiny fraction of time, but an age in terms of communication between neurons. Brainstem responses to sound are organized in predictable patterns, but bad readers present random responses.[606]

The opposite effect occurs in students who have received music classes. Their neurological responses to speech are faster. They process at higher speed,[607] lowering their reaction times.[608] Children with musical training do better on phonological and reading tests.[609] Some therapy programs make use of this link to treat dyslexia and other learning disorders, by including music as a part of the treatment.

THE VESTIBULAR SYSTEM AND DYSLEXIA

The literature emphasizes the relationship between dyslexia and disorders associated with vestibular and cerebellar function: motor skills, balance, muscle tone and rhythm. From its functions we could say that the cerebellum is the vestibular brain,[610] although it does have other responsibilities, such as managing the emotions.[611]

In 1979 the Spanish ENT physician, José Ramón Mozota (mentioned in Chapter 1), published *Chequeo a la dislexia.*[612] His work shows a great parallelism with Tomatis's ideas, highlighting that vestibular tests predict the future development of the dyslexic child.

The cerebellar hypothesis of dyslexia, by Fawcett and Nicolson of the University of Sheffield, published in 2001, is one of the most

---

[606] *Unstable Representation of Sound: A Biological Marker of Dyslexia.* **Hornickel, J. and Kraus, N.** 8, Feb 20, 2013, The Journal of Neuroscience, Vol. 33, pp. 3500-3504.

[607] *High school music classes enhance the neural processing of speech.* **Tierney, A. et al.** 855, 2013, Frontiers in Psychology, Vol. 4.

[608] *Effect of Music on Visual and Auditory Reaction Time: A Comparative Study.* **Prasad, B.K.** 1, 2014, Research and Reviews: Journal of Medical and Health Sciences, Vol. 3.

[609] *The relation between music and phonological processing in normal-reading children and children with dyslexia.* **Forgeard, M. et al.** 4, Music Perception, Vol. 25, pp. 383-390.

[610] *El cerebelo: su implicación en la dislexia.* **Fawcett, A. and Nicolson, R.** 2, 2007, Revista Electrónica de Investigación Psicoeducativa y Psicopedagógica, Vol. 2, pp. 35-58.

[611] *Affective communication deficits associated with cerebellar degeneration.* **Heilman, K.M. et al.** 1, 2014, Neurocase, Vol. 20, pp. 18-26.

[612] **Mozota, J.R.** *Chequeo a la dislexia.* [ed.] Universidad de Zaragoza Instituto de Ciencias de la Educación. Zaragoza : s.n., 1979.

respected ones today.[613] Mozota and Tomatis had already pointed in that direction 20 years earlier, and even they were not even the first. Two Argentinian researchers, Julio Bernaldo de Quirós and Orlando L. Schrager, realized that vestibular deficiencies were abundant among children with learning disabilities. In 1963 they studied 63 cases that presented difficulties in motor development and learning, speech and writing, without any apparent cause. They found abnormal vestibular responses in 52 of them.[614,615] The researchers observed two different syndromes characterized by the following.

1. Motor developmental delay, generalized hypotonia, and reflex alterations.
2. Mild hypotonia and motor clumsiness with frequent falls. At school, these children exhibited constant disinterest and restlessness. They could easily be labeled dyslexic or ADHD.

From 1958 to 1965 they monitored almost 2,000 children, half of them from birth, and observed that the vestibular assessment had predicted subsequent school performance very well. Children with an inefficient vestibule showed posture and muscle tone disorders and delayed motor development.

Another researcher, who has treated more than 20,000 cases of dyslexia and ADHD, is psychiatrist Harold Levinson. He soon realized that motor disorders were a common denominator in these patients. Since 1973 he has published articles and books supporting the hypothesis that both dyslexia and ADHD are vestibular dysfunctions in their origins.[616,617]

Putting his ideas into practice, Levinson treats dyslexia with drugs that regulate vestibular activity, such as motion sickness pills, for which he claims a very high success rate in his books. I am not enthusiastic about using medication if we can regulate the vestibular

---

[613] See note 610

[614] **De Quirós, J.B y Schrager, O.L.** Lenguaje, aprendizaje y psicomotricidad. Buenos Aires : Editorial Médica Panamericana, 1987.

[615] **De Quirós, J.B. et al.** El lenguaje lectoescrito y sus problemas. Buenos Aires : Editorial Médica Panamericana, 1987.

[616] Dramatic Favorable Responses of Children with Learning Disabilities or Dyslexia and Attention Deficit Disorder to Antimotion Sickness Medications: Four Case Reports. **Levinson, H.N.** 3, 1991, Perceptual and motor skills, Vol. 73, pp.723-738.

[617] **Levinson, H.N.** Understanding Attention Deficit Disorder. New York : MJF Books, 1990.

system through exercises, but Levinson's work is capital to understanding the link between learning and hearing system.

French ophthalmologist Patrick Quercia specialized in the treatment of dyslexia, looking for a solution for his son. At first he focused on the visual system, but was unable to solve the disorder. He found the answer thanks to posturology. He states that dyslexia is a sensory dysfunction, a proprioceptive one, which is expressed in the posture, and usually involves the vestibular system.[618] Mouth, sight and hearing form a functional unit, and dyslexia should be treated from this perspective. For example, slight changes in the oral cavity structure can lead to auditory and visual disfunctions.

I do not want to close this chapter without citing Jean Ayres, the creator of sensory integration therapy, and neurosurgeon Temple Fay, whose students Doman and Delacato created a well-known stimulation method. No one has better understood the role of the vestibular system as a neurological harmonizer. They laid the foundations for many of the motor therapies we find today, making us understand the importance of motor skills in the configuration of the nervous system.[619,620] I have had the pleasure of meeting several of the physicians who introduced their work into Spain (J. Moya, V. Casaprima, J. Catalán, J. Ferrer and J. Mombiela).

ANCIENT WISDOM

Plato himself observed the benefits of movement in infancy, which is ultimately a vestibular training, and therefore auditory. In *The Laws*, he explains how an ideal city should work and writes the following in relation to the education of newborns:

*"Let us assume, then, as a first principle in relation both to the body and soul of very young creatures, that nursing and moving about by day and night is good for them all, and that the younger they are, the more they will need it; **infants should live, if that were possible, as if they were always being rocked by the sea** [bold type added]. This is the lesson which we may gather from the experience of nurses [...] for*

---

[618] See note 76

[619] Review *Study on Effect of Stimulation of Vestibular Apparatus on Postural Muscle Tone in Cerebral Palsy.* **Mittal, R. and Narkeesh, A.** 1, 2012, Journal of Exercise Science and Physiotherapy, Vol. 8.

[620] *Estimulación vestibular en Educación Infantil.* **Lázaro, A.** 22,2, 2008, Revista Interuniversitaria de Formación del Profesorado, Vol. 62, pp. 165-174.

when mothers want their restless children to go to sleep they do not employ rest, but, on the contrary, motion-rocking them in their arms [...]"

Plato was no doubt a great observer. He intuitively understood the advantages of vestibular activation in childhood. If the ear does not work well, the information that reaches the brain in relation to the body (limb position, muscle tone, etc.) is poor and requires constant help from other brain areas to compensate for this deficit, hindering learning. Poor posture is also a huge drain on energy, as the anti-gravitational muscles are continually making unnecessary efforts.

LEARNING TO TALK

We know the importance of hearing for language development. That is why we rush to intervene in deaf children, adapting hearing aids or cochlear implants. Beyond hearing impairment, though, scant attention is given to other factors that define the quality of listening and impact, for example, learning at school.

These notions still sound strange to audiology and psychology practitioners. Tomatis's work is not widely known and the evaluation of central auditory processing (APD) is still in its infancy.

A study by an international team, led by Chiara Cantiani,[621] helps us to understand the basis of language. They analyzed the ability of 6-month-old infants to quickly discriminate the duration and frequency of sound by presenting stimuli and monitoring their EEG brain waves. The data confirmed, as previous studies indicated,[622] that the ability to analyze sounds rapidly (e.g., distinguishing phoneme "b" from "p") makes it possible to predict which children will later have language disorders.[623] It is a skill that is born in the brainstem itself and which can determine auditory laterality depending on which hemisphere is faster at processing sound.[624]

---

[621] *Auditory discrimination predicts linguistic outcome in Italian infants with and without familial risk for language learning impairment.* **Cantiani, C. et al.** 20, 2016, Developmental Cognitive Neuroscience, pp. 23-24.

[622] *Infant discrimination of rapid auditory cues predicts later language impairment.* **Benasich, A.A. and Tallal, P.** 136(1), Oct, 2002, Behav Brain Res., pp. 31-49.

[623] *Deficits in speech perception predict language learning impairment.* **Ziegler, J.C. et al.** 39, Sept, 2005, PNAS, Vol. 102, pp. 14110–14115.

[624] *Auditory Brainstem Timing Predicts Cerebral Asymmetry for Speech.* **Abrams, D.A., Trent Nicol, S., Zecker, G. Kraus, N.** 26(43), Evanston : s.n., Oct, 2006, The Journal of Neuroscience, págs. 11131-11137.

The speed of acoustic analysis is a parameter that is independent of the auditory threshold, but equally necessary for good listening. When we are not proficient in a language, we ask our interlocutors to speak to us slowly. If we are slower at listening than our interlocutors are at speaking, we cannot follow the conversation. This is what happens to some children with language disorders.[625]

Advanced phonetics shows us the importance of auditory processing speed. Thanks to this discipline, we know that we recognize consonants by the acoustic characteristics of the adjacent vowels, which are modified according to the preceding or subsequent consonant. The very name suggests this relationship: "con-sonants", that is, those that accompany sounds.

A vowel is defined acoustically by a set of frequencies whose intensity stands out above the rest: the formants. We distinguish between "ba" and "da" because each "a" sound has different formants when we start pronouncing it, since the phonatory organs are in a different position. In "b" the lips are together and the tongue is low down. In "d" the lips are parted and the tongue touches the lower palate.

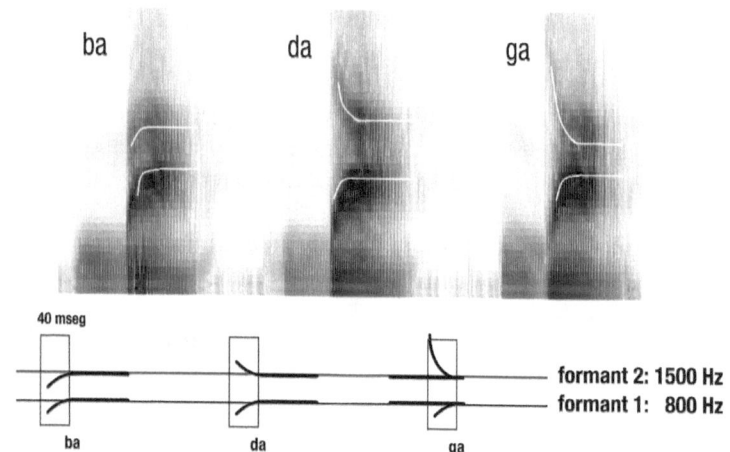

During a short period of time (transient, about 40 msec, the "a" changes until it presents its characteristic formants. We identify "b" and "d", not by their individual sound, but by the transition of the "a", which differs according to the preceding consonant. This takes place

---

[625] *Don't speak too fast! Processing of fast rate speech in children with specific language impairment.* **Guiraud, H. et al.** s.l. : Sonja Kotz, Max Planck Institute for Human Cognitive and Brain Sciences, Germany, Jan, 2018, Plos One.

in a very short time, so we need the hearing system to work at high speed.

If we observe the first two formants of the vowel "a", located about 800 and 1,500 Hz respectively, when pronouncing the syllables "ba", "da", "ga", we see that they are equal at the end, but not at the beginning. In "ba", both the first and the second formant ascend at first. In "da", the first ascends and the second descends. In "ga" the formants are similar, with a steeper descent in the second formant:

The position of the tongue and mouth is different in each case, conditioning the initial frequency and shape of the transition, until the formants are stabilized. This is the key that allows us to distinguish between the three consonants and we do it in those brief 40 msec.

One way to prove this empirically is to suppress the consonant segment, the plosive bar that precedes the vowel:

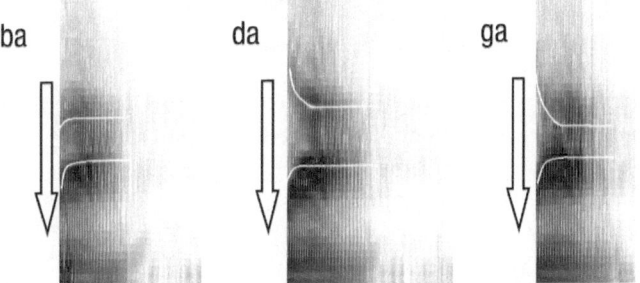

We hear it again and... Nothing has changed! We keep hearing "ba, da, ga". We can hear the consonant just from the vowel segment.

But, if we take off the transients, even if we leave the consonants' bars, we will hear something like "ba-ba-ba". The same syllable, three times:

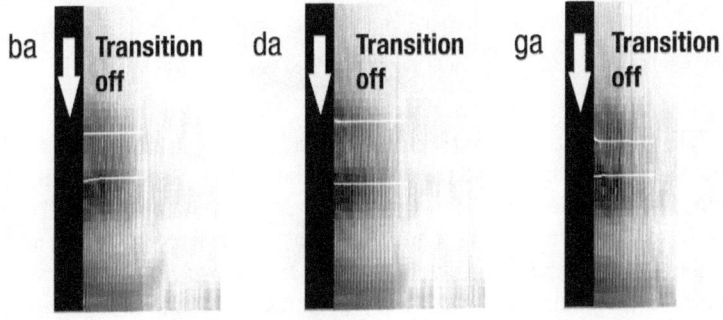

No formant transition: no information about consonants.

We can make fun experiments out of this phenomenon. By minimally manipulating the sound, we will get a person to say something that they never really pronounced. This is the sonogram of the word "say":

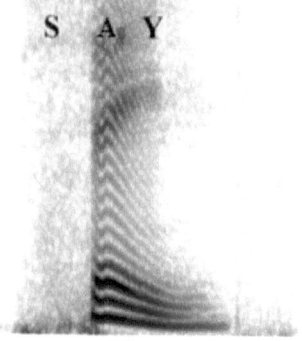

The three segments "s", "a" and "y" are perfectly identifiable. If we insert a silence of about 40 ms between the "s" and the "a", it should sound "s____ay". However, when we hear it, we clearly hear "stay". A "t" has magically appeared:

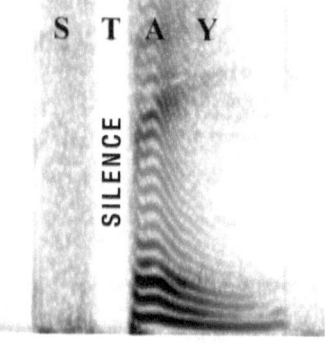

That is because the transient of the "a" is similar after both the "s" and the "t" (tongue and lips are in the same place), but the "t" completely hinders the passage of air for a few milliseconds. By inserting a silence, our brain interprets that the absence of sound, added to the form of the transient, can only correspond to the "t", so we perceive the consonant even if we have not pronounced it. The brain makes up the "t", providing a logical solution to an acoustic dilemma.

Tallal has shown that dyslexic children process slowly and need more than 40 msec to identify consonants. When artificially lengthening the transition time, understanding improves.[626] The *Fast For Word* auditory training program developed by her works this way. EEG records of dyslexic subjects also show a slower response, according to Nina Kraus. Her work points in the same direction as Tallal's.[627]

Children who have trouble understanding in noisy environments may later have problems learning to read.[628] Porges claims that distinguishing the signal from background noise is not just a matter of hearing, but involves the entire autonomic nervous system. According to him, when our vagal system is stressed and we remain on almost constant alert, we trigger defensive responses that prevent the attenuation of noise. Porges highlights that this characteristic is common in different mental disorders. Patients always try to avoid noisy places.[629]

In learning disorders, we often find a slow and imprecise ear. The evidence is old, with references from over forty years ago,[630] but so far, little has been done about it from a practical point of view. Very few underachieving children receive a full auditory evaluation.

I do not mean that language skills depend exclusively on our auditory system. As a psychologist, I still believe that the quality of interactions with adults, especially the parents, makes the difference,[631] but we should make a more detailed assessment of hearing in clinical practice. When we say that a child hears correctly because his hearing thresholds are normal, we are making a partial assessment with a good chance of being wrong, especially if there are language development disorders.

We know that as from a certain degree of hearing loss, we have difficulty in understanding what is being said. Hearing-impaired children also develop speech disorders. Without good self-listening, the pronunciation of the phonemes becomes distorted.

---

[626] See note 227

[627] See note 606

[628] *Auditory Processing in Noise: A Preschool Biomarker for Literacy.* **White-Schwoch, T. et al.** July, 2015, Plos Biology.

[629] See note 151

[630] *An Experimental short form of the Staggered Spondaic Word List for learning disabled children.* **Young, E. and Tracy, J.** 1, 1976, Journal of the ARA, Vol. 9.

[631] *Quality of early parent input predicts child vocabulary 3 years later.* **Cartmilla, E.A. et al.** Dec, 2012, PNAS.

However, several studies show that the ability to listen does not depend only on auditory sensitivity. Some people with normal hearing feel that they have difficulty in hearing, especially because they find it hard to follow a conversation in the presence of noise. These are not isolated cases. About 20% of individuals who believe they have a hearing impairment have a normal audiogram.[632]

Tomatis adds another element to be taken into account: the shape of the audiometric curve. A high sensitivity profile in the bass range, with a drop in the language area or a zigzag curve can indicate difficulty in recognizing sounds quickly, even if there is no hearing loss. As we know, bass sounds have a masking effect, hindering the perception of high frequency sounds. This is a factor that should be considered in children being treated for speech disorders.

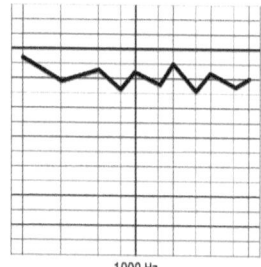 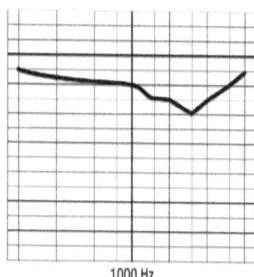

Curves associated with language disorders. On the left, descending curve in the language area. On the right, zigzag curve.

VISION AND HEARING

The case of Felipe

I persuaded my grandfather Felipe to do auditory therapy in a center in Barcelona when he was 89 years old. It was not difficult. He was bored at home and liked the idea of having a new daily occupation.

After a few weeks, he called me. He was overjoyed because his eyesight had greatly improved. He could read the main newspaper headlines: something he could not do months previously. When I went to see him, he rushed to give me a demonstration:

-Look, here it says...

---

[632] *Audiologic Considerations for People with Normal Hearing Sensitivity Yet Hearing Difficulty and/or Speech-in-Noise Problems.* **Beck, D.L.** **et al.** Oct, 2018, Hearing Review.

I do not know what eye-ear connections were reactivated, but I will never forget that phone call. Among other reasons, because I think it was the only one I ever got from him. My grandfather only ever used the phone to receive calls, so this was something very special. He left us at 102 years of age, so he did the therapy when he was still a youngster. Maybe that is why it was so effective.

The auditory system modifies visual perception and vice versa:[633] something to take very much into account when dealing with reading and writing issues. Many optometrists have taken an interest in auditory therapy for this very reason.

The well-known McGurk effect makes it clear that both systems interfere with each other. While watching somebody pronouncing certain phonemes on screen, we actually hear different ones. The power of the visual image is such that we end up hearing what we see, rather than the real syllables that reach our ears. This works like a ventriloquist's doll: we fall for the trick and hear the voice coming from the doll even though we know it is not.

Nerve connections have been discovered which, starting from the visual cortex, modulate auditory processes of the inferior colliculus, a subcortical structure. Phenomena such as the McGurk effect are possible thanks to these connections.[634]

When we see images that refer to sound (a trumpet player, for example), we activate the auditory system,[635] both the afferent and the efferent pathways,[636] and when listening to someone we rely on certain visual cues, such as gestures and gaze shifting, to better understand them. If what we see is not consistent with what we hear, our comprehension is impaired.[637]

When we speak, our facial expression, reflecting our emotions, acoustically modulates the sounds produced. The brain expects this correspondence between what it sees and what it hears[638] and, if its

[633] *Wearing prisms to hear differently: After-effects of prism adaptation on auditory perception.* **Michel, C. et al.** 123-32, 2019, Cortex, Vol. 115.

[634] *Optogenetic auditory fMRI reveals the effects of visual cortical inputs on auditory midbrain response.* **Leong, A. et al.** 8736, 2018, Scientific Reports, Vol. 8.

[635] *When a photograph can be heard: Vision activates the auditory cortex within 110 ms.* **Proverbio, A.M. et al.** 54, Jan, 2011, Scientific Reports, Vol. 1.

[636] *Visual speech gestures modulate e®erent auditory system.* **Namasivayam, A.K. and Wong, W.Y.S.** 4, 2014, Journal of Integrative Neuroscience, Vol. 13, pp. 1-11.

[637] *Audible smiles and frowns affect speech comprehension.* **Quené, H. et al.** 2012, Speech Communication, Vol. 54, pp. 917-922.

[638] *Disgust expressive speech: The acoustic consequences of the facial expression of emotion.* **Chong, C.S., Kim, J. and Davis, C.** 2018, Speech Communication, Vol. 98, pp. 68-72.

expectations are not met, it will try to match what it hears to what it sees, even if this means transforming reality: usually by hearing what our sight is telling us. But vision does not always come out on top. In other experiments, such as temporal tests, it is our hearing that drags us along and makes us see what is not there.[639,640] Visually perceived rhythm improves with auditory training but not with visual training.[641] Some visual tasks are performed better with acoustic stimulation, while others are performed worse.[642] Hearing-impaired children have been observed to be slower in visual tests.[643]

The ear is the cornerstone of our ancestral alarm system, day and night. Unexpected sounds trigger pupillary dilation to identify potential danger.[644] Some children suffer such stress at school that they come to our center with mydriasis (constant pupillary dilation).

DRIVING ON THE SAME HIGHWAY

Language and music share the same ear so, for example, we can predict language proficiency by observing musical skills.[645] Many studies tell us about this relationship. In kindergartens that foster music education, language development is also seen to improve,[646] and this positive influence is maintained in adolescence, favoring cortical maturation.[647]

Nina Kraus' research suggests that this connection helps to delay aging, or at least cognitive aging. She has observed that the

[639] *Auditory dominance over vision in the perception of interval duration.* **Burr, D., Banks, M.S. and Morrone, M.C.** 1, 2009, Exp Brain Res., Vol. 198, pp. 49-57.

[640] *When sound affects vision: effects of auditory grouping on visual motion perception.* **Watanabe, K. and Shimojo, S.** 2, 2001, Psychol Sci., Vol. 12, pp. 109-16.

[641] *Visual rhythm perception improves through auditory but not visual training.* **Barakat, B., Seitz, A.R. and Shams, L.** 2, 2015, Current Biology, Vol. 25.

[642] *Sound enhances visual perception: cross-modal effects of auditory organization on vision.* **Vroomen, J. and de Gelder, B.** 5, 2000, J Exp Psychol Hum Percept Perform., Vol. 26, pp. 1583-90.

[643] *Visual perception in acoustically deprived and normally hearing children.* **Thannhauser, J. et al.** 5, 2009, Child Neuropsychol., Vol. 15, pp. 507-16.

[644] *Human Pupillary Dilation Response to Deviant Auditory Stimuli: Effects of Stimulus Properties and Voluntary Attention.* **Liao, H. et al.** 43, 2016, Frontiers in Neuroscience, Vol. 10.

[645] *Links between early rhythm skills, musical training,and phonological awareness.* **Moritz, C. et al.** 26, 2013, Reading and writing, pp. 739-769.

[646] **Blank, T. and Adamek, K.** *Singen in der Kindheit.* Münster : Waxmann Verlag GmbH, 2010.

[647] *Music training alters the course of adolescent auditory development.* **Tierney, A.T., Krizman, J. and Kraus, N.** 32, London : s.n., Aug 11,2015, PNAS, Vol. 112, pp. 10062-10067.

responses of the brainstem to speech sounds are slower as we get older, but this is not the case among musicians. She gathered a group of elderly people to give them piano lessons, half an hour a day, and found that in three months their processing speed and memory had significantly improved.[648] Other researchers have published similar findings.[649]

If the elderly make rapid progress, young children are even faster. Twenty days of musical training are enough for them to get better scores in verbal intelligence tests.[650]

The sense of rhythm is a skill that is already developed at birth. Christina Zhao, a professor at Washington University, has researched the musical qualities of babies, emphasizing that the ability to detect patterns is a cognitive tool that can also be applied to language.[651]

Rhythm is linked to later grammatical competence, which highlights the neurological overlap between musical and linguistic structures.[652] Rhythmic perception conditions word recognition and reading.[653] A. Brandt et al. go so far as to say that "without the ability to listen to music, it would be impossible to learn to speak".[654]

At the Budapest Institute of Psychology, they played rhythmic patterns from rock music to a group of newborns, occasionally omitting some element, in order to check if the babies noticed something missing in the sequence and, indeed, their brain waves reacted every time the expectations were not met.[655]

Another team, from Italy this time, played music to newborns less than three days old, while they monitored their brain waves, sneaking in the odd dissonant note from time to time. The babies were not

---

[648] *Music Training: An Antidote for Aging?* **Kraus, N. and Anderson, S.** 3, 2013, The Hearing Journal, Vol. 66.

[649] *Effects of music learning and piano practice on cognitive function,mood and quality of life in older adults.* **Seinfeld, S.et al.** 810, Barcelona : s.n., 2013, Frontiers in Psychology, Vol. 4.

[650] *Short-Term Music Training Enhances Verbal Intelligence and executive function.* **Moreno, S. et al.** 11, 2011, Psychol Sci., Vol. 22, pp. 1425-1433.

[651] See note 277

[652] *Musical rhythm discrimination explains individual differences in grammar skills in children.* **Gordon, R.L. et al.** 2014, Developmental Science, pp. 1-10.

[653] *Cross-Modal Priming Effect of Rhythm on Visual Word Recognition and Its Relationships to Music Aptitude and Reading Achievement.* **Fotidzis, T.S. et al.** 210, 2018, Brain Sci., Vol. 8.

[654] *Music and early language acquisition.* **Brandt, A., Gebrian, M. and Slevc, L.R.** 327, 2012, Frontiers in Psychology, Vol. 3.

[655] *Newborn infants detect the beat in music.* **Winkler, I. et al.** 7, 2009, PNAS, Vol. 106.

fooled. The waves indicated that they identified the mistakes made in the music being played.[656]

S. Koelsch posed the question of whether young people with language disorders showed similar difficulties when analyzing musical structures. To investigate this, he observed their brain waves as they listened to music in normal or altered patterns. The waves precisely marked out each wrong note but their latency was greater than expected, indicating that they noticed the errors a little later than their unaffected peers.[657] These results match those obtained by Nina Kraus's team in the USA[658] and by Stephan Sallat, in Germany.[659]

INTELLIGENCE

Some studies have raised the possibility of a relationship between musical education, language competence and intelligence.[660] The latter requires good language development, which in turn depends on the auditory system.

Until barely fifty years ago, Spanish commercial law forbade deaf people from working in business unless they had express judicial permission, the reason being that they were often mentally handicapped also. Deprived of a structured language during childhood, the development of their intelligence had also been impaired. Today that is just history, at least in Spain, but it is still true that language depends on the auditory system and intelligence needs language to develop.

In New Zealand, 711 children from three to fifteen years old were evaluated, with data being obtained regularly on the development of their intelligence, language and behavior, and on their audiometric test results.[661] Those with better hearing scored higher in IQ, language

---

[656] *Functional specializations for music processing in the human newborn brain.* **Perani, D. et al.** 2010, PNAS.

[657] *Children with Specific Language Impairment also show impairment of music-syntactic processing.* **Jentschke, S. et al.** 11, 2008, Journal of Cognitive Neuroscience, Vol. 20.

[658] *Dyslexia risk gene relates to representation of sound in the auditory brainstem.* **Neef, N.E. et al.** 2017, Developmental Cognitive Neuroscience, Vol. 24, pp. 63-71.

[659] *Music Perception Influences Language Acquisition: Melodic and Rhythmic-Melodic Perception in Children with Specific Language Impairment.* **Sallat, S. and Jentschke, S.** 2015, Behavioural Neurology.

[660] *Associations between music education, intelligence, and spelling ability in elementary school.* **Hille, K. et al.** 1-6, 2011, Advances in Cognitive Psychology, Vol. 7.

[661] *Variation in the Normal Hearing Threshold Predicts Childhood IQ, Linguistic, and Behavioral Outcomes.* **Welch, J.D. and Dawes, D.** 6, Dunedin, New Zealand : s.n., 2007, Pediatric Research, Vol. 61, pp. 737-744.

skills and behavior. Once more, audiometry appears to reveal more than just hearing thresholds.

The same scientists carried out another study comparing the audiograms of almost a thousand people with their height. They concluded that the better the hearing, the greater the height, demonstrating that there is also a close physiological relationship. The authors hypothesized that the insulin growth factor IGF-1 might be the common link.[662]

Could this have anything to do with verticality, as we discussed in the section on phylogenesis? (See Chapter 3). Tomatis goes a little further when he accredits speech with the ability to "sculpt" body shape:

"The voice we assume could have an effect on the structure of our body. I'll give you a very simple example. Let's take a short Italian from the Naples region, a skinny Englishman and a stout, thickset German, and move them to the United States. After a while, everyone's head is the same shape.

By changing their languages, they change their face. If you look at them you will see that their head is flatter and they are tall, like the native Indians. The determining element in this mutation is sound, which shapes each being in its totality. In my opinion, the sounds we emit selectively touch the endocrine glands [...]" [663]

Among older people, this link between intelligence and hearing continues. In a large-scale study with a sample of more than half a million people, it was found that people with the lowest cognitive test scores had the most difficulty listening in noisy places.[664]

In 1997, M. Zurrón and F. Díaz, from the University of Santiago de Compostela, in Spain, published a study that linked auditory evoked potentials with intelligence.[665] They found that the latency of the P300 wave decreased when the IQ was higher and when the subject performed tasks that implied a certain cognitive activity.

The authors emphasized that the P300, in addition to being a cortical response, is linked to the limbic lobe and thalamus.

---

[662] *Childhood Hearing Is Associated With Growth Rates in Infancy and Adolescence.* **Welch, D. and Dawes, P.J.D.** 4, Dunedin, New Zealand : s.n., 2007, Pediatric Research, Vol. 62.

[663] *Son et structure du corps.* **Gerber, A. and Tomatis, A.** 1973, Son Magazine, Vol. 40.

[664] *Relation between Speech-in-Noise Threshold, Hearing Loss and Cognition from 40–69 Years of Age.* **Moore, D.R. et al.** 9, Sept, 2014, Speech Hearing in Middle Age, Vol. 9.

[665] *Conditions for correlation between IQ and auditory evoked potential latencies.* **Zurrón, M. and Díaz, F.** 2, 1998, Person. individ. diff., Vol. 24, pp. 279-287.

Intelligence is mixed in with emotions and sensory integration. It is not an isolated unit.

I MOVE, SO I HEAR

What role do motor skills and the vestibular system play in language? The classic answer to this question is that speech requires precise and orderly control of a large set of muscles. In children with speech delay, we often observe generalized motor retardation. But maybe we should consider a new factor.

What if movement itself had a leading role in language perception? What if sounds woke up the necessary motor patterns to be able to speak and the brain recognized them, attributing meaning not only to sound, but also to the motor sequence silently unleashed within us?

This question was addressed by professors Skipper, Devlin and Lametti.[666] The title of their publication defines it very well: The hearing ear is always found close to the speaking tongue. They conclude that theoretical language models should take account of both the cerebral auditory areas, and the motor ones.

When we listen to someone, the brain simultaneously recognizes the sequence of movements that is required for these sounds to be pronounced. Inwardly, we repeat what we hear. Motor areas are activated as much as sensory areas. We imitate our interlocutor. Listening involves all our audio-vocal equipment as a whole, including phonation.

I suspect the mirror neurons are very much involved in this. Tomatis explains this same concept with an anecdote:

"To hear someone else play an instrument, sing or speak is, in some way, to let yourself go, to let them take control of your actions. Inevitably, we integrate the way our interlocutors use their body. That's what explains why, in the presence of a stutterer, we sometimes end up stuttering like them. And this imitation can even go further!

A few years ago, I participated in a very instructive consultation in South Africa. There were seven or eight of us, counting the interpreter, around an extremely brilliant young man with a stutter who presented, from the moment he began to speak, a very curious dynamic: his body launched into a series of

---

[666] See note 144

uncoordinated movements. After a while, I realized that everyone except my wife and I were imitating the same gestures without being aware of it! The most agitated of all was the interpreter, which was totally normal as he was the one most directly involved with what the subject was saying.

Two interlocutors facing each other (or a speaker and a listener) are like two pianos placed in the same room: if the keys of the first one are touched, the second one immediately starts to vibrate. That said, I do not want to "blow my own trumpet" for making an impressive discovery. In truth, I have done nothing but rediscover and verify very ancient intuitions. The founder of Taoism, Lao Tse, expressed this idea as far back as the sixth century BC, using the example of two harps."[667]

Babies provide us with another lesson about the unity of the audio-vocal circuit. As part of a singular investigation, some babies performed a phonetic discrimination task. Later, they were prevented from moving their tongue freely. In those conditions they were no longer able to identify the sounds.[668]

The indissoluble link between listening and speaking will help us to understand and resolve some language or even psychiatric disorders, such as the mysterious misophony syndrome, a rare dysfunction that consists of perceiving everyday sounds with intense aversion: someone chewing, scratching, brushing their hair, and so on. The patients suffer serious discomfort that prevents them from leading normal work and family life, as these unbearable noises are all around them.

It is surprising that they are always affected by sounds produced by people, not by machines or natural elements such as rain or wind. They ignore the washing machine as it spins, but they get desperately irritated next to someone eating soup, even if they do not look at them. I suspect the noise from a machine does not activate the motor areas of the brain, but human sounds do. This is how the mirror neurons work.

These patients tolerate sounds much better, to the point of not being affected by them, if they control their emission. They cannot stand hearing someone brushing their teeth, but they do not feel any discomfort when brushing their own or their children's. In other

---

[667] See note 3
[668] *Sensorimotor influences on speech perception in infancy.* **Bruderer, A.G. et al.** Sept, 2015, PNAS.

words, it appears the noise is unbearable for them when the inner imitation happens automatically, without their conscious involvement, with the auditory and motor areas being activated independently.

Among the auditory delusions, we find the phenomenon of subvocalization. In the 1940s, Louis Gould was the first to record electrical activity in the speech muscles of these patients, even being able to hear the hallucination by using a microphone.[669] Silent phonation also accompanies the imagined voice, remaining faithful to the unity of the audio-vocal circuit.

APD

Some people have poor listening without any auditory pathology. The disorder can take many forms: inability to learn music or languages, to concentrate, to remember oral information, to understand speech in noisy environments, etc. Other researchers, in addition to Tomatis, have studied the processing of acoustic information regardless of the degree of deafness.

This is the case of Teri James Bellis, one of the most respected voices in this field. Bellis, after a car accident, was herself a victim of one kind of this disorder. She was able to hear, but could not help feeling assaulted when people talked to her.[670] She lost the ability to perceive the communicative intent of her interlocutor.

The accumulation of evidence in this regard led to the creation of an ASHA working committee in 2005 and the subsequent official adoption in 2007 of the term CAPD (central auditory processing disorders), which would later be simplified into the acronym APD.

To diagnose APD, the ASHA makes some recommendations but does not specifically state which tests should be used. In fact, there is still no reliable test battery, let alone one calibrated for different languages. However, many audiologists already offer this service.

APD syndrome is still being debated. Its definition is imprecise, generating confusion and contradictory data. Its incidence in children, for example, is either 0.2 per cent,[671] or 2–3%,[672] depending on the authors consulted. In adults it is believed to be higher, although the

---

[669] **Bentall, R.P.** *Medicalizar la mente.* Barcelona : Herder Editorial, 2011.

[670] **Bellis, T.J.** *When the Brain can't hear.* New York : Atria books, 2002.

[671] *Prevalence of Auditory Processing Disorder in School-Aged Children in the Mid-Atlantic Region.* **Nagao, K. et al.** 9, 2016, J Am Acad Audiol., Vol. 27, pp. 691-700.

[672] **Chermak, G.D. and Musiek, F.E.** *Central Auditory Processing Disorders: New Perspectives.* San Diego : Singular Publishing Group, 1997.

percentages vary across such a wide spectrum that we are clearly dealing with subjective judgments. In fact, the lack of rigorous criteria can lead to prevalence rates anywhere between 7.3% and 96%, which gives an idea of the diagnostic chaos in which we find ourselves today.[673]

It is often difficult to distinguish APD from other syndromes, such as ADHD. Disturbingly, both affect children from poor backgrounds more. They are usually attributed to genetic causes, but we mainly find them among the underprivileged classes.[674] Something does not fit.

The tests that are carried out, following ASHA guidelines, focus on the ability to discriminate, to listen in adverse conditions, to integrate information from both ears (binaural fusion), auditory laterality (dichotic listening), etc.; but I am afraid that APD tests do not yet meet the criteria of validity and reliability to a sufficient degree. They barely consider the assessment of rhythm or musical competencies—key elements, in my opinion, when talking about learning disorders.[675]

I do not find the adult batteries to be very accurate either. Patients with problems in auditory memory, language learning or singing in tune can easily pass APD tests for adults, such as the Santiago battery (developed at the University of Chile). It is not that this is a bad test: more likely, we have differing ideas on what good listening is. The Tomatis perspective offers a different approach, in which I feel more comfortable, as it contemplates the whole patient and allows me to obtain a great wealth of information. I use APD tests as a complementary diagnostic tool. Auditory assessment should not be limited to audiometry anyway, because there are multiple auditory skills.

APD tests should be integrated into a test battery that encompasses the whole person. We analyze the degree of motor development, rhythmic control, primary reflexes, emotion management, functional quality of vision, etc. I do not believe it is appropriate to suggest a particular therapy just because some APD test results have not been satisfactory.

---

[673] *Using different criteria to diagnose (central) auditory processing disorder: how big a difference does it make?* **Wilson, W.J. and Arnott, W.** 1, 2013, J Speech Lang Hear Res., Vol. 56, pp. 63-70.

[674] *Low Socioeconomic Status Linked to Impaired Auditory Processing.* **Kraus, N. and Anderson, S.** May, 2015, The Hearing Journal.

[675] *Awareness of Rhythm Patterns in Speech and Music in Children with Specific Language Impairments.* **Cumming, R. et al.** 672, 2015, Frontiers in Human Neuroscience, Vol. 9.

For a few years now, I have been using a screening test for children, which indicates the degree of automation of the hearing system. I get them to listen through headphones to a fragment of a story, narrated at a speed of about 70 words per minute and I ask them to repeat what they hear, while the story is being told, as if they were acting as a simultaneous interpreter in their own language.

Those who read well do this task with total ease. The audio-vocal loop works automatically and they can talk while listening. Fluent reading requires this same unconscious control, just as professional pianists play without thinking about where to place their fingers at any given moment. If we need to bring our conscious attention into play, we will slow down and stumble. When we learn a new language, we again read clumsily until, little by little, it becomes an automatic process.

I have noticed that most children with reading problems are not able to pass this test. Their usual response is unintelligible speech. Suddenly they do not seem to know how to talk. Others try a stratagem, such as memorizing a fragment and then saying it quickly, but as they speak they are not paying attention to the story and no longer remember the next sentence. Clearly, their difficulties are not limited to reading. Their hearing system needs help from voluntary control, like the novice driver who cannot talk while driving.

From the conscious level we are not able to do two tasks at the same time. When asked to calculate 5+3 and 4+2 we do one operation first and then the other The child with an immature hearing system either listens or speaks, but cannot perform both together. Automation is the liberation of consciousness. Other parts of the brain take on the task. When this happens, we can read effortlessly and, in the meantime, we can think about what the text is telling us.

As I mention above, it is also important to check if patients have any sense of rhythm or if it is random in their case; if they can distinguish between the A and the C notes or they both sound the same; if they can sing in tune or not. Language is music too. In my opinion, tests like these provide much more valuable information than whether the patient understands words with high pass filters at different frequencies or passes the Staggered Spondaic Word Test (SSW). The Tomatis way of interpreting the listening test provides us with elements that go unnoticed in a classical audiometric reading.

In 2007, D. Ross-Swain assessed the application of Tomatis's techniques under ASHA criteria. She diagnosed 41 subjects with several classic APD tests: Wrat, Lact, etc. After 90 hours of Tomatis's therapy, she repeated the tests. The results showed progress in short-term memory and discrimination, and a significant reduction in auditory latency time. Their reactions were faster,[676] which harks back to the work of Tallal and Kraus.

In Poland, Tomatis's protocols have been widely used in public schools to improve hearing skills,[677] in a program closely monitored by the Department of Speech Therapy of the University of Lublin.[678]

OTITIS

Official statistics tell us that otitis episodes are the most frequent cause of visits to the pediatrician, apart from periodic check-ups.[679] In a study carried out in the Valencian Community,[680] in Spain, 60% of children were recorded as having suffered at least one episode of acute otitis by the age of three. Taking the first five years as a reference, there were on average over two cases of acute otitis per child.

Considering that these episodes then lead to serous otitis lasting more than one month in 40% of cases and three months in 10%,[681] the impact on learning can be considerable. If we also include the cases of serous otitis that will never be seen by a doctor because it does not hurt, but will still interfere with listening, the issue is worrying.

A few years ago, a school asked my team to screen all their pupils. We determined that 20% of the audiograms were compatible with serous otitis. Practically all of it had previously gone unnoticed. The effects of these pathologies could explain many cases of ADHD. The child's listening is distorted, but not so much as to suspect deafness. They just seem absent-minded and inattentive.

A longitudinal study (with monitoring from childhood to age 18) carried out on a sample of almost one thousand schoolchildren found a relationship between the otitis episodes suffered and certain

---

[676] *The Effects of Auditory Stimulation on Auditory Processing Disorder: A Summary of the findings.* **Swain, D.R.** 2, 2007, The International Journal of Listening, Vol. 21.

[677] *Tomatis auditory stimulation and learning difficulties: an overview of recent studies.* **Ożańska-Ponikwia, K.** 7, 2016, Konteksty Pedagogiczne, Vol. 2, pp. 39-45.

[678] **Kurkowski, Z.M.** Tomatis Method applied in the diagnosis and speech therapy. [book author] Lublin University. *Logopedia.* 2013, Vol. 42.

[679] *Propuestas sencillas para el tratamiento de la otitis media.* **Saz, P. et al.** 1, 2010, Medicina Naturista, Vol. 4, pp. 33-43.

[680] *Epidemiología e impacto de la otitis media aguda en la Comunidad Valenciana.* **Garcés-Sánchez, M. et al.** 2, 2004, An Pediatr (Barc), Vol. 60, pp. 125-32.

[681] **Roland, P.S. and Scoresby, T.W.** Tympanostomy Tubes and Otorrhea. [book author] R.B. Mitchell and K.D. Pereira. *Pediatric Otolaryngology for the Clinician.* s.l. : Humana Press, 2009.

variables determining academic performance, such as IQ, reading level and, of course, grades.[682]

Repeated otitis can seriously compromise learning,[683,684] and it is not enough to administer antibiotics and antihistamines. Tomatis insisted on proper nutrition. He said that when he was a young doctor, there was hardly any otitis and cases started to go up considerably when the American Pediatric Association recommended the early intake of fruit juices in the 1960s, Tomatis advised against acidic food: too many citrus fruits, dairy products and sugars, carbonated drinks, etc.

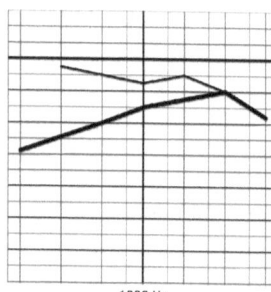

1000 Hz

Typical serous otitis audiogram. The gap between bone and air curve in the bass range is remarkable. The curve inversion extends into the mid-range and even the trebles.

Today the situation is more complex, as pollution, food intolerances and allergies increase the risk of otitis.[685] It is common to see children with a constant excess of mucus.

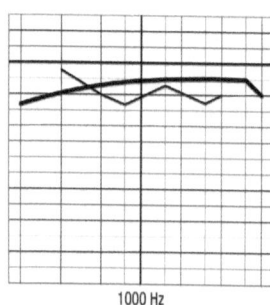

1000 Hz

Typical audiogram of a child under 7, or an older one with motor development problems. This characteristic is also common in ADHD. The be curve rises in the bass range, unlike the air curve, which usually falls.

[682] *Behaviour and developmental effects of otitis media with effusion into the teens.* **Bennett, K.E. et al.** 2001, Arch Dis Child 2001, Vol. 85, pp. 91-95.

[683] See note 291

[684] *Otitis media in language impaired and normal children.* **Tallal, P., Curtiss, S. and Allard, L.** 4, Dec, 1991, JSLPA, Vol. 15.

[685] *Recurrent otitis media with effusion and food allergy in pediatric patients.* **Arroyave, C.M.** 5, 2001, Rev Alerg Mex., Vol. 48, pp. 141-4.

As I mention above, Tomatis relates the activity of the hammer muscle to the audiometric curve, between 125 and 1,000 Hz. In ADHD and also in psychomotor immaturity, the bone curve is usually above the air curve (curve inversion) in that area.

ADHD

I suspect this is over-diagnosed,[686] but I will not go into details as this is not the purpose of this book. I will only mention auditory issues linked to it.

When the term ADHD did not yet exist, we talked about "minimal brain dysfunction" and even then there were claims that this diagnosis included a history of above-average episodes of otitis.[687] Two later studies came to the same conclusion,[688,689] but there was never any large-scale follow-up, as far as I know, and that line of research was virtually abandoned.

Since APD was first discussed as an independent diagnostic unit, its relationship to ADHD has been debated, to the point of doubting whether they are two separate nosological entities or not.[690]

From the year 2000 on, when a group of experts laid the groundwork for the APD diagnosis,[691] the links with ADHD have once again been a recurrent topic of study. Both syndromes share so many characteristics that publications have even appeared to help develop a differential diagnosis.[692]

A compilation of these papers concludes that sensory processing disorders are more frequent in children with ADHD and that includes

[686] *Las otras verdades del Tdah.* **Alós, C. and Ruiz, C.** 2013, Aula de Infantil, Vol. 70, pp. 27-31.

[687] *Minimal brain dysfunction and otitis media.* **Hersher, L.** 3, 1978, Percept Mot Skills. 1978 Dec, Vol. 47, pp. 723-6.

[688] *An association between recurrent otitis media in infancy and later hyperactivity.* **Hagerman, R.J. and Falkenstein, A.R.** 5, Clin Pediatr (Phila)., Vol. 26, pp. 253-7.

[689] *Otitis media in children with learning disabilities and in children with attention deficit disorder with hyperactivity.* **Adesman, A.R. and al., et.** 3 Pt 2, 1990, Pediatrics., Vol. 85, pp. 442-6.

[690] *A Preliminary Study of the Relationship Between Central Auditory Processing Disorder and Attention Deficit Disorder.* **Cook, J.R. et al.** 3, 1993, JPsychiatr Neurosci, Vol. 18.

[691] *Report of the Consensus Conference on the Diagnosis of Auditory Processing Disorders in School-Aged Children.* 9, 2000, J Am Acad Audiol., Vol. 11, pp. 467-74.

[692] *Aetiology and clinical presentations of auditory processing disorders—a review.* **Bamiou, D.E., Musiek, F.E. and Luxon, L.M.** 2001, Arch Dis Child, Vol. 85, pp. 361-365.

auditory and vestibular impairments.[693] Coincidentally, the incidence of ADHD is higher among deaf children.[694]

Although the model cannot be directly extrapolated to humans, it has been proven that mice with vestibular deficits present, in addition to motor clumsiness, hyperactivity, disorientation and anxiety,[695] typical characteristics of ADHD.

ADD means attention deficit disorder, which implies that the main feature of these children is that they fail to be attentive. However, careful observation suggests otherwise. They pay attention to everything that happens around them, but cannot concentrate on a single point of reference. They cannot be selective. Everything stimulates them at the same time.

In the listening test they usually show the well-known alert antenna:

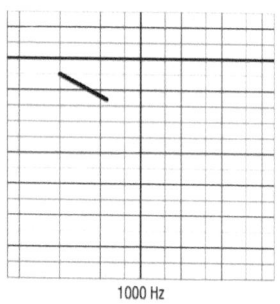

1000 Hz

Hyperreactivity often occurs. They act as if they receive constant sensory overstimulation, so their responses are also oversized. They usually avoid physical contact and are bothered by clothing, noise, light or abrupt movements. Sometimes we find the opposite case, the hyporeactive ones, although these are less frequent. All of this generates a state of anxiety, which is not necessarily very high but permanent, unsuitable for exercising the attention that learning demands.

From an auditory point of view, they do not regulate filtering mechanisms well. They cannot listen carefully for long. Soon another sound distracts them. They respond as if the background noise were as

---

[693] *Sensory Processing Problems in Children with ADHD, a Systematic Review.* **Ghanizadeh, A.** 89-94, 2011, Psychiatry Investig, Vol. 8.

[694] *The Severity of Vestibular Dysfunction in Deafness as a Determinant of Comorbid Hyperactivity or Anxiety.* **Antoine, M.W. et al.** 20, May 17, 2017, The Journal of Neuroscience, Vol. 37, pp. 5144-5154.

[695] *Mice with vestibular deficiency display hyperactivity, disorientation and signs of anxiety.* **Avni, R. et al.** 2009, Behavioural Brain Research.

interesting to them as the signal, failing to distinguish the relevant information. However, a certain (constant) level of noise has been seen to favor their cognitive performance.[696] Does it have to do with the immaturity of the efferent system or of the muscles associated with the ossicular chain, which are in charge of selecting the sounds? That would explain the beneficial effects of auditory therapy on these children.

This lack of control prevents these children from focusing on what really matters. They are overwhelmed by everyday noises, such as the refrigerator motor, the computer fan or traffic. Paradoxically, we often need to repeat things two or three times to get them to understand us.

Although their audiogram usually presents a normal HAIC level, peaks and scotomas abound throughout the curve, as do selectivity and spatialization mistakes, which Tomatis regarded as an indicator of immaturity of the hearing system.

Recent studies also confirm alterations in sound discrimination and spatial location.[697] They do not usually pass the "repeat what you hear" test either. If focusing on one point is hard for them, two are totally impossible (remember that this test consists of reproducing, in real time, what we are hearing through a headset).

When we add the H to ADD, it means that the syndrome is accompanied by hyperactivity. In ADHD there is a peculiar motricity, with an insecure balance that suggests a vestibular dysfunction.[698] Patients have greater instability in postural control tests.[699,700,701] If we place them on a balance platform and ask them to perform some cognitive task such as an auditory memory test, we will see that they have to make an effort not to fall down, which leads them to move around more than children without ADHD.

---

[696] *Listen to the noise: noise is beneficial for cognitive performance in ADHD.* **Söderlund, G., Sikström, S. and Smart, A.** 8, 2007, Journal of Child Psychology and Psychiatry, Vol. 48, pp. 840-847.

[697] See note 693

[698] *Characteristics of the sensory-motor, verbal and cognitive abilities of preschool boys with attention deficit/hyperactivity disorder combined type.* **Iwanaga, R. et al.** 2006, Psychiatry and Clinical Neurosciences, Vol. 60, pp. 37-45.

[699] *Postural control among children with and without attention deficit hyperactivity disorder in single and dual conditions.* **Shorer, Z. et al.** 2012, Eur J Pediatr.

[700] *Stability and Psychophysiological Support of Upright Posture in Children with Attention Deficit Hyperactivity Disorder.* **Guseva, E.A. et al.** 6, 2003, Biomedical Engineering, Vol. 37.

[701] *Sensory Integration in Attention Deficit Hyperactivity Disorder: Implications to Postural Control.* **Hassan, D.M. and Azzam, H.** 2014, Contemporary 4 Trends in ADHD Research.

Rhythm and motor coordination disorders are their sign of identity too. They fail in temporal tasks, such as perceiving the duration of sounds or moving to the beat, as dyslexics do.[702] Other clues also point to this lack of temporal precision, which links to the auditory system.[703] In fact, vestibular stimulation has been proposed as a therapy for ADHD,[704] not only to develop motor skills, but also verbal ones.[705]

A recent study postulates a direct link between hearing disorders and behavior, which may be related to ADHD. Jean Hebert's team has discovered that some inner ear injuries can cause molecular changes in the brain, resulting in typical ADHD behavior:

They discovered a gene that caused hyperactivity in mice and thought that it encoded a brain structure associated with behavior. Much to their surprise, though, they saw that the gene was not linked to motor areas of the brain as they suspected, but to the ear.

Neither dyslexia nor ADHD have specific biomarkers. They cannot be diagnosed by an X-ray or blood test. However, some proposals have already been submitted that involve the ear,[706] which compare auditory evoked potentials (such as wave P1) obtained in children with ADHD to those of control groups.

In her doctoral thesis, psychologist Liliana Sacarin, studied the effect of Tomatis's auditory therapy on children diagnosed with ADHD, with satisfactory results despite the therapy group only carrying out 30 hours of sessions, a third of what a normal schedule usually lasts.[707]

---

[702] *Children and adults with Attention Deficit/Hyperactivity Disorder cannot move to the beat.* **Puyjarinet, F. et al.** Sept 14, 2017, Scientific Reports.

[703] *Auditory temporal processing in children with attention deficit hyperactivity disorder (ADHD).* **Leite, A.C., Capellini, S.A. and Figueiredo, A.C.** 2, Sao Paulo : s.n., Apr, 2015, Rev. CEFAC, Vol. 17.

[704] *Vestibular Stimulation for ADHD: Randomized Controlled Trial of Comprehensive Motion Apparatus.* **Arnold, L.E. et al.** 5, 2008, Journal of Attention Disorders, Vol. 11, pp. 599-611.

[705] *A possible correlation between vestibular stimulation and auditory comprehension in children with attention-deficit/ hyperactivity disorder.* **Haghshenas, S. et al.** 2, 2014, Psychology & Neuroscience, Vol. 7, pp. 159-162.

[706] *Neural Biomarkers for Dyslexia,ADHD,and ADD in the Auditory Cortex of Children.* **Serrallach, B. et al.** 2016, Frontiers in Neuroscience, Vol. 10.

[707] **Sacarin, L.** Early Effects of the Tomatis Listening Method in Children with Attention Deficit. [ed.] Antioch University Seattle. Jan, 2013.

WITH AN EYE
ON THE FUTURE 11

ULTRASOUNDS

We can read in any audiology textbook that the human ear can hear frequencies up to 16,000–20,000 Hz, but are we sure that is true?

High-frequency sounds provide very precise information. Bats and dolphins use them to locate obstacles and generate a three-dimensional image of their environment. Some blind people use echoes to detect objects. A trained blind person acquires amazing skill through echolocation, discriminating on the horizontal plane with an accuracy of little more than one degree, almost like a bat.[708] Blind babies emit clicks (charged with high frequencies) and the bouncing sound wave tells them the position of objects.[709]

As early as 1951, Pumphrey and Ackroyd claimed we could hear ultrasounds up to 50,000 Hz, or even 150,000 Hz in young subjects, as demonstrated to them by Maass, from Bremen, in 1945.[710] We pick them up by bone conduction. It is not feasible by air. In 1962, Haeff and Knox explained how they were perceived from different parts of our body.[711] However, we are not aware of most ultrasounds that impact us.

They penetrate from different points,[712] mostly through the eyes, being transmitted across the intracranial soft tissue.[713] Incidentally,

---

[708] *Ultrafine spatial acuity of blind expert human echolocators.* **Teng, S., Puri, A. and Whitney, D.** 2011, Exp Brain Res.

[709] **Bower, T.** *El mundo perceptivo del niño.* s.l. : Ediciones Morata, 1982.

[710] *Upper limit of frequency for human hearing.* **Pumphrey, R.J.** 1950, Nature, Vol. 166, p. 571.

[711] Perception of ultrasound. **Haeff, A.V. y Knox, C.** 1963, Science, Vol. 139

[712] *Measurements of vibration at the external auditory meatus and the upper limb in the living human body caused by distantly presented bone-conducted ultrasound.* **Ogino, R., Otsuka, S. and Nakagawa, S.** SGGE12, 2019, Japanese Journal of Applied Physics, Vol. 58.

audiograms can be obtained by placing the vibrator on the eyeballs, with similar results to those obtained from the mastoids.[714]

Ultrasounds activate brain areas even in deaf people.[715] Vinyl nostalgics may be right in preferring their LPs to CDs. They contain ultrasounds that affect the brain, even though they are not audible sounds.[716] This can be seen in brain images. Why does our brain react to them? Is it useful to us? Where do we process them? Do blind children use only the audible band of their clicks, or do they also use ultrasound?

Evoked otoacoustic emissions can be suppressed by applying an ultrasound via bone conduction. How is it possible for a high-frequency sound to change the cochlea's physiology in this way?[717]

M. L. Lenhardt, who taught at Virginia Commonwealth University, wrote several articles on ultrasonic perception.[718] He noted that even people with profound deafness could clearly hear words when these were modulated in the ultrasonic range.

In 2002, he even patented an ultrasound hearing aid that works by bone conduction, though in a way radically different from any conventional hearing aid, since it does not amplify sound, which instead is encoded in ultrasonic waves that the brain translates (it is not well known how) into audible sound.

At the 2007 International Acoustics Conference in Madrid, a Japanese team presented a prototype of this type of hearing aid.[719] It is not yet available commercially, since the problems of noise produced by the device have not been solved. Further research is being carried out and it will probably one day replace conventional amplifying hearing aids.[720]

---

[713] *Eyes as Fenestrations to the Ears: A Novel Mechanism for High-Frequency and Ultrasonic Hearing.* **Lenhardt, M.L.** 1, 2007, International Tinnitus Journal, Vol. 13, pp. 3-10.

[714] *Eyes as windows on brain pressure.* **Sinha, T. and Lenhardt, M.L.** 2, 2011, International Tinnitus Journal, Vol. 16, pp. 130-4

[715] *Ultrasound activates the auditory cortex of profoundly deaf subjects.* **Imaizumi, S. et al.** 3, 2001, Neuroreport, Vol. 12.

[716] *Inaudible High-Frequency Sounds Affect Brain Activity: Hypersonic Effect.* **Oohashi, T. et al.** 2000, Journal of Neurophysiology, Vol. 83, pp. 3548-3558.

[717] **Martin, J.A.** Bone-Conducted Ultrasonic Hearing: Can Distortion Product Otoacoustic Emissions Confirm Cochlear Involvement? [ed.] Chalmers University of Technology. Goteborg, Sweden. : s.n., 2011. Master Thesis.

[718] *Human Ultrasonic Speech Perception.* **Lenhardt, M.L. et al.** 5015, 1991, Science, Vol. 253.

[719] *Assessments of bone-conducted ultrasonic hearing-aid (bcuha): frequency-discrimination, articulation and intelligibility tests.* **Nakagawa, S., Okamoto, Y. and Fujimoto, K.** 19th International Congress on Acoustics, Madrid, Sept 2-7, 2007.

[720] *Development of a Bone-Conducted Ultrasonic Hearing Aid for the Profoundly Deaf: Evaluation of Sound Quality Using a Semantic Differential Method.* **Nakagawa, N., Fujiyuki, C. and Kagomiya, T.** 7S, Japanese Journal of Applied Physics, Vol. 52.

The vibrational spectrum does not end with ultrasounds and it has more surprises to offer us. In the corporate magazine of Airborne Instruments Laboratory, New York, dated October 1956, D. B. Williams wrote:

"Back around 1947 [...], several of us at AIL were working on the antenna of a large ground radar, when we noticed an interesting phenomenon that does not seem to be generally known. We found that it was possible to hear repetition rate of the radar when we were standing close to the antenna horn. It became obvious from simple tests that sound was produced in the head without any direct acoustic input".[721]

It is one of the first historical references to the *Frey effect*. Microwave signals between 200 MHz and 3 GHz cause the brain tissue to warm up at each pulsation, triggering a pressure wave that travels through the skull to the cochlea. Military applications of this phenomenon were investigated in order to transmit messages remotely or to harm the enemy. At certain intensities it causes sickness and headaches.[722]

One of the most common ultrasounds in our environment in recent years is the 2100 MHz frequency. I am talking about cell phones. The safety of these devices, as far as health is concerned, is a topic of recurring debate.[723] Several studies suggest that they can have harmful effects, but they have become so essential to our daily lives that we are reluctant to listen to any talk of limiting their use, unless faced with undeniable evidence (and maybe not even then).

Other studies have been published that recommend keeping ultrasound scans to a minimum during pregnancy. In laboratory mice, exposure to ultrasounds has been found to impact the neural development of the embryo.[724]

A great specialist in this field, Mostafa Fatemi from the Mayo Clinic, presented a paper in 2001 at the American Society of Acoustics Conference, in which he stated that at the point where the ultrasound is focused it can reach between 100 and 120 dB. This is a

---

[721] *An observation on the detection by the ear of microwave signals.* **Williams, D.B.** [ed.] Airborne Instruments Laboratory. Oct, 1956.

[722] *Auditory Response to Pulsed Radiofrequency Energy.* **Elder, J.A. and Chou, C.K.** 2003, Bioelectromagnetics Supplement, Vol. 6.

[723] *Health risks associated with mobile phones use.* **Naeem, Z.** 4, 2014, Int J Health Sci (Qassim), Vol. 8

[724] *Prenatal exposure to ultrasound waves impacts neuronal migration in mice.* **Ang, E.** et al. 34, 2006, PNAS , Vol. 103, pp. 12903–12910.

dangerous intensity, which decreases sharply as we move away from the excited region, but which means we should avoid focusing the ultrasound on the auditory areas.[725]

To be clear, I am not questioning the competence of healthcare staff here. I am referring rather to the ultrasound machines that allow the mother to see her child for a few seconds by inserting some coins, as if they were vending machines.

SOUND AND DNA

In a few years, L. Montagnier went from glory to exile from the scientific community. Having won the Nobel Prize for discovering the AIDS virus, he was harshly criticized for subsequent research work that got too close to the "pseudosciences". Now aged 87, he works in China. In 2009 he published an article that constitutes an authentic Copernican revolution in biology.[726] The experiment is well described, so any research team could replicate it and draw their own conclusions. You can see the story in this video:

Montagnier detected low-frequency electromagnetic waves in cultures of certain microorganisms, which could also be obtained from their DNA. He recorded the waves with a microphone as a WAV file (yes, the same one we use for songs) and sent it over the internet to an Italian laboratory. There they placed two loudspeakers and let an amino acid mixture listen to the waves in the file for a few hours. The amino acids arranged themselves in accordance with the structure they were listening to. Miles away in Italy they had just obtained a very similar DNA. This experiment shakes the very foundations of biology. Something so transcendental, that defies deep convictions, should already have been accepted or rejected by the scientific community, but not ignored.

As an audiologist, Montagnier's research raises many questions for me. For example, when speaking, does sound also impact at the

---

[725] *"Quiet, Please!" Says the Fetus.* **Fatami, M.** Fort Lauderdale, Florida : s.n., 2001
[726] *Electromagnetic Signals Are Produced by Aqueous Nanostructures Derived from Bacterial DNA Sequences.* **Montagnier, L. et al.** 2009, Interdiscip Sci Comput Life Sci.

molecular level, in our DNA, in the same way that it modulates our brain waves, as in Nina Kraus' experiment?[727] (See Chapter 9). Will we be able to modulate biological processes by acting on the nervous system through waves, as suggested by Maksymov and Pototsky?[728]

COSMIC VIBRATION

While concluding the last pages of this book, I have had the opportunity to read a magnificent book: *Biocentrism*, in which Robert Lanza[729] offers a new approach to humanity's eternal questions: topics that Tomatis also addressed in his final work, *Listening to the Universe*.[730] The enigmas of the ear are not far-removed from the mystery of life—from the two great questions whose answers have eluded us ever since our consciousness arose to pose them: "What is our origin?" and "What is our destiny?" or, if preferred: "Where do we come from?" and "Where do we go when we die?"

Tomatis and Lanza introduce two original hypotheses. Tomatis suggests that, since everything is vibration, the Big Bang must have been a vibratory phenomenon as well, which would place sound at the origin of the cosmos. Lanza reflects on the consequences of quantum phenomena, in particular the interference caused by the observer in the behavior of particles, and states that the only way to understand consciousness–matter interactions is to accept our ability to "create" external reality.

We have known for some time that what we perceive is nothing more than an illusion. What we see is a recreation by our brain based on certain electromagnetic waves, located within a specific wavelength range, which we call light. But, in fact, there is no light out there as we know it: just immaterial vibrations.

What we hear is also an invention of our neurons. There is no such thing as sound as a physical entity. When air molecules move in a characteristic pattern, we have an acoustic experience, very different from the visual one; but light and sound are nothing more than displacements of particles. Perceiving is, in short, capturing movement.

Not even the word "particle" responds to a solid, well-established construct. According to the discoveries of quantum physics, which

---

[727] See note 563

[728] *Excitation of Faraday-like body waves in vibrated living earthworms.* **Maksymov, I.S. y Pototsky, A.** 8564, 2020, Scientific Reports, Vol. 10

[729] **Lanza, R. and Berman, B.** *Biocentrismo.* Málaga : Editorial Sirio, 2017.

[730] See note 39

tries to explain the behavior of the smallest things that can be observed, the world around us is far from being tangible matter. It is not composed of identifiable microscopic elements. What we call atoms, represented by a hard and compact nucleus, orbited by little balls, are bundles of vibratory energy, waves of probability that, far from solving unknowns, add in a few more.

Scientists have had to accept, very reluctantly, that in the quantum universe matter is not subject exclusively to specific pre-established physical laws, but its behavior is determined by the presence of the observer. Is light a wave or a particle? It depends. If we try to measure the phenomenon, we will see particles. If not, they will be waves. It is not that the measuring instruments get in the way: it is the act of observing that changes the situation. It is our own consciousness that is exerting its influence, in a permanent dialogue with the energy that makes up matter.

Science has systematically dodged the issue of consciousness, not willingly but because, as an object of study, it shows itself to be intractable. Where does our will or our capacity to love reside? Even psychology flees from these questions, following conduct-centered models and avoiding the question of what ultimately generates our behaviors and thoughts wherever possible. However, we cannot just hide consciousness when it suits us and it has shown itself, in all its magnitude, where it hurts the most: in the sanctuary of the unbreakable laws of physics.

In an attempt to cling on to Newton's laws, we might hope that consciousness only acts at quantum level and not in our everyday reality, but that would be a new illusion. It is not so easy to remove from the equation.

If we could, for example, observe what happens at the subatomic level in a case of depression; descend to that still unknown level and understand the behavior of each electron, each quark, perhaps we would discover the mechanisms of illness. But, having reached that point, we should remember that the observer's consciousness instantly interferes with the observed. Will this be the way to heal in the future? Will we enter the quantum universe with our mind, reorganizing the energetic structure in its final link?

Just as vibrational energy manifests itself in the form of objects that seem tangible to us, it could also crystallize in other phenomena, such as language and music, and these could store in each note, in each syllable, a complex vibrational energy structure. Perhaps these are the "objects" that our quantum body emits to interact with other quantum systems or with itself. Because, what lies behind a wonderful symphony? Merely neurons transmitting electricity? Avicenna said that in the art of healing, first comes the word. Was he not referring to the same thing? Could speech and music not be instruments used by consciousness to engage with the vibration that shapes matter and the biofield? When I am moved by that Mozart work, what influence is it having on the quantum level of my cells? From the biocentric perspective, perhaps it is consciousness that determines harmony, beauty or aesthetic pleasure in music, and matter obeys those wishes.

Tomatis regarded the ear as a vector for development, which facilitates the appearance of language and consciousness. I believe there is sufficient reason to justify that kind of thinking. The scientific evidence invites us to reflect on an ear that is much more than a perceptive system.

We must continue to explore its secrets. It offers a great opportunity. I am confident that, in the near future, audiological research will adopt elements from audio-psycho-phonology. This would be a great step forward, which patients would appreciate.

We are advancing towards a medicine that is progressively moving away from chemistry in favor of physics. I do not know how long it will take, but I have no doubt that, in the future, diagnoses and treatments will be based on doctors' knowledge of our bioelectric and biomagnetic makeup.

As measuring instruments are perfected and evidence accumulates, the ancestral energy therapies will be accepted. Someday, doctors will incorporate the chakras and acupuncture meridians into their everyday vocabulary, and vibrational therapies using light and sound will become as popular as antibiotics today.

When this new paradigm is consolidated, all the information contained in these pages will become obsolete and will have to be reinterpreted. I am afraid that from a biophysical approach at quantum level it will be difficult to even identify an auditory system as such. We will doubtless discover that auditory therapy acts on our biofield and we will have to reposition all the pieces of the puzzle again.

Until that happens, I hope this book has helped you to look at the ear from another perspective. If that is the case, I will be satisfied.

Alfred Tomatis (1920-2001)
In memoriam

GLOSSARY OF TERMS

- **Afferent.** Information that travels to the brain. Efferent, in the opposite direction.
- **ANS.** Autonomic nervous system. It includes the sympathetic and parasympathetic systems.
- **Audiometric test.** This is the main audiological test. With it we detect the hearing thresholds, that is to say, the minimum intensity of sound necessary for us to be able to hear, by means of a device called an audiometer. The test evaluates different frequencies, from bass to treble, which are quantified in hertz (Hz). In this way we determine the patient's hearing capacity in the whole range of audible sounds, or frequency spectrum. Both ears are tested, and both air and bone conduction. In the air-conduction test, we use headphones. For bone conduction, we use a vibrator placed on bone, usually the mastoid, the bone behind the ear. With the results we obtain audiometric curves that allow the detection of auditory pathologies, in their conventional interpretation. From the A. Tomatis perspective, other parameters are also considered.
- **Brain map.** A graphical representation of brain activity, obtained by computerized processing of the electrical impulses it generates.
- **Brain waves.** In the brain, the activity of neurons generates electrical impulses that can be recorded. These discharges are not chaotic, but follow certain patterns. Groups of neurons respond in unison, in a coordinated manner. Depending on our state of attention, relaxation or sleep, the electrical activity presents different cycles that we can measure: alpha, beta, theta and delta waves.
- **Branchial arches.** Small fissures that appear in the developing embryo, which in fish will form the gills, but which in mammals give rise to auditory and phonatory structures. Those arising from

the first branchial arch are innervated mainly by the trigeminal nerve or fifth cranial pair, while those from the second arch are innervated by the facial nerve, the seventh pair.

- **Circadian cycle.** Throughout the day, organisms present cyclic physiological activities, which are repeated. The best known is wakefulness and sleep, but other systems also follow these patterns in their metabolism. The continuous alteration of the habitual circadian cycles generates stress and metabolic disorders that can lead to disease.

- **Decibel.** In audiology, the measure of sound intensity. A whisper reaches about 30 dB, the spoken voice, around 60 dB and a great opera singer can exceed 100 dB. It is not a linear but a logarithmic variable, in which one plus one is not two. If a loudspeaker is producing 60 dB and we place an identical one next to it, the sound level meter will mark 63 dB. When the sound source is doubled, the increase is only 3 dB. The level of 0 dB does not mean absence of sound, but the threshold, the weakest sound we can hear. The intensity of a sound of 30 dB is 1,000 times greater than one of 0 dB and one of 60 dB is 1,000,000 times more intense.

- **Dyslexia.** Disorder of the learning of reading and writing, characterized by a great difficulty in the recognition of words or their graphical representation in spite of having normal intelligence, and which is not overcome by applying pedagogical methods. It is considered to be a neurological disorder, although its actual cause is still under debate.

- **Ear (anatomy).** Divided into three different parts for study purposes: the outer ear, made up of the auricle and the auditory canal; the middle ear, made up of the eardrum and the ossicular chain (hammer, anvil and stirrup). Finally, the inner ear, with the vestibule and the cochlea.

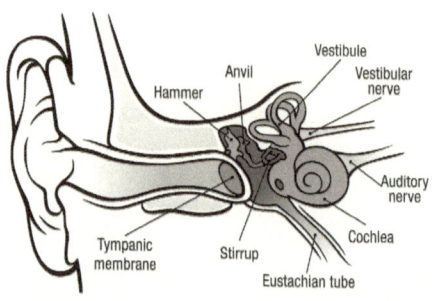

- **Efferent.** Information that travels from the brain to other parts of the body. These are orders that regulate different systems. In the auditory system, the efferent innervation modulates the perception of sound. Efferent pathways are also called centrifugal pathways.
- **EMDR.** Eye Movement Desensibilization Reprocessing. Psychological technique designed by Francine Shapiro for treating post-traumatic stress through bilateral stimulation. It has seen great development worldwide in recent years due to its effectiveness and relatively simple implementation.
- **Evoked potentials.** Brain waves that appear in response to a stimulus, in our case an acoustic one. They allow the response of the hearing system to be established without the need for patient collaboration, making them particularly useful in the auditory diagnosis of young children. They are designated by the letter P and a digit indicating their latency time (the milliseconds between the stimulus and the appearance of the potential).
- **Facial nerve.** The seventh cranial pair, responsible for moving all the muscles of the face (except the eyelid elevator). It also innervates the muscle of the stirrup and the eardrum, which is why it is deeply involved in the auditory system.
- **Fundamental note.** When an object vibrates, such as the string of a violin, a set of sounds is produced, a harmonic series whose lowest note we call the fundamental note. The rest of the sounds that accompany this note are the harmonics, whose frequency is a natural multiple of the fundamental. For example, if we play A_2 on the violin, whose frequency is 220 Hz (fundamental), we will find harmonics at 440 Hz (x2), at 660 Hz (x3), at 880 Hz (x4), and so on. The same will occur when playing any musical instrument or with our own voice. The relative intensities of the different harmonics will change, which distinguishes the sound of one instrument from another.
- **Graphical representation of sound.** Sound has three components: intensity, frequency and duration. Its graphic representation allows two of these three variables to be located on the X axis and on the Y axis. If we show time on the X axis and the frequencies in the Y axis, we obtain a sonogram, which shows us the frequencies that make up the sound

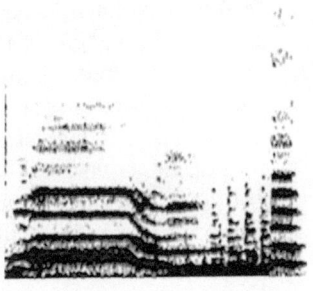

and how it changes over time. The differing intensity of each frequency is also displayed, with a lighter or heavier stroke. In this way the sonogram records the three components of sound. It is the most complete graphic representation.

- **Hair cell.** In general, any cell provided with cilia, but in audiology we use this term for the auditory cells inside the cochlea.
- **Harmonics.** Set of frequencies that accompany a fundamental sound and allow the nature of that sound to be identified. Thanks to the harmonic structure we can distinguish a harp from a violin or a trumpet, even if they play the same note. It is the same with the voice. Great harmonic richness is a sign of a great singer.
- **Hertz.** Standard measure of the frequency of a sound. The higher the frequency, the higher the pitch of the sound and the shorter the wavelength. The reference note that an orchestra tunes itself to, A_4, has a frequency of 440 Hz. Beyond 16,000-20,000 Hz, we are dealing with ultrasounds, which the human ear is no longer able to hear. Infrasounds below 20 Hz are also inaudible to us.
- **Intracochlear pressure.** Liquids (endolymph and perilymph) circulate inside the inner ear. Their pressure is constantly regulated. If altered, this causes auditory and balance dysfunctions.
- **Labyrinth.** Synonym for inner ear. It is made up of the vestibule and the cochlea. Its name derives from its irregular shape.
- **Lagena.** Inner ear of reptiles and birds, ancestor of the cochlea of mammals.
- **M100.** Evoked field that appears at 100 msec. Similar to an evoked potential, but obtained by magnetoencephalography.
- **Meniere's disease.** Syndrome whose cause is still unknown and for which there is no effective treatment. A triad of hearing loss, vertigo and tinnitus (noises or ringing in the ears) appears suddenly. It is a disease that completely disables the patient. In mild cases, it disappears within a few days. In others, symptoms recur periodically.
- **MMN.** MisMatch Negativity. An electrical response of the brain, an evoked potential of long latency that occurs when a novelty is introduced into a repetitive and constant series of equal auditory stimuli, at a rate of several per second (oddball paradigm). It is the signal that indicates that the brain has noticed the change introduced, even if the subject is not conscious. It appears about 100 msec after the stimulus, and fades 150 msec later. Due to its characteristics, it is widely used in research, as it is altered in several pathologies and experimental situations.

- **Olivocochlear bundle.** One of the main pathways of the efferent auditory system. As its name suggests, its fibers project from the superior olivary complex, located in the brain stem, to the cochlea.
- **Ossicular chain.** A series of tiny ossicles that, in mammals, connect the eardrum to the inner ear. These are the hammer, the anvil and the stirrup. Traditionally it has been believed that sound is transmitted through these bones, although this is a widely contested opinion today.
- **Otoacoustic emissions.** The set of sounds that are obtained when inserting a microphone in the ear and are made by the activity of the hair cells. Their origin and function remain a mystery, but they are very useful in detecting possible cases of deafness in young children. Otoacoustic emission testing is routinely applied to newborns.
- **Otosclerosis.** Degeneration of the ossicular chain due to an imbalance in bone metabolism. It can cause considerable hearing loss, usually in the bass range, and the ability to understand what is being said can be significantly altered, especially in noisy places.
- **Otoscopy.** Inspection of the ear canal and tympanic membrane through the otoscope, a small flashlight attached to a magnifying lens.
- **P50, P100, etc.** See evoked potentials.
- **Saccule.** Part of the vestibule that, in evolution, appears after the utricle. It is responsible for capturing gravity in vertical displacements, such as when we go up in an elevator.
- **Scotoma/peak.** In an audiometric curve, a drop in sensitivity at a given point is called a scotoma. The opposite is the peak, a noticeable increase in sensitivity in a particular area.
- **Spectral analysis.** Graphical representation of sound, which allows us to visualize its intensity, its duration and its frequency composition.
- **Stapedial reflex.** Involuntary reaction of the stapedial muscle to an intense noise. Its characteristics (latency, reflex intensity, etc.) can be determined by means of a device called an impedance meter, which is of great help in the investigation and detection of auditory pathologies.
- **Stapedial.** Relating to the stirrup or stapes.
- **Statocyst.** Organ of balance, the primeval vestibule of the invertebrates, which contains a set of hair cells among which

seawater circulates. A calcareous stone, the otocyst, located in its interior, provides gravitational information. Its inertia, the reverse of the movement of the animal, provides the hair cells with the positional reference.

- **Supporting cells.** Hair cells are not found in isolation within the cochlea, but embedded in structures that give them physical support, formed by the Deiters, Hensen and Claudius cells.
- **Trigeminal nerve.** This is the fifth cranial pair, responsible for the sensitivity of the face and movement of the jaw. It also innervates the tensor tympani muscle.
- **Tympanometry.** An audiological test to check the mobility or stiffness of the tympanic membrane. Of great help in the detection of auditory pathologies.
- **Utricle.** The most archaic part of the vestibule. It is charged with capturing gravity in horizontal displacements.
- **Vagus nerve.** The tenth cranial pair. It innervates the eardrum and adjacent areas of the auditory canal. Responsible for the parasympathetic nervous system, it is closely related to stress management and activation of the viscera.
- **Vestibular nuclei.** They most probably constituted the primordial brain. They are groups of neurons, which manage the information provided by the vestibule, relating to control of balance and muscle tone.
- **Vestibule**: Organ of balance. It corresponds to the most primitive part of the ear. It is composed of the utricle, saccule and semicircular canals. It is a gravity sensor that provides the necessary reference point for executing body movements.

ANNEX

SOME CONSIDERATIONS ON THE LISTENING TEST

Content collected in the 3rd International Congress of Audio-Psycho-Phonology. Antwerp, 1973.

Interview with Professor Tomatis.
Unknown author*

*This document was included in the materials that A. Tomatis distributed in his training courses, and is therefore completely authentic, although it has not been possible to identify its author.

Interpretation of the listening test

Could you define what you mean by a listening test and indicate the fundamental differences between a listening test and an audiogram?

I think there is an important difference between an audiogram and a listening test. The material provided by the latter on different planes allows a considerable number of elements to be grouped together to give the expert therapist valuable information to establish the diagnosis.

This test differs from the simple audiogram, which measures the subject's hearing, so to speak. We are certainly interested in this, but it is not the essential element we are looking for. Indeed, let me repeat once again that it is important to distinguish between hearing and listening. Hearing does not imply the presence of a field of consciousness. To hear is, in a way, to pick up a sound or a message that is addressed to us. To listen is to try to apprehend that sound or that message. These are two different postures.

Audiometry is certainly not something to be overlooked, but the spirit in which it is conducted can lead to differing interpretations of the clinical or psychological contribution that it can make. This testing continues to be essential in hearing research. For the otologist it is a fundamental test from which the etiological data of an auditory function disorder are drawn. The prognosis that will guide medical or surgical therapy, or prosthetic or re-educational therapy, among others, depends on it. It will therefore be possible, on the basis of these data, to apply the protocol of care for restoring an impaired function.

The listening test integrates these data within the framework of a psychological process that will make it possible to understand whether or not the subject wishes to make use of the resources available at the perceptual level. Everyone is familiar with such commonly heard popular sayings as: "They have ears and do not hear; they hear but do not know how to listen". There is a gradation between hearing and listening and the listening test allows us to learn what use a subject is able to make of his hearing. The audiogram gives us a certain curve but does not indicate whether the individual being examined really knows how to use this curve to communicate with others through self-control. We find the same gradation in vision. You can come across a perfect eye, with the best retina in the world;

that does not allow you to know if the subject can aim a rifle well or paint. There is, therefore, a dimension of gnosis that provides complementary data. In audio-psycho-phonology we see that a bad curve can be very well used: providing the subject with listening possibilities that many of those who hear perfectly are deprived of. I have seen people who, based on their hearing, are considered to be deaf but who nevertheless are able to hear by focusing their attention. So there is a dimension of attention, of adhesion that is instituted in listening, a raising of awareness that embeds itself into hearing itself. The listening test is therefore at a higher level than the audiogram itself. Above all, it is a psychological test, while the audiogram is a test of a physiological, or even an anatomical nature.

Do you therefore consider that there is an essential difference between hearing and listening?

Yes, I think it is necessary to be able to distinguish between these two essentially different functions, even though they apparently develop on identical terrains. Both run through the same territory, but differ in their mode of action, depending on the underlying motivations. Hearing is the result of a perception that responds to a stimulus from outside. Listening is based on an external stimulus, certainly, but one that must be sought internally, with intentionality. Here is where the notions of sensor, choice and filter come into play. The conscious element thus becomes the essential factor that explains the difference between these two activities which evolve in parallel and one of which, listening, is placed on a higher plane because it calls on a specific characteristic of man in his evolution. Seeing and trying to see are two totally different mechanisms, with the latter making use of the former. Trying to see is aiming. With hearing and listening it is the same. Listening results from trying to hear and is the equivalent of aiming. Listening is to the ear what aiming is to the eye. The distinction must be constantly present in the mind of the audio-psycho-phonologist. It is up to him to use the results offered by pure audiology to safeguard the psychological data that will allow him to make his diagnosis and determine his mode of action.

-Several of your publications speak of an ideal curve, towards which every ear should tend in order to listen well. This curve would look like this.

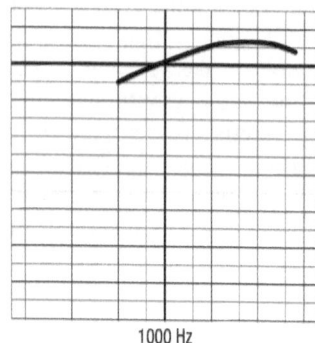

1000 Hz

We see an ascending curve between 500 and 2,000 Hz, which corresponds to an approximate slope of between 6 and 18 dB per octave, then a dome between 2,000 and 4,000 Hz, and then a slight descent. We find this curve in your book "L'oreille et le langage" (The Ear and Language) when you talk about the musical ear. Perhaps you could explain to us what this curve corresponds to on the physiological level?

At the level of pure physics, it indicates the responses of the ear when it functions well. It actually corresponds to Wegel's "lemon-shaped curve", but inverted. Indeed, Wegel's curve is the response curve obtained when the frequencies are placed on the abscissas axis and the intensities on the ascending ordinates. An initial threshold is obtained, in the lower part, starting from a minimum that begins in the low frequencies around 40–50 dB, then approaches the curve of the abscissas between 2,000 and 3,000 Hz and rises again to 40–50 dB in the trebles between 8,000 and 10,000 Hz. This curve is completed and adopts the shape of a lemon when sounds of increasing intensity are sent, obtaining a curve of maximum thresholds that determine the point where the ear begins to suffer: the "pain thresholds".

These thresholds also start in the bass range at 50–60 dB, returning to the first curve, then reach 120–130 dB between 2,000 and 3,000 Hz, only to fall in the trebles and rejoin the first curve.

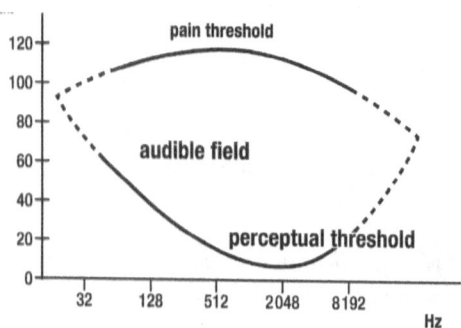

The median line of about 50–60 dB represents an area called the "Munsen Zone", which responds to the dynamics of the ear or, in other words, its optimal area of operation without distortion. In all other areas, as you can see, the ear acts as a filter whose slopes are variable depending on the intensity, with a rotation point between 1,000 and 2,000 Hz. In order to reduce these distortions, which are always difficult to integrate into the reading of graphs, the Americans have standardized the audiograms of the type that we all use, by inverting Wegel's image, and straightening out the minimums to obtain a straight line. However, these standards maintain a preferential zone between 1,000 and 2,000 Hz (the hump or dome that we know) in spite of the compensations of 30–40 dB that modify the curve in the bass and treble ranges.

There is therefore a kind of ideal physiological curve to look for. But do not think that when you acquire it, you reach the conscious field. Anyway, it is certain that if you are not gifted with that exceptional ear, you are very unlikely to be musicians, able to produce sounds of high quality. If a cellist does not have that ear, he will not be able to play. In other words, it is indispensable in order to reach a certain level, but not sufficient.

I believe, then, that this is a physical–acoustic response curve that is necessary for the elaboration of listening processes. Why does it not exist in all individuals? In fact, when children come into this world, they have the potential for it. But the dramas of life—affective upheavals, parental and social prohibitions and sometimes physiological suffering—make them close out the world of listening, the universe of communication. In their desire not to listen again, they introduce distortions, disconnections, and reductions; they lengthen their response circuits in order to be able to distance themselves from those who make them suffer and avoid contact with them. But they end up entrapped by the tricks they use to defend themselves against the aggressions of the outside world: locked up in a chamber, with no escape. In the listening test, distortions or imperfections then appear with respect to the underlying ideal curve that remains present in every individual. There is therefore a need to smooth out these distortions, to remove these imperfections, by using appropriate techniques to free the self from the chains of non-listening.

The acquisition of this ideal curve corresponds to the harmonization of the interplay between the two muscles of the middle ear that make it possible to permanently regulate the internal pressures of the labyrinth by causing the intervention of the phenomena of least impedance. In electro-acoustics or mechanics, impedance is the name we give to the process of minimum resistance. Along the path of sound through the ear, we need to find points of minimum impedance that allow the ideal response to be obtained. Then we discover that the entire auditory system, from the external canal to the internal vesicle, responds to this ideal curve. That is a wonder of nature: yet another! The human ear is therefore made, adapted, shaped to hear and to listen. The distortions that occur, the blockages, the weaknesses that appear are there only to slow down motivation, to prevent exchange, to disrupt dialogue, to make communication difficult. Those who have not felt, have not enjoyed, true listening cannot fully realize what they are missing as they conserve their distortions. It is so easy to hear, to communicate when the ear is harmoniously open to the outside world, while it is so difficult to interact with the environment when, at the level of the cortex, we are constantly having to eliminate the distortions that complicate life.

If you listen in this ideal way, which corresponds to a certain tension of the muscles of the hammer and stirrup, you obtain, according to your texts, a damping of bass sounds and a fine-tuned perception of the trebles. What is the role of the eardrum in these listening processes?

The eardrum is placed in a certain state of tension to play the role of tuning fork, making the cranium vibrate by means of the "sulcus tympani". It is the whole cranium that vibrates and transmits sound to the labyrinth, not the ossicular chain, which is commonly thought to be the vehicle of sound. The ossicular chain plays the role of adapter or regulator, not transmitter.

The conduction of sound through the air and then through the bone should also be studied therefore, at the same time, so that the listening posture of the subject can then be determined.

What is the difference between the air curve and the bone curve?

You are right to ask me this very important question. I will say straight away that the air curve makes it possible to specify the form in which the subjects listen to the outside world, and in particular to the other person, to the interlocutor. The bone curve gives information on the way in which the subjects listen to their inner life, their vegetative universe, their consciousness. It is the curve of self-listening, self-control, inner listening.

In fact, there should only be one curve corresponding to the union of the two listening types: external listening and internal listening. The ideal curve is actually a single one. We have voluntarily separated the arrangement of the two curves (air and bone) in order to be able to distinguish the different responses and interpret the distortions. When the listening is perfect, the curves are joined together but, to facilitate analysis of the results, parallel curves have been established: the air curve should be above the bone curve, as seen in this diagram.

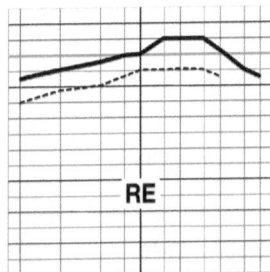 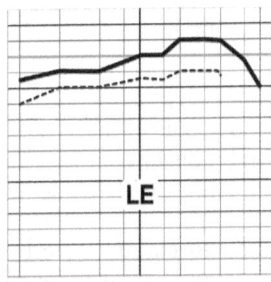

Obviously, this result is rarely found. Distortions can usually be seen between the two curves and these gaps are very interesting to observe. I truly regret that hearing specialists—most of them anyway—do not pay attention to these differences, which nevertheless provide marvelous elements for establishing the diagnosis. When there are distortions between the two listening types, when there are problems within the self, there are irregularities between the two curves that indicate that the subject hears the outside in a different way to his inner life. There is a mismatch. There is a dilemma. We may find a very good external listening curve (air conduction) together with a self-listening (bone conduction) curve with significant distortions, or vice versa: we see perturbations in air conduction while bone conduction indicates internal listening of high quality. It is important to study the relative position of one curve with respect to the other, as the gaps between air curve and bone curve represent compensations.

How should we approach the interpretation of a listening test? What information can the air curve and the bone curve provide us and what conclusions can be drawn from studying the graphs for each ear: right and left?

It is clear that this analysis can be done globally, almost instantaneously, but only on the basis of great experience. This is true of all the other tests as well as the listening test. Leaving aside the data accumulated, a long, patient, meticulous learning path must be followed before even beginning to acquire the global vision this test can offer us. In fact, with time, the experienced tester should be able to capture, at a glance, all the successive levels depicted by the curves obtained in order to produce a synthesis and draw the necessary conclusions. But isn't that the case with any test used in psychology?

With any listening test, you have to consider several parameters and establish the connections between them. Let us start by analyzing some in depth, to learn from specific examples. We have various data, as follows:

- air curve (AC)
- bone curve (BC)
- relationship between AC and BC for each ear
- relationship between AC and BC from one ear to the other.

In order to take this work of interpretation to a deeper level, we will incorporate new elements of analysis that will lead us, on the one hand, to the meaning of the graph of the left ear (the one on the right in our diagrams) and that of the graph of the right ear (on the left in the diagrams) and, on the other hand, to the tripartition of each one of the graphs according to the frequencies.

1) Meaning of the graphs on the right and left:
   - Everything concerning the left ear corresponds to affectivity, adhesion to the past, to the mother. The left ear is the mother, as you have known for a long time.
   - Everything concerning the right ear corresponds to dynamics, to the future, to the father. The right ear is the father, as you also know well.

2) Definition of the different sectors within each graph.
   Each graph can be divided into three sectors that we are going to study in turn, from 125 to 8,000 Hz. These sound bands are distributed as follows:

   1) from 125 to 1,000 Hz
   2) from 1,000 to 2,000 Hz
   3) from 2,000 to 8,000 Hz

This corresponds to different factors that are described briefly here:

1) the sector that goes from 125 to 1,000 Hz is the one that corresponds to the bodily element and more especially to the visceralization of the self, to the ego, to the unconscious.
2) the sector that goes from 1,000 to 2,000 Hz. is essentially that of language, of communication with the other.[1]
3) the next sector, which goes from 2,000 to 8,000 Hz, and is therefore located in the region of high frequency harmonics, corresponds to spirituality, to intuition, to the subject's ideals and aspirations.

These are summarized in the following diagram:

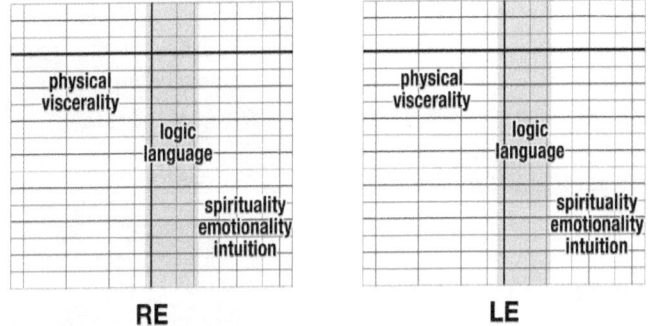

RE   LE

At the time of interpretation, this distribution at the level of the two ears and in the relationship between one ear and the other must be taken into account, since the meaning of the analyses of the left ear will be different from the right ear on a symbolic level. Thus, the right-hand part of the right-ear graph (spirituality) should be considered, so to speak, in relation to the same part of the left-ear graph (although this also corresponds to spirituality). In order to better understand what I am trying to explain, we will use some examples. But first I would like to make some clarifications with regard to the area called "viscerality", which corresponds to bass sounds. We will distinguish different territories: at 125 Hz is sexuality, 250 Hz is the large intestine, 500 Hz the small intestine, 1,000 Hz the stomach. Let us move on to the examples. If you find this kind of curve:

---

[1] AN: Later, he considered that this zone was between 1,000 and 3,000 Hz

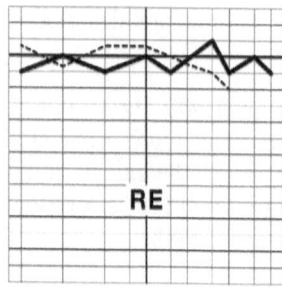 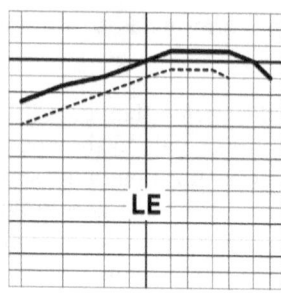

With peaks on the left and not on the right, we can already conclude that the subject is undergoing a dynamic that does not follow his affectivity. He lives almost outside himself, outside his deep self. That can happen under certain circumstances.

Suppose a subject has entered a room where there is suffocating gas and has had a sudden asthma attack because of this temporary intoxication. You may notice a change in his voice and, if he takes a listening test, an alteration to his curves like the following:

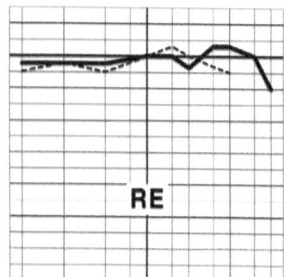 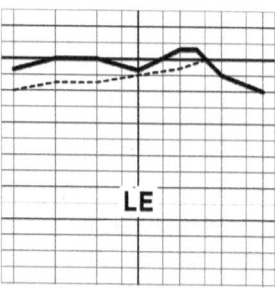

You can see a peak at 1,500 Hz in the right ear but nothing has happened in the left ear, but if there was also that peak at 1,500 in the left ear, you would know that this was an asthmatic state (or at least an allergy) on top of an affective blockage. There is a problem with the mother. Being unable to attack her, the subject traumatizes in himself what he has integrated as being the mother, in this case the respiratory tree. He can get pulmonary asthma (shortage of breath), laryngeal asthma (dry cough, especially at night) or nasal asthma (rhinitis, hay fever, etc.).

Let's take another example.

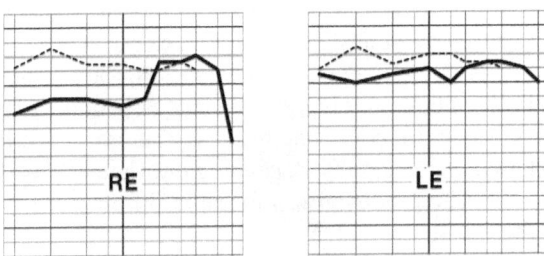

I can see a peak at 250 Hz on the right and left, so this is a disorder of the colon in a subject who is somatically experiencing (RE) a colitis of affective origin (LE).

If this peak at 250 Hz appears only in the LE and not in the RE as in the following case:

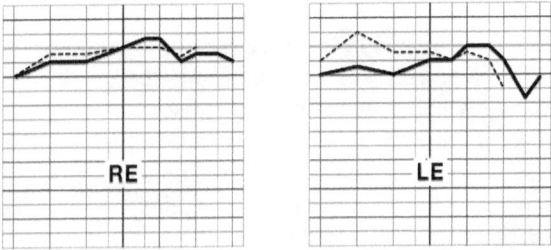

it means that there is an underlying colitis of affective origin (vulnerability at colon level) that for the moment has not manifested itself, since the peak is not present in the right-ear graph, but can appear at any time.

If, on the other hand, this peak at 250 Hz appears only on the graph of the right ear, it simply means that the subject has eaten badly the previous day and has stomach pain.

He does not feel this disturbance at the affective level. It is not a deep reaction.

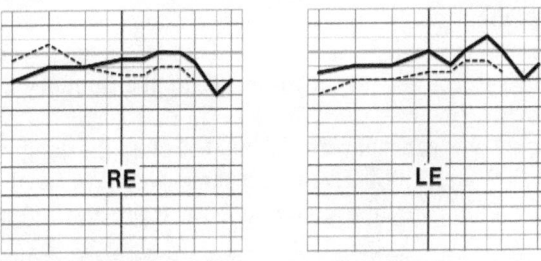

Third example: a curve with a peak at 500 Hz. I therefore know this subject has a small-intestine problem. I can interpret the curves in the same way as in the previous case depending on whether the peak appears in both graphs, only in the left ear or only in the right ear.

It is interesting to note that there is therefore a difference in reactions shown on the graphs, depending on whether it is the large or small intestine. There is even a noticeable difference at vocal level related to these disturbances. When you have a trained ear, you can tell, just by listening to the subject's voice, whether he suffers from the colon or the small intestine. This is normal since they are different passing bands, at audio–vocal level. Together with some gastroenterologist colleagues I did some experiments by tape-recording their patients' voices. Listening to them, I could tell unmistakably what their digestive complaints were, so it occurred to me that modifying a subject's voice could certainly improve digestion. But that's another issue I won't dwell on today. I'll continue with the examples.

If we have a peak at 1,000 Hz we are in the presence of a disorder that affects the stomach. We will also study the graph of the left and right ear to see whether this is an acute disorder (RE), a chronic one (RE + LE) of an affective nature, or a vulnerable area (LE) that can manifest itself at the slightest weakness of the organism.

This has been an overview of the so-called "visceral" sector: the area of the body, the area of the ego. When there are peaks in this region we cannot say that this is a visceral person, but one who cannot get rid of his organic universe, the noise of his viscera, the messages that his ego interprets as a signal. Such a person often hears his swallowing, his heart or his breathing; in this way he experiences a whole universe of anguish which forces him to remain too concerned about himself. What if his heart suddenly stops? Is he breathing differently? Why does his intestine make that noise? His organic life takes on such importance that dialogue with the other takes second place. On the other hand, these are people who do not know how to listen to what they are being told, who talk about themselves constantly, about their illnesses, about their boo-boos. So these indications are interesting. They allow us to know the psycho-somatic state of the subject and to be informed of the auditory universe in which he lives.

Of course, we can analyze the next sector, the language sector, between 1,000 and 2,000 Hz in the same way. We need to look at what is happening in this region in both right and left ear, to see whether there are scotomas or, on the contrary, peaks expressing an aggressiveness that is more or less contained, more or less expressed, depending on whether the peak is in the left ear only or both ears. This is an important element when it comes to making a prognosis. Indeed, you can warn the mother that, throughout the audio-vocal education to which the child is subjected, the child is going to have this or that reaction. For example, if in the left ear there is a peak at 1,500 Hz, I can say that the reaction will be of the respiratory type. The child will feel breathless, give the impression of breathing badly; sometimes even an asthma crisis appears (nasal, pharyngeal or pulmonary). If the peak is at 250 Hz in the left ear, you can tell the mother that the child has abdominal problems. She will be surprised by this, but in the course of the sessions she will tell you that her child has been suffering from diarrhea or constipation for a few days. When I see a peak at 500 Hz, I cannot tell what the digestive problem will be but I am sure there is a problem at this level. I know the child's belly speaks to him; it is the famous internal dialogue and it is there where there will be a reaction during the treatment at somatic level.

Another interesting phenomenon shows whether this aggressiveness is expressed or not: opened or closed selectivity. When you see in the graph some enormous peaks of aggressiveness, but with a closed selectivity, you can deduce that it is all incubating, but the surrounding universe is so dominant that the child seems to shrink: unable to speak up and docile as a lamb. When I tell the mother or the family that the child is aggressive, the reply is "That's not possible, he is the sweetest child you can find". If the mother is very powerful, we see throughout the therapy that the inner organization improves little by little, that the curves are modified, but nothing happens because the curtain of selectivity has not been opened. On the other hand, aggressiveness manifests itself as soon as selectivity is opened before all is in order; then we notice strong reactions towards the mother, since she is still the focal point the child turns to first, blaming her for all his ills. Then it will be necessary to solve his issues with her before tackling other dialogues, especially the one he must establish with his father.

If, for example, you have a listening test showing selectivity closure on both sides, you know immediately that the subject is not in contact with his mother and has therefore not connected to his father. The patient should immediately be placed in filtered sound with maternal voice until selectivity is opened. It will first open in the left ear (that of the maternal image, graph on the right) and you will rush to discover the dialogue with the father, but as long as the selectivity has not been opened in the right ear (graph on the left) and there are still blockages in the trebles, the problem with the mother will still not have been solved. In summary, we can say that the image of the mother as far as selectivity is concerned is distributed on the one hand over the whole set of frequencies of the left-ear graph and, on the other hand, in the treble region in the right-ear graph (which nevertheless corresponds to that of the paternal image).

Let us look at a few examples:

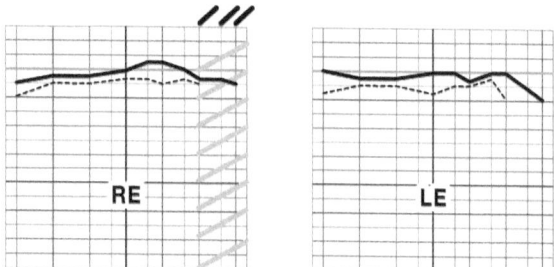

After 40 sessions of maternal voice

The graph indicates that the left ear has been opened, in terms of selectivity, but that the right ear remains blocked as from 4,000 Hz. In this case, we can say that the maternal problem has not been completely solved and that therefore, the encounter or dialogue with the father is not yet possible.

When I say that the maternal relationship is not normalized, I do not mean that the mother has been rejected or that the child is fighting against her; we simply have to conclude that the subject continues in a buried intrauterine universe, that he has not resolved his situation, and

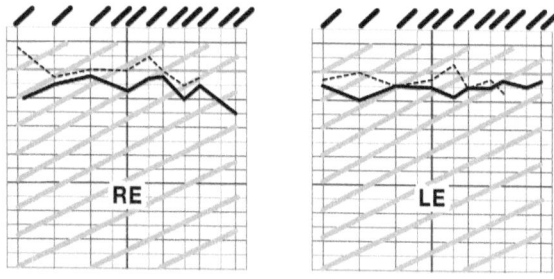

Selectivity closed on both ears

his present is still impregnated with his past. We find these reactions of maternal attachment represented by resistances at the level of selectivity opening in certain children, such as those with a mental disability, who remain very tied to their mother and who are so dependent on her that they do not want to leave their former state.

Could you explain why it is that when, during a selectivity study, a subject makes an error for example between 500 and 1,000 Hz, it is said that selectivity is completely blocked from that value onward?

Indeed, when there are deficiencies of analysis in an area located in the bass range, there is a good chance that the capacity for selectivity in the trebles is non-existent. I can confirm this from my experience, but it is still hard for me to say why. What is certain is that the subject cannot use bands located above the non-selective zone. It is a kind of barrier that keeps the subject in the bass region. In addition, we can emphasize that his voice is low and he lacks high harmonics.

In other words, whether there is a total blocking of selectivity or only between 500 and 1,000 Hz for example, the result is the same. There is certainly no possibility of selective analysis in the areas above the blocked frequencies. In therapy, it will be easier and faster to achieve opening when the closure is partial. When the barrier is raised between 500 and 1,000 Hz, to continue with the example, all other areas will then quickly light up and the subject will be able to benefit from all the underlying vitality that was until now in a state of somnolence. When selectivity is blocked across all frequencies, the work takes longer. It is necessary to clear the uncultivated areas little by little, to give them new life.

With selectivity it works in the same way as with certain scotomas located in the bass range. They constitute a veritable barrier that prevents the individual from going beyond the "scotoma zone". The subject does not use the range of treble sounds. He will speak in a low pitch, and if he sings he will have difficulties in "going up" as they say in the business. Here, you will be able to intervene quickly because, once the scotoma has been filled in, all the underlying possibilities will burst into life and you will see the voice light up in a surprising way.

This phenomenon is more easily observed in the singing voice than in the spoken voice. When we have a scotoma of 15 decibels at 500 Hz, the subject can have two voices when singing. He can express himself in the bass region perfectly and then, at a given moment, he jumps over the scotoma and is in another register.

I have had the opportunity to meet opera singers who came to consult me because, suddenly, when trying to produce an G they came out with a E. It was due to a scotoma. I put them under the Electronic Ear and when they recovered their quality control (eliminating the scotoma) they were able to sing again without such unpleasant surprises.

In the selectivity test, we often find children who do not understand what is being asked of them. We explain the basses and the trebles but they still respond randomly without perceiving the distinction. What can we do then?

First of all, we have to go back to the basics regarding this test. I realize that many of you make your patients happy by sending the sound to them several times until they recognize the difference. In reality, you are making yourselves happy but you are falsifying the test and are not helping the subject.

The most important thing is that at a given moment and quite quickly, the subject perceives one piece of information and then another that he must contrast with it. If he gets it wrong, it does not matter, just keep a record of it. Of course, if you start over thirty times, he will end up getting it right, but that is not what happens when an individual receives one word and then another in real life, when he will need to analyze them quickly within the verbal chain. Naturally, if you repeat the words ten times, he will understand in the end, but sentence dynamics do not work that way.

It is normal for children to find the test more difficult than adults, but this is a question of pedagogy. You have to learn to express yourself so that the child understands what is being asked of him. If he does not understand the instructions, it is because in life itself he does not perceive the subtle difference between one word and another. He does not know what "higher" or "lower" means because he does not have an image of his body, because he is de-lateralized. His answers show that he is not able to analyze the information reaching him. Some centers deal with children with mental disabilities and educators sometimes complain that they cannot pass on the instructions. "They don't understand what's being asked of them, what higher or lower is," they say, talking about the children to be tested. Then one day, during a check-up, they realize that the child has perceived a difference between 500 and 125 Hz. It is because, at that moment, he is beginning to integrate what is asked of him, to understand what is being said.

So what you have to do is write down the answers they give you that differ from their initial ones. The chain of speech is made up of thousands of phonemes that must be distinguished for the word to reach its true meaning. The selectivity test is specially made to reveal the subject's auditory possibilities with respect to a pure sound, which is an enormous simplification compared to a word. A "pure" sound as its name indicates is a sound stripped of ambiguities that should be easy to distinguish from another by comparison. If an individual cannot make this distinction between pure sounds, how can he distinguish the subtleties, the infinite variations, the multiple colors that wrap a word inside a sentence?

The human ear has exceptional analytical possibilities. It can perceive a difference of 3 Hz at 1,000 Hz; it can also decipher the direction of that variation, recognizing whether it is a sound of 997 Hz or 1,000 Hz, by placing it on the frequency scale. Consequently, it can easily distinguish one octave from another; indeed, there is a world of difference between the two pure sounds that are sent to the subject's ear.

Until now we have spoken mainly about children, but very often we find the same difficulties in adolescents and adults. They answer "Higher" or "Lower" randomly in the selectivity test as if they did not want to understand what is being asked of them. Should we change the instructions we give them?

No. We should stick to what we have been taught as to how to run the test. Whatever the cost, nothing should be done to get right answers. There is no point in restarting the test on the pretext that the person did not understand what was being asked of them. Some adults, so as not to look foolish, act as if they can distinguish one sound from another, and respond haphazardly in the test. In reality they do not know how to distinguish the difference, often confusing pitch with intensity. They have few selection options with respect to certain sounds, especially in the treble area which is the most subtle. But they do not want to admit it. Just leave them to their own devices and record the mistakes.

The most surprising thing I have seen in this type of investigation is the type of responses collected from certain singers, musicians or dancers. A tenor has different selective possibilities from those of a bass, and a violinist moves in different areas from those of another instrumentalist. As far as dancers are concerned, they generally have a relatively poor ear. They practically never hear, in terms of selectivity, above 500–1,000 Hz. They only perceive the rhythms inherent to the body. Some become famous dancers precisely because they actually cut out the area of the melody. They are not great musicians; they have a great sense of rhythm.

-*What is the test by which you were able to determine that children have a musical ear?*

By counter-reaction at the voice level. All children sing, and sing in tune, reproducing the music immediately. Naturally I am talking about normal children who have not had major emotional trauma. If you observe how children react to a tune, they integrate it, they reproduce it by singing or playing an instrument, they dance to it, they mime to it, they live it. They are the music. It is an integral part of their body. That is why education through music, especially in kindergarten, is so important. So often today we forget this basic principle because we try first and foremost to intellectualize education. We try to turn children into beings full of knowledge. That is when the difficulties begin. Intelligence ripens gently in a body ready to receive language.

Children at first have a musical ear, without distortion, without deformation. Our mistake is to take that still overly fragile nervous system and burden it with knowledge, with a semantics that will introduce disturbances of a psychological nature. The problems, the complexes, then arrive with great speed. The least vulnerable children are those with mental disabilities. Unable to access the world of intelligence, they continue to be children who are sensitive to music, which they appreciate very much and which they reproduce easily. The more gifted child will want to go further, will want to enter more quickly into the linguistic universe that attracts him and to which adults (parents and teachers) will try to lead him. From that moment on, the distortions appear. In order not to hear certain unpleasant things, certain voices, the child will produce scotomas, will break his auditory diaphragm, will move away from communication by choosing the longest circuits. He will adopt a left-ear lead, losing all possibilities of listening to language and, of course, music. He will start singing out of tune and, as he will then be laughed at, will stay silent for a long time.

-Do the aggressiveness peaks mentioned previously appear in the air curve or in the bone curve?

In general, we find these distortions on the two curves, but in some cases the air curve compensates for the bone curve. As I have said many times, one can die inwardly while giving the impression, at least for a certain time, of coping with the present. But this mask ends up falling and then the drama unfolds. You have to be wary of people who compensate, because one day they break down. This situation can be predicted by studying the subject's curve: how the bone curve and air curve relate to each other.

-What references, what information can a flat, rectilinear curve give us? Since the ideal curve should have a fairly steep upward slope, it seems that when it is not so, when it does not appear on the graph, there is an abnormality. Faced with a flat curve, can we conclude that frequencies are perceived with the same intensity? Does this not imply a lack of nuances, of sensitivity? Does it affect the analysis of sounds and the timbre of the voice eventually?

A straight curve does not allow for analysis. It seems to indicate an inability to distinguish between one octave and another. In order for an ear to be able to distinguish such variations, there have to be intervals, steps that make it possible to decipher the different heights of the sounds. On the physiological level, one can try to explain this phenomenon in the following way. The slightest low-frequency noise masks the other sounds. The inner ear is a device that works at constant pressure; it is a manometer, an accelerometer, but when there is a low frequency and therefore, there is not enough tension to suppress it, this low frequency erases the other frequencies. This is a masking phenomenon.

The subject who presents a flat curve actually hears only the bass frequencies and cannot make an analysis at the treble level. You will see that this curve is found in people who have a flat voice, without a timbre. We find it quite often in subjects with mental disabilities, who have few possibilities of analysis at cortical level. As they are unable to use high-pitched sounds to charge the cortex, their difficulties of integration and comprehension can be understood to a certain extent.

The presence of an ascending slope is necessary so that the ear can block the low frequencies, attenuate them, allowing the proximal part of the cochlea to be used, specifically in the language area. This is specific to the human ear. The hearing of certain animals, in terms of the passing bands, is more developed than in our ear: the dolphin, for example, hears up to 200,000 Hz, some vampire bats up to 150,000 Hz, a dog up to 45,000 Hz. But these amount to very little compared to the human ear's faculty of hearing language. This area of fine-grained analysis is disrupted by any excessive perception of low frequencies.

Why is this language region so important? Because it actually represents the image of the body. If you make a frequency table, you will notice that the deepest sounds (16 to 20 Hz) correspond to the height of the human body.[2]

If you continue this analysis in language you can see that each wavelength touches, informs on a part of the body, from the feet to the head. The bass sounds correspond to the lower part and the treble sounds (short waves) to the higher part. Distributed in this way, the frequencies of language are thus adapted to the human body in order to be able to shape it completely.

Is it language that has sculpted the human body? Or is it the human body that has forced language to install itself in the frequency zones that allow it to control the body schema? I would opt for the first hypothesis, remembering that man is born of sound and reflecting on one of the great maxims of Hermes Trismegistus: "It is sound that has made the ear. If you want to know sound, study the ear first". In terms of language, men sculpt their bodies according to the sounds they emit. Furthermore, these sounds are strongly influenced by the acoustic characteristics of the location. I often have cause to evoke the phenomenon of the inhabitants of the USA: made up of a highly varied mixture of peoples from England, Germany, France, Italy, etc., each with quite pronounced linguistic differences.

In the common acoustic atmosphere of the North-American continent, the speech of all these peoples becomes nasalized (although Italian and English, in particular, have no nasal sounds) like the local Indian. They adopt the same psycho-morphology as the Indian: their face flattens and they grow larger; in other words, they take on a different body image based on the sounds that they emit.

There is therefore a very important counter-reaction between language and body schema. This is why the image of the integrated body can be read on a listening test, from the feet (low frequencies) to the head (high frequencies).

-Can you give us further details about the analysis of body posture based on the listening test, and involving the spinal column?

---

[2] AN: The wavelength of a 200 Hz sound is 1.72 m.

Yes. Posture itself is affected by auditory counter-reactions, by the interplay of the nerve fascicles emanating from the utricles and the saccules in the direction of the anterior roots of the spinal nerve. It is through two pathways that each motor root, which controls all the body musculature, is itself cybernetically dependent on vestibular control.

These fascicles, citing from memory for the sake of brevity, are, I remind you, the homo-lateral vestibular-spinal or Deitero-spinal fascicles and the hetero-lateral vestibular-spinal fascicles emerging from Roller's nucleus. Let us also take note in passing of a fact that I consider essential and which is too often forgotten: the homo-lateral fascicles, that is to say the direct and therefore not decussated ones, are by far the most important. This is of capital importance in terms of laterality.

Thus, thanks to the vestibular circuits, a dynamic and static action will be reflected onto the overall posture of the spine. To this function of permanent vestibule–body dependence is added another, no less important, with its source in the vestibule, which, starting from the same point, the Scarpa ganglion, radiates upwards towards the roof nuclei, of Schwalbe and of Betcherew.

Thanks to this last set, the ocular-cephalogyric pathways are under the control of the vestibule. You can see the importance of this. I am not going to dwell on the subject for the time being, but I will emphasize that the third, fourth and fifth pairs are bound together in their activities, on which closely depends the performance of the second cranial pair: the optic nerve.

These body dynamics and statics are even more under the control of the vestibule, and consequently reflected in our tests, if we consider that all the neurological elements we are referring to have their protopathic sensory counter-reactions (that is, in the field of unconscious mechanisms) at the level of the archaic parts of the cerebellum, through the Fleschig and the Gowers sensory fascicles.

The corticalization of this whole, that is, the awakening of the epicritic awareness of this underlying image, unconsciously directed and deliberately pulled into mechanisms that shape its contours, appears with the cochlear system. The audiometric profile then takes on another dimension, the one we know, since this indispensable complement that is the cochlea is there to transform the analysis of the mechanical impulse received by the labyrinthine vesicle into acoustic-sonorous activity. Which the deaf person cannot do, as you will remember, because he is unable to perform that transformation.

Thanks to the cortex, in its recent part, and the force of the cerebellum of the same temporal level, these neo-formed stages evolve concomitantly with the neo-ear: the cochlea.

To those who know how to decipher it, any reading of the listening curve will reveal in some way the mechanisms of psychosomatic counter-reaction, through muscle and bone interplay. One could write a book on the subject but we will just give an outline here. Let us remember first of all that we can adopt various types of interpretation of the fact that each part of the body represents the whole at its own scale. This topic can be developed in as many ways as there are elements to be analyzed. Let us take for example the work of Nogier de Lyon, who established auriculotherapy based on the auricular pavilion. This doctor discovered a set of points on the auricle corresponding to different parts of the body and, thanks to acupuncture, was able to act with great precision on the body as a whole. The same goes for the cochlea, which has a metameric and segmental representation of the whole body.

Today we will deal with the representation of the spinal column and that of the head. I will add a quick analysis of internal vagal activity, remembering that the vagus, or pneumogastric nerve, or tenth cranial pair, is highly bound up with the tension of the eardrum, and therefore with listening.

The curves are read in terms of the pattern of the air curve and the bone curve. However, we are going to focus on the bone curve regarding the body's bone conduction, which in a way marks an "interiority".

Starting from the bass region, moving towards the trebles, we find the following points:

- 125 Hz: pelvis, feet, genitals
- 250 Hz: junction of the pelvis with the lumbar spine, colon, knee
- 500 Hz: dorsal-lumbar junction, intestine, elbow
- 1,000 Hz: medial-dorsal region, stomach
- 1500 Hz: dorsal-cervical part, lung
- 2,000 Hz: cervical-occipital region
- 3,000 Hz: upper part of the cranium

One could certainly read all the pathology inherent to the phenomena that show us the psychosomatic impacts of colitises, disorders of the small intestine, stomach ulcers, eczema of the knee or elbow, or asthmas, in short, so many psychological points of attachment to the body, which, in this case, has become the regulating valve for psychic disorders that cannot be dissolved and resolved in any other way.

It would be interesting to prepare a new graph of the listening test taking into account these different considerations. In order to be able to study the position of the body based on the frequencies, a vertical rather than a horizontal reading could be envisaged. Man would thus be represented in his general bodily attitude, so closely bound up with his psychic attitude. But this is only an idea that can be explored in more depth so that each one of you can propose a new graph.

As for the position of the head, here too the bone curve taken as a whole reveals the positioning of the cranium relative to the listening posture. If the bass sounds are dominant up to 500 Hz, for example, the front part will be higher than the occipital part. In other words, the plane passing through the culminating point of the forehead is higher than the vertex. On the other hand, if the curve is ideal, ascending to 6 dB/octave the vertex takes its place and becomes the culminating point, as its name indicates.

Here is, in general terms, what we should remember from the interpretation of the listening test in relation to the subject's posture. Whenever you come across these patterns, you should think about the close relationship between an individual's posture and his listening, with the latter governing the body that serves as its instrument.

-Could you give us some details about organic deafness and deafness of psychic origin?

Indeed, it is necessary to clearly distinguish between these two types of hearing loss. Certainly, it is sometimes difficult to know whether it is really a listening difficulty due to organic handicap or a refusal to hear of psychological origin. But to avoid the risk of missing something serious, it is good to be cautious in making a diagnosis.

When a unilateral or bilateral deafness is found, that is to say when an important deficit is observed, either in air conduction, in bone conduction or in both, you should immediately consider having the ear checked by an ENT specialist, unless the patient has a clear history of diseases and interventions that justify the deafness.

I will examine schematically the different cases of hearing impairment of organic origin, which are grouped into three types of deafness:

- transmission deafness
- perception deafness
- mixed deafness

Transmission deafness:

This corresponds to a modification of the so-called "transmission" system. All the elements whose function is to transmit sounds coming from outside to the labyrinthine vesicle are grouped under this denomination. It is therefore a question of searching for the obstacles that may arise in this sound pathway, which is traditionally deemed to pass through the outer ear, then the middle ear and then the inner ear. Personally, I consider that there are only two blocks: the outer ear and the inner ear. The middle ear is the intermediate place between the mechanisms of the outer ear and those of the inner ear. The so-called "transmission" disturbance will intervene at these two levels.

The obstacles that can appear can be of various types and affect the following.

- External auditory canal: wax plug, osteoma of the canal, otitis externa with boils, eczema, etc.

- Eardrum, due to thickening or loss of tissue.

- Tympanic cavity: otitis media, serous otitis, bloody, purulent or dry otitis.

- Annexes: Eustachian tube (tubal catarrh) and mastoid cavities (mastoiditis).

The graphs corresponding to these different clinical patterns are identical. It goes without saying that there may be diversification, depending on the context, which means studying the pathological description. Let us look at the general graph:

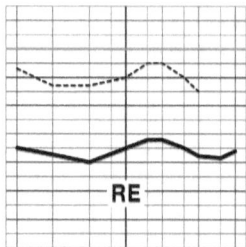 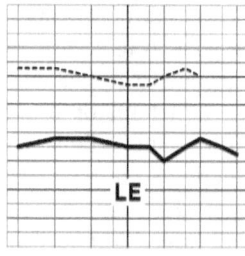

In this case the bone curve remains normal while the air curve plunges, remaining in general parallel to the bone curve. It is plotted horizontally here, like the latter. The air curve/bone curve relationship is inverted. In other words, Corti's organ functions well—as revealed by bone conduction—but the system for transmitting sound to the internal level is defective.

There is hardly any other solution than to remove the obstacle. It is up to the otologist to initiate the treatment, which, after the simple removal of the wax plug, could include anything up to mobilization of the stirrup. Deafness surgery is currently very good and has excellent results. You should not hesitate, if confronted with an otosclerosis, to refer the patient to a specialist capable of unblocking the ear.

There is no use trying to re-educate an otosclerosis sufferer. However, help can be given when the bone conduction has begun to drop, so that the subsequent intervention is more effective. It is possible to help after the intervention—two or three months later—allowing the liberated ear to learn to listen, to analyze, to discern the sounds that it had not heard for years. I will point out some problems that appear after the intervention, especially when the left ear is operated on before the right. I would remind you that otosclerosis is often a bilateral hearing impairment. When the surgeon intervenes, he first operates on one ear, generally the most deficient one, and a few weeks, or months, later, the other.

It is important to operate first on the right ear, which is, as you know, the most important one in terms of control of language, memory, concentration, etc. But when, for a particular reason, the specialist starts with the left ear, the patient can be helped by putting him under the electronic ear, until the right ear is liberated. After the intervention on their left ear, patients will naturally report hearing better with that ear, but that they have not fully regained balance or they have migraines or memory gaps, they cannot concentrate, or they have several of those symptoms at once. Your mission will be to create a bespoke program to allow them, on the one hand, to harmonize their left-side hearing and, on the other, to sustain their right ear until it is operated on. If for one reason or another that ear cannot be operated on, i.e. if the patient must be satisfied with hearing mainly through the left ear, it is possible to intervene under the electronic ear with regular sessions, making the right ear in particular work with filtered music and certain sibilants. For the texts it will be good to set the balance to 10 or to 7 so that the person perceives the phrases well and does not become discouraged.

That is what can be said briefly about transmission deafness and the means to deal with it. It is true that in this eventuality the otologist has to be involved. We should not encroach on his territory—quite the opposite. In many cases, he is the only one qualified to take charge of matters. However, it would be desirable for him in turn to consider the various ways of adding to the usual investigations. Indeed, beyond his therapeutic armory, there are techniques that can help the patient, either before or after the operation, with the aim of improving listening capacity. Many times, I have referred a patient with otosclerosis to a great specialist in Béziers who operates remarkably well and obtains exceptional results. As soon as the patient's hearing is working, I can round off the work on listening through some sessions of auditory education, teaching the newly operated subject to aim at sounds, to analyze them and make them converge, so to speak, and to use his ear for communicative purposes.

Our techniques may also be useful when it comes to fitting an otosclerosis patient with a prosthesis. In addition to the operation we just talked about, there is another way to help the patient hear: the hearing aid. For some people whose curves present enormous distortions, it is good to undertake some training sessions under the electronic ear in order to harmonize the curves and raise the thresholds. The subject can then be more easily fitted with the hearing aid, since the distortions have disappeared. Some audiologists send us their clients so that they can benefit from our techniques before buying a device. This prevents them from being dissatisfied with their hearing aids and angry at not hearing well.

Perception deafness

This is the second kind of deafness we are going to study. The disturbance in this case will not act on the air curve/bone curve relationship but on the shape of the curve itself, which is globally modified by alteration of the high frequencies. Here is an example of perception deafness:

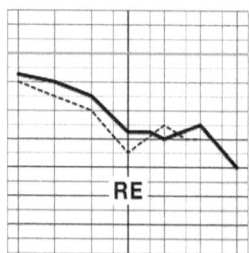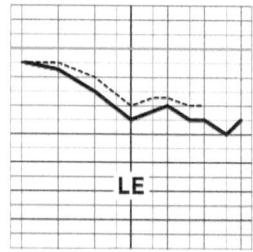

In this type of hearing loss, it is the perception apparatus that is affected. There is a cochlear deficiency. There is one exception to this, however: an alteration to the stapedial mechanics (stirrup) through lack of tone in the stirrup muscle can produce a curve of the same type. This needs to be verified, as it affects the chances of recovery, which is a serious matter.

This category of deafness includes all alterations caused by toxins, drugs (streptomycin, kanamycin, etc.) or other factors (tobacco, alcoholism, syphilis, virus, rubella, etc.) and sound trauma with the onset of occupational deafness characterized by a scotoma at 4,000 Hz, which you know well and which I reproduce here:

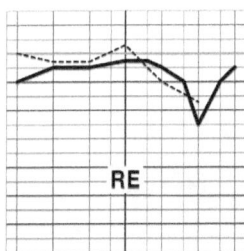 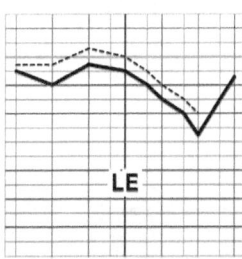

This alteration, little by little, will evolve and will affect the middle frequencies, modifying the possibilities of listening at language level. The person will end up hearing but no longer able to understand what is being said. Here is an example of progressive occupational deafness:

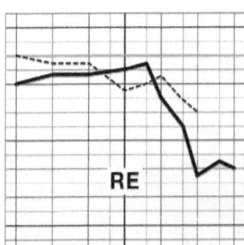 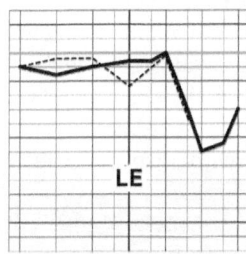

Well, the deafness is gaining ground, and we get the following curve, showing that it has become very pronounced, difficult to reverse not even with hearing aids:

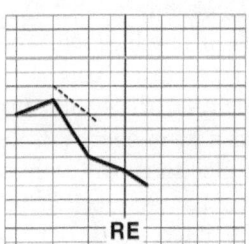 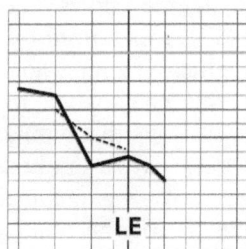

Mixed deafness:

This represents the third category of deafness. As its name indicates, it is a hybrid of the two previous cases of otological pathology. Its characteristics reveal, indeed, disorders of transmission mechanisms together with alterations of perception phenomena. The conjunction of these two disturbances can easily be seen in the graph in an inversion of the air and bone curves—as we have described in the study of transmission deafness—and by the fall in the treble region in both curves, air and bone, which remain parallel of course, as dictated by transmission deafness:

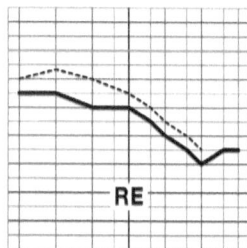 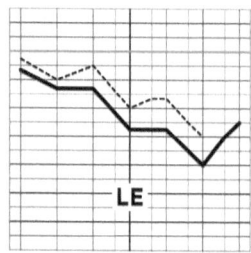

We have thus far approached the study of so-called organic deafness. I have merely offered you some key principles from which to identify the main characteristics of such anomalies, which fall outside the educator's remit, so you can refer the patient to a specialist. However, you should know that in certain cases it is possible to act with our techniques, but we can only make differential diagnoses with respect to these anomalies on the basis of lengthy experience.

Around twenty auditory education sessions under the electronic ear can constitute one of the best means of eliminating the causes of error. The rapid modifications that can appear in the two curves, or in one of them, will tell us whether the organic origin is determinant or not. Thus, in some cases of transmission deafness, not characteristic of otosclerosis, the curves "move" which proves that the ossicular chain can still be mobilized by means of re-education. This is often seen in children, among whom cases of otosclerosis are moreover very rare. This could point to a deafness of psychic origin, to a rejection of listening that diminishes as a consequence of the psycho-sensory process carried out under the electronic ear with the help of specially adapted programming. But if the ossification process has gone too far, it will be impossible to intervene in air conduction, which will remain blocked, although bone conduction, as I said before, can sometimes improve very clearly, thus allowing the usual remedies, surgery or hearing aids, to have a greater effect.

Before talking about the other types of deafness, those of psychological origin, I would like to say a few words about the difficulties associated with them: headaches, ringing or other noises, vertigo, nausea, etc. In all cases, the patient can be relieved, which is no small matter. Nine times out of ten, well-managed training should eliminate these various discomforts by rebalancing the entire vestibular apparatus and toning the eardrum.

Now let us look at psychological deafness. "There is no one deafer than he who does not want to hear", is a saying you all know, and one that you relive every day as you re-educate children and adults who have deliberately decided not to listen, who have cut off communication with their environment. I remind you that a human being has several means to disconnect his listening. You will see it when you study the graphs corresponding to this non-communication policy.

Let us look at some broad features.

a. First, the subject can lower his hearing threshold in order not to hear very distinctly anymore. We find a slight or already quite pronounced hearing loss, affecting both ears or one. Knowing whether the left or right ear is affected gives us some early clues about the affective problem of parental origin that is at the base of this hearing loss.

b. The individual decides to close the curtain so as not to see what is happening outside. Selectivity is blocked either on all frequencies to right and left or only on a part of the sound spectrum, in one ear or in both. When discussing selectivity, we already touched on this subject.

c. A third "trick" is to shuffle the cards, not knowing where the sound is coming from, living in confusion. This is the characteristic tangle of spatialization difficulties that is the object of the third part of the listening test.

d. Finally, there is the possibility of putting the other at a distance by choosing the longest circuits: by taking the left-side auditory path. We see this on the audiolaterometer. The left audio-vocal circuit becomes dominant.

That is what we can say today, in the framework of this conference, about the different types of deafness that show an organic origin or a psychic origin. This is obviously just a broad outline. We should probe more deeply into these issues in future meetings, to conduct specific case studies.

-*What can be done with a person who, after an operation, continues to hear an accordion?*

First of all, it is necessary to specify whether the internal noises that the person hears are really characteristic of a tune played on the accordion, which would make us think in terms of a fantasy, or a sound hallucination, or whether it is a tinnitus, perhaps vaguely reminiscent of the sound of an accordion, but closer to the buzzing or whistling that we regularly find in some cases of deafness. Sometimes the intervention succeeds in restoring auditory function but does not completely suppress associated troubles like tinnitus or vertigo. This means that the regulation of the different levels of the ear is not perfect.

I advise immediately performing auditory education so that the subject learns to stretch his eardrum with the aim of suppressing his internal noises and restoring the labyrinthine function. These symptoms should not be allowed to remain after the intervention, because one day or another the hearing loss will reappear. The poorly regulated ear will succumb again and its chances of recovery will then be much lower.

We have techniques at our disposal that allow us to alleviate listening difficulties considerably. We must not let this opportunity pass us by and we must get down to work so that these difficulties disappear. In your own activity you have probably come across people who suffer from tinnitus, vertigo, etc. and you know the hell they are going through. It is absolutely terrifying to hear internal noises permanently and to live in a constant state of vertigo.

If we consider the other hypothesis, that of acoustic hallucination, we must naturally adopt a different approach and continue to investigate on the level of psychology. A psycho-sensory process under the electronic ear can also be very effective by giving the individual back the desire and the possibility of communicating with the outside world, of establishing a dialogue with his environment, of thinking about others and not just shutting himself up in an egocentric attitude that conjures some quite unexpected interpretations.

This question reminds me of an experiment done in Sainte Anne, about fifteen years ago. I had asked to examine the hallucination sufferers in order to learn about their auditory faculties. I was surprised to find that these mentally ill people actually had two hearing thresholds. The first one, very subtle, very fine, led to responses like "Wow, that's it, I recognize the voice that speaks to me every afternoon and tells me this and that". Then, on going further to reach a more intense threshold, I would get reflections like "Ah! Wow, I hear a noise", sometimes followed by "It's light", "It's dark", "It's blue", "It's red" or "It's fat", etc.

For these patients, therefore, there are two types of auditory references that, in fact, all of us have, but which we do not interpret in the same way. The first threshold, so subtle, so tenuous, is that of molecular noise, of Brownian movement that can be reached by putting oneself in the listening posture. It is the one that recharges us, the one that we need to reach certain zones of thought but that is not essential to us. The second, heavier, more material, is situated at a lower level and connects with the common concerns of the world of sound.

I learned a lot by living with the insane and re-educating some of them. Their different reflections on what they heard allowed me to take great strides in research. When they said to me: "It's a bell sound", "It's the village bell ringing", "It's the noise of the sea", "It's the noise of the waves"... I thought they were right and that they perceived things that our reason no longer allows us to hear. So I was able to dialogue with them on a totally different level to the one we usually have in the conversational universe and, always thanks to our techniques, lower their thresholds in such a way that they could be brought to the level of common mortals. When the connection was made, their alienation disappeared naturally, as the references became the same. I helped several of them to be discharged from the hospital.

The problem of sound hallucinations based on a noise, and sometimes on a pure sound, made me think then of a test, of which I already spoke years ago in one of my lectures, and which a Swiss psychologist carried out and published. If you wish I can give you the bibliographic reference. The idea was to make a kind of sound-based Rorschach from certain noises determined beforehand and noting down the different interpretations. The results were very revealing of the individuals' psychic universe. You must have wondered what was happening on hearing a noise during the night, and it must have given you a good scare, although in fact it was just a door banging or a joist creaking.

I think there is great work to be done, then, in that direction and I invite you all to think about this sound test that can give some extraordinary insights into the inner world of the patients in our charge. All suggestions are welcome so that we can establish a complete battery that allows us to compile statistics from the results obtained in each center.

-What should we think when we are faced with a subject who has an excellent right ear but on the other hand a deficient left ear, with an air curve that begins to descend from 3,000 Hz to 60 dB and with a bone curve located above it that zigzags?

If you first eliminate the hypothesis of an organic problem in the patient's history (an old case of otitis with paracentesis, ear trauma, etc.), you should surely think in terms of a psychological origin.

The first reaction could be: "It's the left ear, so it isn't serious because the right ear is intact". We all know that the right ear is essential in all control processes but that does not mean that the left ear is unimportant. There must always be harmony, let me repeat, between right and left. This is the problem of laterality, arising once again, with its symbols and multiple implications.

Since this is the left ear, you should immediately think about a possible maternal relationship problem. There is an adhesion to the mother, to the extent that the dynamics, the future, the father represented by the right ear remains a myth. There is a blockage, a fatigue. As soon as the individual tries to move forward, make projects, launch himself into a new task, he is stopped, he is held back. He starts everything but finishes nothing. It is the policy of failure. He remains locked up in his maternal problem and until he has solved it, he cannot go any further.

When I say that there is a blockage at the level of the mother, it means a problem of internal relationship, a matter of ego, of the self, of the unconscious as opposed to the transcendental "I", the "I" of the "In truth, in truth I say to you" of full consciousness. We are in the world of "I can't move forward, I'm tired, I'm this, I'm that". These are eruptions of the unconscious emerging. It is the unconscious that is expressing itself and not consciousness. As soon as the latter appears, the two curves take on the shape that we know well and which have occupied us so often during these work sessions.

What to do in the face of this? The importance of the maternal problem naturally demands that we first undertake education in intrauterine hearing based on the mother's voice. The sonic births should follow this fetal period and we should distribute them quite intensively so that the subject can at last detach himself from the maternal core.

The next phase should not consist of making the left ear "rise" by keeping the balance at 7 (with the cable to the right) or placing the cable to the left with the balance at 1. On the contrary, we should quickly lateralize to the right and then, to our surprise, we will see the left ear improve noticeably. In fact, it is necessary to understand that there are enormous biauricular counter-reactions, especially due to medulla oblongata- pons connections, such as Rasmussen's fascicle, which bridges the two cochleas.

-I think I have understood that children lose part of their perception of high frequencies very quickly after birth. Is this the reason why the father's voice is filtered in a region of pretty low frequencies, between 300 and 800 Hz, I think?

The diaphragmatic opening of the child's hearing is achieved very gradually. It is true that at birth, or to be exact, from the 10th day, from the moment when the Eustachian tube gets rid of its liquid, the child is immersed in a sound "shadow" which no longer allows him to hear the high frequencies that he perceived perfectly in his fetal life. He still does not know how to use his musculature in the aerial environment in order to recover his perception of the high trebles and his ear will have to spend years working on accommodation, on convergence, to regain the heights of communication. Not until the age of four or five will he be able to pronounce the sibilants properly.

As far as the encounter with the father is concerned, in an approach that does not yet correspond to the real dialogue that the child will establish much later, we take into account this progressive diaphragmatic opening and we filter the paternal voice[3] so that it will appear first in the band that goes from 300 to 800 Hz, then from 300 to 2,000 Hz, then from 300 to 4,000 Hz; finally we will open the curtain completely when the previous stages have not caused any dazzlement or strong reactions in the child.

I remind you that this period of re-encounter with the paternal voice marks a very important stage on the way to self-realization.

---

[3] AN: Tomatis soon stopped using the father's voice in therapy

If the maternal problem is completely solved and if, after a linguistic preparation carried out with the help of a skillfully constructed program, the dialogue with the father can be established, the game is won. The being thrown into an exceptional life dynamic will be able to face all the difficulties of existence with surprising strength.

But we all know that things do not always turn out so well and that this famous "paternal" stage is one of the most difficult to get through. It must be approached by the educator with great caution so that the confrontation is not dramatic and does not bring about a phenomenon of regression, of inward withdrawal that would waste time. In addition, I think the first step should be done with the paternal voice filtered at 8,000 Hz, at that high altitude where problems are solved on another level. But this is nothing more than a hypothesis that I will talk about once we have experimented with it.

Given that children lose their high frequencies at birth and only hear the low ones, how do they come to have a high-pitched or even very high-pitched voice?

We should not confuse a high-pitched voice with a fragile, shrill, thin voice. The child actually has a "small" voice that is restricted to a narrow band. There are few harmonics in a child's voice. You can tell when you hear young singers try to "go up" to the high notes. Their high notes are sometimes a bit stiff and lack that rich, dense, harmonic spray that we find in some adults.

The child's voice is mono-harmonic or mono-band. It shows a still narrow auditory diaphragmatic opening similar to that of the "hautes-contres", who are, as you will know, singers who can "go up" very high in frequency. I knew one who had an exceptional voice and when I heard him I thought he would burst my cathode tubes while analyzing his voice. But he did not go above 1,500 Hz. He sang Mozart divinely but did so within a narrow band that corresponded to his register.

-What happens when testing a subject who has the proper posture for hearing the high frequencies? Are the answers different according to the patient's posture?

Yes, naturally, but when you give a listening test to an individual it is to find out their posture towards ordinary life, which is very often one of non-listening. Obviously, his answers will be different if you ask him to place himself in an upright posture, with his head at a certain angle, which corresponds to the fine perception of the trebles, etc. But since this is not his normal stance, this way of proceeding will only have the value of an experiment.

You yourself will have noticed, no doubt, in a concert for example, how different the music sounds if you listen in a "treble posture" as opposed to slumped in the seat. Let us go back to the comments we made about the placement of the head during the listening test. The perception of the trebles determines a particular curve while the perception of the bass determines another. The first, corresponding to the maximum tension of the stirrup muscle, is found in the experiments done by the Americans Moller, Schmitt and Reger,[4] with a curve of 12 dB/octave, while the second corresponds to a relaxation of the stapedial muscle (of the stirrup) and submerges the self in the depressive universe of low-frequency sounds.

The ideal, of course, is to be constantly in a posture for listening to high-pitched sounds. That requires some training. I have just mentioned the work carried out by a team of researchers who demonstrated that the human ear can be conditioned to hear in various ways, which is what I have been trying to say for 25 years. They discovered that, by pulling on the hammer and stirrup muscles, they could achieve a slope of at least 15 dB between 250 and 1,000 Hz.

This tension of the muscles of the middle ear must therefore be sought permanently and in all circumstances. If you are immersed in a sound universe that is unpleasant, disharmonious, rich in low frequencies, if you are obliged to hear things without interest or spoken aggressively, you will have to adopt the posture for listening to the high frequencies in order to be able to recharge and benefit as much as possible from the sound environment, while at the same time avoiding the negative side. Personally, I always do this when flying, in order to arrive fresh as a daisy at the place where, most often, I have to immediately give a consultation or a lecture. I always manage to put myself in a posture for listening to the high frequencies during the journey while I see around me people who have wilted, annihilated by the low frequencies and vibrations transmitted by the plane.

Why are bass sounds so dangerous? Because they require the body to expend more energy than the cortex receives from stimuli. Sounds

---

[4] AN: *Effect of middle ear muscle action on certain psychophysical measurements.* **Reger, S.** 1960, Ann. Otol. Rhin. Laryngol., Vol. 69, pp. 1179-98.

like those of the tam-tam, for example, are precisely meant to move the body and put the individual in a daze, in a kind of hypnosis that places him at the mercy of the medicine man. High-pitched sounds, on the other hand, such as those found in Gregorian chant, recharge the subject, lead him towards consciousness, without, however, having to mobilize the body. Finally, I should mention martial songs, which combine both procedures: they recharge individuals by making them march as if they were just one man.

-Is there a characteristic curve for depressives?

Yes, just as there is a characteristic curve for paranoia sufferers, those with compulsive traits, etc. The depressive one has this general shape, which you know well:

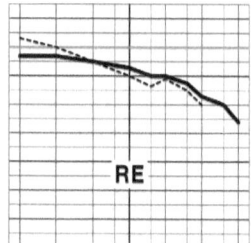 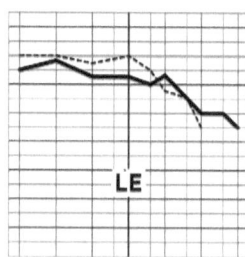

It is the inverse of the recharge curve. Several eventualities may occur, of course, depending on whether or not the individual compensates for his depressive state. Then you can find the following graph:

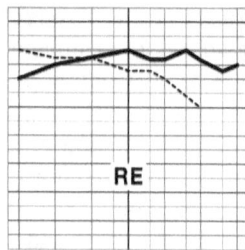 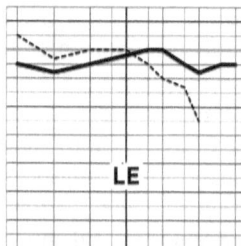

The depressive state can be seen at the level of the bone curve, but the air curve is deceptive and allows the subject to weather the storm apparently.

Depression and fatigue should not be confused. You will often get someone who comes to you because he feels depressed. In fact, this person is exhausted and do not know how to recharge any more.

Then you get a pattern of this kind:

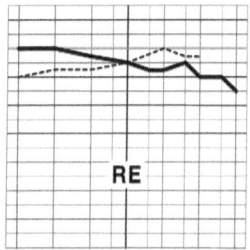 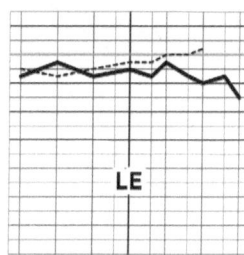

The bone curve is not a falling one.

As a general rule, the presence of a depressive state can be inferred when the bone curve falls from the basses to the trebles.

-What kind of support can all this provide as a whole? Is it neural support or psychological support?

That is a tricky question to answer, and it would be impossible to do so without getting into a philosophical-psychological-physiological diatribe that leads nowhere. It brings to mind the endless dialogue between Aristotle and Anaxagoras over the predominance of the brain and the hand. Which of the two organs allows man to be what he is? No one can answer.

In this case, it is the same. From the perspective in which the question places us, the psyche is as necessary as the nervous system, its instrument, just as the violin is necessary for the violinist. Each needs the other to respond to a higher instance which, in this case, would be music. For us, it is the call towards transcendence that focuses our attention on listening, pulling man towards his field of consciousness.

Driven, as it were, by a complex neural organization from which he cannot escape, the human being thus finds that he must respond, at his own scale, to motivations that will be manifested in him through a desire to communicate, to understand, to know. In fact, these motivations are hardly more than interferences from who knows where, veritable incursions of consciousness acting as the first manifestation of the life that animates the being.

www.ingramcontent.com/pod-product-compliance
Lightning Source LLC
Chambersburg PA
CBHW021351210526
45463CB00001B/60